MOLECULAR TECHNIQUES FOR THE STUDY OF HOSPITAL-ACQUIRED INFECTION

MOLECULAR TECHNIQUES FOR THE STUDY OF HOSPITAL-ACQUIRED INFECTION

EDITED BY

STEVEN L. FOLEY
National Farm Medicine Center, Marshfield Clinic Research Foundation, Marshfield, Wisconsin, USA

ANNE Y. CHEN
Division of Infectious Diseases, Henry Ford Hospital, Detroit, Michigan, USA

SHABBIR SIMJEE
Elanco Animal Health, Eli Lilly and Company, Basingstoke, Hampshire, UK

MARCUS J. ZERVOS
Division of Infectious Diseases, Henry Ford Hospital, Detroit, Michigan, USA

WILEY-BLACKWELL
A John Wiley & Sons, Inc., Publication

Published by John Wiley & Sons, Inc., Hoboken, New Jersey
Published simultaneously in Canada

For general information on our other products and services or for technical support, please contact our Customer Care Department within the United States at (800) 762-2974, outside the United States at (317) 572-3993 or fax (317) 572-4002.

Wiley also publishes its books in a variety of electronic formats. Some content that appears in print may not be available in electronic formats. For more information about Wiley products, visit our web site at www.wiley.com.

Library of Congress Cataloging-in-Publication Data:

ISBN: 978-0-470-42085-0

Printed in Singapore

eISBN: 978-1-118-06382-8
oISBN: 978-1-118-06384-2
ePub ISBN: 978-1-118-06383-5

10 9 8 7 6 5 4 3 2 1

To Missy and our kids, Colin, Riley and Ava, and to my parents

Steven L. Foley

To my husband Merwin and our children, Brandon and Kathryn

Anne Y. Chen

To my mother Farida, wife Saida, and son Usman

Shabbir Simjee

To my wife Ellene and children Mary, John, and Tommy

Marcus J. Zervos

CONTENTS

CONTRIBUTORS

Ngolela Esther Babady, M.D., Mayo Clinic, Rochester, Minnesota 55905

Faiqa Alam Cheema, M.D., Division of Infectious Diseases, Henry Ford Hospital, Detroit, Michigan 48202

Anne Y. Chen, M.D., Division of Infectious Diseases, Henry Ford Hospital, Detroit, Michigan 48202

Franklin R. Cockerill, M.D., Mayo Clinic, Rochester, Minnesota 55905

Louise-Marie Dembry, M.D., Division of Infectious Diseases, Yale University School of Medicine, New Haven, Connecticut 06519

Steven L. Foley, Ph.D., National Farm Medicine Center, Marshfield Clinic Research Foundation, Marshfield, Wisconsin 54449

Beilei Ge, Ph.D., Food Science Department, Louisiana State University, Baton Rouge, Louisiana 70803

Richard V. Goering, Ph.D., Department of Medical Microbiology and Immunology, Creighton University School of Medicine, Omaha, Nebraska 68178

Sonja Hansen, M.D., M.P.H., Institute of Hygiene and Environmental Medicine, Charité—University Medicine Berlin, Campus Benjamin Franklin, 12203 Berlin, Germany

Vanthida Huang, Phar M.D., Department of Pharmacy Practice, College of Pharmacy and Health Sciences, Mercer University, Atlanta, Georgia 30341

Aaron M. Lynne, Ph.D., Department of Biological Science, Sam Houston State University, Huntsville, Texas 77341

Robin Patel, M.D., Mayo Clinic, Rochester, Minnesota 55905

Eli N. Perencevich, M.D., Department of Internal Medicine, The University of Iowa, Iowa City, Iowa 52242

Hiren Pokharna, M.D., M.P.H., Division of Infectious Diseases, Henry Ford Hospital, Detroit, Michigan, 48202

Johann D. D. Pitout, M.D., Division of Microbiology, Calgary Laboratory Services, Calgary, Alberta, T2L 2K8, Canada

Carl M. Schroeder, Ph.D., Office of Public Health and Science, USDA Food Safety and Inspection Service, Washington, DC 20250

Sanjay K. Shukla, Ph.D., Clinical Research Center, Marshfield Clinic Research Foundation, Marshfield, Wisconsin 54449

Shabbir Simjee, Ph.D., Elanco Animal Health, Eli Lilly and Company Limited, Hampshire, RG24 9NL, United Kingdom

Mary E. Stemper, M.S., Division of Laboratory Medicine, Marshfield Clinic, Marshfield, Wisconsin 54449

Carlos Torres-Viera, M.D., Division of Infectious Diseases, Yale University School of Medicine, New Haven, Connecticut 06519

Jose A. Vazquez, M.D., Division of Infectious Diseases, Henry Ford Hospital, Detroit, Michigan 48202

Ralf-Peter Vonberg, M.D., Institute for Medical Microbiology and Hospital Epidemiology, Medical School Hannover, D-30625 Hannover, Germany

Marc-Oliver Wright, M.T. (ASCP), M.S., Department of Infection Control, Evanston Northwestern Healthcare, Evanston, Illinois 60201

Marcus J. Zervos, M.D., Wayne State University School of Medicine and Division of Infectious Diseases, Henry Ford Hospital, Detroit, Michigan 48202

FOREWORD

Nosocomial infections continue to be an issue of increasing importance, especially in light of the fact that many of these pathogens are becoming increasingly resistant to our effort to treat them, resulting in infections that have significant morbidity, mortality, and cost. With the emergence of strains with increasing levels of resistance to multiple antimicrobial agents, along with limited new drugs, we are faced with formidable diagnostic, prevention, and treatment challenges for nosocomial pathogens. Despite these challenges, our understanding of epidemiology, mechanisms for pathogen control, and measures for detection and characterization has also progressed.

Much has been written recently about the problems of healthcare-associated infections and the development of antimicrobial resistance in the causative organisms. *Techniques for the Study of Hospital-Acquired Infection* is, however, a unique and concise text providing state-of-the-art information. It provides the infection control practitioner, clinician, epidemiologist, and microbiologist a practical tool to understand the mechanism and implementation of a comprehensive program to study and control healthcare-associated infections.

The text of the book is divided into three parts. Part I is an introduction to healthcare-associated infections and their control, while Part II focuses on the techniques to characterize nosocomial pathogens; Part III examines the application of techniques to characterize predominant nosocomial pathogens focusing on representative Gram-positive, Gram-negative, and fungal pathogens.

The text is written by an internationally recognized team of contributors. Importantly, it is the clinical perspective that distinguishes this book from other publications, and it is the coordination of infection control, laboratory methods, and exploration of clinical practices to control pathogens that will be of interest to readers and will help the healthcare practitioner develop improved strategies to minimize the impact of nosocomial infections on patients.

BARBARA E. MURRAY, M.D.

J. Ralph Meadows Professor and Director,
Division of Infectious Diseases Houston, Texas
December 2010

PREFACE

Nosocomial infections are a significant cause of morbidity and mortality. Each year it is estimated that 2 million patients develop a healthcare-acquired infection in the United States. Put another way, this represents nearly 5% of all hospitalized patients, and these infections directly contribute to approximately 88,000 deaths and add an additional 4.5 billion dollars to healthcare costs. Because of the importance of these infections, we were invited to edit this book exploring the techniques for the study of hospital-acquired infections. The book is divided into three general parts: Part I is an introduction to healthcare-associated infections and their control, Part II discusses molecular techniques to characterize nosocomial pathogens, Part III describes the application of techniques to characterize predominant nosocomial pathogens focusing on representative Gram-positive, Gram-negative, and fungal pathogens.

Major themes that are examined in this book include the characteristics of healthcare settings that allow for the development and spread of nosocomial pathogens, the implementation of effective infection control programs, the epidemiological methods to study nosocomial disease, and the elimination of pathogens and the development of resistance to these treatments. These topics are followed up by sections that focus on the molecular techniques used to study hospital infections, as well as by an exploration of the characteristics of some of the major nosocomial pathogens that are currently plaguing healthcare settings in the context of best practices to deal with these pathogens.

Why is it important to examine the techniques for the study of hospital-acquired infections? There a number of good reasons; these include the fact that there are increasing numbers of healthcare-associated infections that are caused by multidrug-resistant pathogens, which, in addition to the infection-associated pathology, leads to difficulty in treating infected patients. These more commonly resistant pathogens include Gram-positive pathogens such as methicillin-resistant *Staphylococcus aureus* (MRSA), glycopeptide (vancomycin) intermediate, and resistant *S. aureus* and glycopeptide-resistant enterococci (VRE). Some of the primary concerns among the Gram-negatives include fluoroquinolones-resistant *Pseudomonas aeruginosa* and *Escherichia coli* and the extended spectrum beta-lactamase (ESBL)-producing strains of *E. coli* and *Klebsiella pneumoniae*. Because of their importance in causing healthcare-associated infections, individual chapters have been dedicated to antimicrobial resistance, as well as to *S. aureus* and *E. coli.*

There are many known risk factors that associated with the development of nosocomial infections, including suffering from underlying conditions such as cancer, diabetes, or renal failure, prior antimicrobial therapy, the presence of indwelling catheters, surgical procedures, and having extended hospital stays. The examination of the transmission of pathogens from the healthcare environment and/or personnel to the patient is also very important to explore and as such has been explored thoroughly in the Part I of the book. The determination of the sources and relatedness among pathogens is important to understanding the epidemiology of nosocomial infections, which will aid development of rational pathogen control strategies. Many of the bacterial species that are prominent causes of nosocomial infections are also readily found as normal commensal organisms on the human body, including the staphylococci, enterococci, and *E. coli.* Because these commensal strains are not typically associated with human infection, it is important to be able to determine whether strain isolated from a patient is pathogenic and the likely source of the infection or part of the normal flora.

To assist in the determination of the strain type, infection control practitioners and molecular epidemiologists typically rely on pathogen subtyping to determine if strains are likely pathogens and to decipher whether isolates that are epidemiologically related are also genetically similar. Traditionally, much of the strain typing was done based on the phenotypic characteristics of isolates, including methods such as biochemical profiles, serotyping, phage typing, and antimicrobial susceptibility profiles. However, these techniques typically lack the specificity to more closely link isolates from patients to likely sources. Thus as molecular typing methods became more readily available, many hospitals and other healthcare organizations began to rely more on DNA-based technologies to characterize pathogens. These molecular methodologies include polymerase chain reaction (PCR)-based rapid identification and typing methods as well as restriction-enzyme-based methods such as pulsed-field gel electrophoresis (PFGE). Many of these methods are covered extensively in chapters in the Part II of the book. The molecular methods allow for a deeper assessment of strain interrelationship, which is important to establish genetic links that provide evidence which aids in determining the source of organisms that cause disease and distinguish them from commensal strains; this is important in the development of treatment strategies to minimize the health impact of the infections. Part III of this book explores some of the major groups of nosocomial pathogens with representative Gram-positive, Gram-negative, and fungal pathogens, examining their characteristics and methods for characterization and study of hospital-acquired infections caused by these organisms. We hope that you find this book helpful as you tackle the difficult problems associated with healthcare-associated infections.

Steven L. Foley

Anne Y. Chen

Shabbir Simjee

Marcus J. Zervos

PART ONE

Introduction to Healthcare-Associated Infections and their Control

CHAPTER ONE

The Hospital and Ambulatory Care Environment

HIREN POKHARNA AND ANNE Y. CHEN

Introduction

HEALTHCARE-ASSOCIATED INFECTIONS (HAIs): THE EVOLUTION

Although the modern-day concepts of prevention and control of hospital-associated infections originated in the middle of the nineteenth century, the history regarding knowledge about hospital-related infections dates back to the sixteenth century. Ambroise Pare (1517–1590), a surgeon at Hotel-Dieu in Paris, was one of the first physicians to describe increased frequency and severity of wound infections in hospitalized patients compared to nonhospitalized patients. The phrase "hospital disease" was first used in the eighteenth century. Hungarian physician Ignaz Philipp Semmelweiss (1818–1865) introduced the concept of hand washing while Sir Joseph Lister (1827–1912), a British surgeon, pioneered the concept of asepsis. Over the years, the Center for Disease Control and Prevention (CDC) has published several sets of definitions for Nosocomial Infections. Definitions used during the Comprehensive Hospital Infections Project (CHIP) (1969–1972) and in the National Nosocomial Infectious Study (NNIS) (1970–1974) were first used in the *Proceedings of the First International Conference on Nosocomial Infection* organized by CDC in 1970 (1). Definitions were further extended in 1974 for hospitals participating in NNIS (2). Definitions for nosocomial infections were again modified by CDC in 1988 (3). The term HAI (4) was officially introduced in 2008 to reflect infections

Molecular Techniques for the Study of Hospital-Acquired Infection, First Edition. Edited by Steven L. Foley, Anne Y. Chen, Shabbir Simjee, and Marcus J. Zervos.

acquired by patients while receiving treatment for any surgical or medical conditions. It was defined as a localized or systemic condition resulting from an adverse reaction to the presence of an infectious agent(s) or its toxin(s) without any evidence that the infection was present or incubating at the time of admission to the acute care setting. HAIs can occur in acute care settings within hospitals or in ambulatory outpatient care settings, including same-day surgical centers or dialysis center. HAIs are increasingly associated with long-term facilities such as nursing homes and rehabilitation centers.

Healthcare-associated infections (HAIs) are a major cause of morbidity and mortality in the United States. It is estimated that there were 1.7 million HAI in 2002 which resulted in around 99,000 deaths, making it among the most common healthcare-associated adverse event (5). HAIs can occur in patients at any age and in any healthcare setting, but the most common infections are seen among adults and children in the non-ICU setting. According to National Nosocomial Infections Surveillance (NNIS) system data from 1990 to 2002, out of an estimated 98,987 deaths associated with HAI in the United States hospitals, 35,967 were due to pneumonia, 30,665 were related to bloodstream infections, 13,088 were related to UTIs, 8205 were due to for surgical site infections (SSI), and 11,062 due to infections from other sites.

HAIs have significant economic implications as well. They increase the healthcare burden on the society by $35.7–45 billion every year (6).

PATHOGENS

Bacteria remain the most common pathogens and source of HAIs (7, 8). HAI are typically associated with Gram-positive pathogens including methicillin-resistant *Staphylococcus aureus* (MRSA) (9–13), coagulase-negative *Staphylococci* (14), and glycopeptide (vancomycin)-resistant *Enterococci* spp. (15–20). More recently, there are increasing reports of glycopeptide intermediate and glycopeptide-resistant *S. aureus* (21). *Clostridium difficile*, a normal intestinal flora in 3% of healthy adults and 20–30% of hospitalized adults (22), is responsible for 25–30% of antibiotic-associated diarrhea and is being increasingly recognized as a major nosocomial pathogen (23–27). There is increasing resistance among Gram-negative organisms. Among *Enterobacteriaceae* pathogenic isolates, resistance to fluoroquinolones, extended-spectrum cephalosporins, and carbapenems is increasing (14). There is also an increasing carbapenem resistance among *Acinetobacter* spp. (14, 28) and *Klebsiella pneumoniae* (14). MDR *Pseudomonas* spp., *Klebsiella* spp. *and Enterobacter* spp. are concerning as well. Emerging resistance to carbapenems conferred by New Delhi metallo-B-lactamase 1 (NDM-1) in countries such as India, Pakistan, and United Kingdom is a potential global health problem that will require coordinated international surveillance (29).

Candida species remain the most common healthcare-associated pathogens among fungi (14, 30); and although less common, viruses including Adenovirus, Rotavirus, Norovirus, and hepatitis B have been recognized as nosocomial pathogens.

Common HAIs

URINARY TRACT INFECTION (UTI)

UTIs are the most common HAIs in both acute care setting and long-term care facilities. A major cause of septicemia and mortality, rates are similar in adult and pediatric patients (31) and account for 36% of all HAIs (5). Intrinsic risk factors associated with UTIs include: advanced age, female gender, and severity of underlying illness (e.g., diabetes mellitus (DM)) (32). Duration of indwelling catheterization is by far the most important extrinsic risk factor for UTIs (33). Indwelling urinary catheters are used in nearly all hospital nursing units, unlike ventilators and many other devices. Various studies have emphasized that catheter use is frequently inappropriate; inattention to both the proper indications for catheter use and catheter status in patients seems to be an important factor (34–39).

The most common etiologic agents for catheter-associated UTI (CAUTI) as reported to the NHSN at CDC, 2006–2007, are *E. coli* (21%), *Candida* spp. (20%) [*C. albicans* (14%)], *Enterococcus* spp. (15%), *P. aeruginosa* (10%), *K. pneumoniae* (8%), *Enterobacter* spp. (4%), coagulase-negative *Staphylococci* (3%), *S. aureus* (2%), *A. baumannii* (1%), and *K. oxytoca* (1%) (14).

Hospitals and Long-Term Care Facilities (LTCF) should develop, maintain, and propagate policies regarding indications for catheter insertion and removal. Education of staff, use of condom catheters where appropriate, and consideration of intermittent catheterization and suprapubic catheterization as an alternative to short-term or long-term indwelling urethral catheterization have all been recommended to reduce the risk of nosocomial UTIs (40).

PNEUMONIA

Pneumonia is the third most common HAI, the second most common in the ICU, and the most common cause of mortality among all HAIs (5). It is associated with considerably increased healthcare costs and hospitalization days (32, 41). Hospital-acquired pneumonia (HAP) is defined as pneumonia that occurs 48 hours or more after admission, which was not incubating at the time of admission (42, 43). Ventilator-associated pneumonia (VAP) refers to pneumonia that arises more than 48–72 hours after endotracheal intubation (44, 45). Healthcare-associated pneumonia (HCAP) includes any patient who was hospitalized in an acute care hospital for two or more days within 90 days of the infection; resided in a nursing home or long-term care facility; received recent intravenous antibiotic therapy, chemotherapy, or wound care within the past 30 days of the current infection; or attended a hospital or hemodialysis clinic (43, 45, 46). Most current data, including microbiological, have been collected from patients with VAP but can be extrapolated to HAP and HCAP patients as well (47). Tracheal intubation and mechanical ventilation are the strongest risk factors, with 3- to 21-fold increase in risk for nosocomial pneumonia (48).

Among etiologic agents, *S. aureus* (24%) is the most common pathogen, followed by Gram-negative organisms: *P. aeruginosa* (16%), *Enterobacter* spp. (8%), *A. baumannii* (8%), *K. pneumoniae* (7%), and *E. coli* (5%) (14).

Various infection control measures can help modify the risk factors for pneumonia. Intubations and reintubations should be avoided if possible, and noninvasive modes of ventilation should be used whenever possible. Orotracheal intubations and orogastric tubes, semirecumbent position rather than supine position, continuous aspiration of subglottic secretions, adequate endotracheal cuff pressures to prevent leakage of bacterial pathogens into the lower respiratory tract, and passive humidifiers or heat-moisture exchangers can all help decrease the risk for VAP (47).

SURGICAL SITE INFECTIONS (SSIs)

SSIs are second only to UTIs in frequency, accounting for 22% of all HAIs (5). It is estimated that SSI develop in 2–5% of the 27 million patients undergoing surgical procedures each year (49, 50). Healthcare personnel and operating room environment have been implicated as common sources of pathogens for SSIs. Prolonged preoperative stay, preoperative shaving, length of surgery, and skill of surgeons are well-documented risk factors for SSIs (51). Intrinsic host-related risk factors include: severity of underlying illness (e.g., high American Society for Anesthesiology score, DM), obesity, advanced age, malnutrition, trauma, loss of skin integrity (e.g., psoriasis), and presence of remote infections at time of surgery (32).

Most common etiologic agents are: *S. aureus* (30%), coagulase-negative *Staphylococcus* (14%), *Enterococcus* spp. (11%), *E. coli* (10%), *P. aeruginosa* (6%), *Enterobacter* spp. (4%), *K. pneumoniae* (3%), and *Candida* spp. (2%) (14).

Various pre-, intra- and postoperative measures will help minimize the risk of SSI (51). Preoperative bathing with an antimicrobial has been advocated to reduce skin colonization (52). Removing hair from the site of surgery and preoperative skin preparation reduces contamination of the operative site (53). Clipping with clippers or using cream to remove hair results in fewer surgical site infections than shaving (54). Intraoperatively, appropriate barrier devices, good skills, adequate hemostasis to prevent hematomas and seromas, and adequate debridement of dead tissue are some ways to reduce transmission of microorganisms (55). Postoperatively, adequate wound care will help prevent infections.

BLOODSTREAM INFECTIONS (BSIs)

Bloodstream infections (BSIs) are the fourth common cause of HAIs (5). Both the incidence and prevalence of BSIs have increased over the past several decades. An estimated 350,000 nosocomial BSIs are reported in the United States every year (56). Differentiating a clinically significant BSI from a blood culture contaminant remains a constant challenge for physicians (57). Because many patients receive home healthcare, including intravenous infusions and chemotherapy that until the recent past would have been administered in inpatient settings, the distinction between nosocomial and community-acquired BSIs has been difficult. Friedman et al. (58) and Siegman-Igra et al. (59) described 37% and 39% BSIs, respectively, that occurred in settings traditionally classified as community acquired and could be more accurately classified as healthcare-associated. The term "nosohusial" has been proposed to describe infections occurring in homecare subjects (60).

Various automated blood cultures systems that are reasonably comparable to each other are being used by most laboratories. To ensure appropriate identification of the pathogen, all efforts should be made to avoid contamination of the sample. Skin preparation plays a major role. Various methods have been used for skin preparation. This includes cleaning venipuncture site with alcohol followed by an iodophor or iodine tincture and povidone iodine. More recently, Mimoz et al. (61) showed that alcoholic chlorhexidine may be more efficacious in preventing skin contamination compared to povidone iodine. Reliability of blood culture results also depends on various other factors including amount of blood volume sampled, timing of blood cultures, and site from where blood cultures are obtained (57).

Bloodstream infections (BSIs) are associated with various risk factors. In the past, 75% of healthcare-associated (nosocomial) BSIs were secondary to SSIs, UTIs, intra-abdominal infections, pneumonia, or skin and soft tissue infections (62, 63). Over the years, the proportion of primary nosocomial BSIs has increased and most episodes without an obvious source are thought to be related to intravascular catheters (57, 64). Age (<1 year and >65 years) is a known predisposing factor for BSI (32, 57, 65–67). Patients with underlying malignancies and/or neutropenia are long known to be at risk for BSI (68–70). Notably, patients with hematologic malignancies are at higher risk than those with solid tumors. Other risk factors include patient with chronic liver disease (71), hemodialysis patients (72), burn patients (73), spinal cord injury patients (74, 75), transplant patients (76), and patients admitted to the ICU (77).

The pathogens differ in patients with various risk factors. Based on most recent studies, the common pathogens associated with central line associated BSI are coagulase-negative *Staphylococcus* (34%), *S. aureus* (15%), *Enterococcus* spp. (12%), *Candida* spp. (11%), *E. coli* (10%), *P. aeruginosa* (8%), *K. pneumoniae* (6%), *Enterobacter* spp. (5%), and *A. baumannii* (3%)(14).

Various recommendations have been made to prevent catheter-related BSI (78). Use of an all-inclusive catheter cart kit and barrier devices, chlorhexidine-based antiseptic for skin preparations, disinfecting catheter hubs, needleless connectors, and injection ports before accessing the catheter and appropriate surveillance are a few of the recommendations made by the Society for Healthcare Epidemiology of America/Infectious Disease Society of America (SHEA/IDSA).

Epidemiology of Infectious Disease and the Hospital and Ambulatory Care Environment

Epidemiology is defined as the study of the determinants and distribution of health and disease in populations. It is well recognized that health and disease occur due to the complex interactions between an agent, the host that is the target of agent actions, and the environment. In relation to HAIs, agent refers to the various healthcare-associated microorganisms, the host comprises the patients or/and the healthcare workers, and the environment would include different healthcare components such as acute care hospital, intensive care units, hemodialysis centers, ambulatory clinics, and so on.

Various models and equations have been used to describe these multifarious interactions. The simplest epidemiologic model described is the triangle model (79) (Figure 1.1). It signifies, in the most simplified manner, the complex yet close interaction between the agent, host and environment. The Seesaw model (Figure 1.2) is another way by which the interplay between the three components (agent, host, environment) has been described (80). By introducing the Seesaw model, Fox et al. (80) has illustrated the role that environment plays to keep an equilibrium between the agent and the host. Conversely, any disequilibrium results in adverse events. Therefore, the environment provides platform upon which the interaction between host and agent takes place. An "equation of infection" has been used to determine the probability of a microbial agent to cause infection in the host (81):

$$IP = \frac{D \times S \times T \times V}{Hd}$$

where *Ip* is the probability of infection, *D* is the dose (number of microorganisms) transmitted to the host, *S* is the receptive host site of contact with the agent, *T* is the time

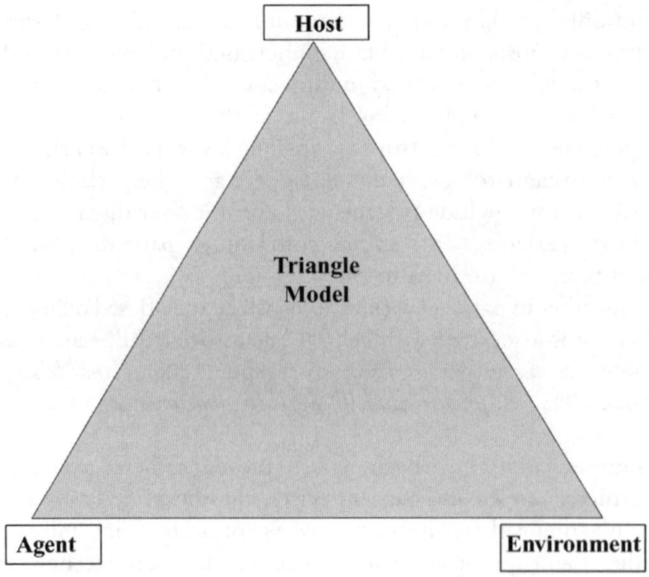

FIGURE 1.1 Triangle model for epidemiological relationships. The simplified model demonstrates the complex yet close interaction between the agent, host and environment.

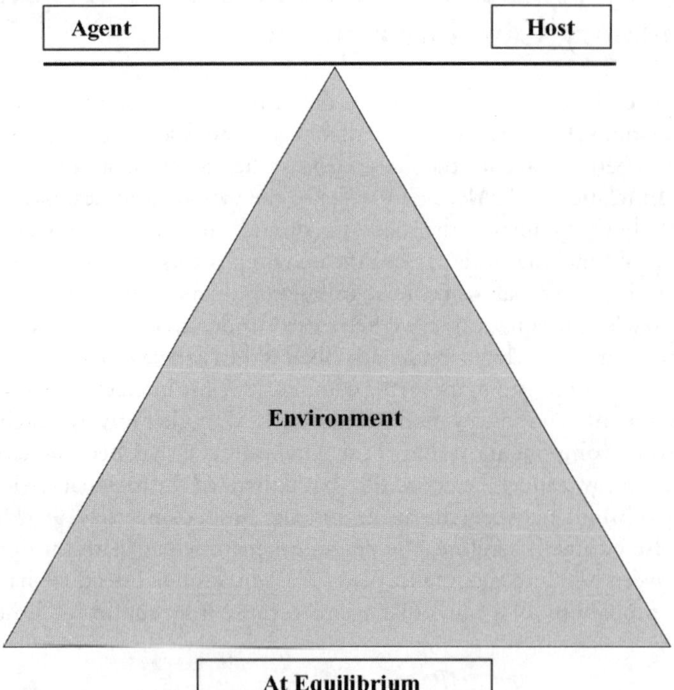

FIGURE 1.2 Seesaw model for epidemiological relationships. A second simple model to demonstrate the epidemiologic balance between the agent, host and environment.

of contact (sufficient for attachment and multiplication or not), *V* is the virulence (the intrinsic characteristics of the microorganism that allow it to infect), and *Hd* is the force of the combined host defenses attempting to prevent the infection. Thus, if there is any compromise in the host's defense system, as may happen in the case of an immunocompromised patient, there may be a propensity to cause infection with lesser quantity of the microorganisms. Similarly, the host site may be one that may have otherwise been an unlikely site. The time required for the agent to cause infection and the virulence of the agent may be variable as well. For example, in a patient with febrile neutropenia secondary to chemotherapy, an organism such as *Propionebacterium acnes* may be able to cause a BSI compared to an unlikely possibility of the same agent to cause an infection in a healthy host.

The Agent, Host, and the Environment

The healthcare environment provides the platform for the complex interactions between agent and host that eventually results in disease.

AGENT

Various bacteria, fungi, and viruses act as agents causing HAIs (32). These microorganisms are necessary, but by themselves they are not sufficient to cause an infection. The healthcare environment plays a pivotal role in aiding the disease process. The healthcare setting provides the required reservoir for these microorganisms to blossom. These reservoirs are numerous in the hospital environment. Humans are the most common reservoirs. These include healthcare workers (82–93), patients (94–102), the household members, and visitors of the patients (103–108). Healthcare workers are frequently colonized with MRSA (109). It is also known that clothing (including uniforms and lab coats) and personal protective equipment may get contaminated with potential pathogens after taking care of patients colonized with organisms including *A. baumannii* (29), MRSA, VRE, and *C. difficile* (110–113). Although these have not been implicated directly as sources of infections, there is definitely a potential for same that remains. Healthcare workers, patients, and visitors will transmit pathogens from their hands (114, 115). The bedrails, doors, and other objects in the patient's room are colonized with microorganisms; if appropriate hand hygiene is not followed, the organisms will get transmitted among patients. Commonly used patient care devices such as electronic thermometers, infusion sets, glucose monitoring devices, and blood pressure cuffs, if not cleansed properly, may transmit pathogens (116–119). *Legionella* spp. can survive in the air-conditioning humidification systems, *C. difficile* will remain in the rooms of patients treated for *C. difficile* for an extended time, and *Burkholderia* spp. and *P. aeruginosa* are known to be transmitted from patient to patient in adult and child clinics for patients with cystic fibrosis (120, 121).

HOST

As seen in the "equation of infection," the agent has a major role in disease occurrence. The virulence of organism, the number of organisms, and the duration of contact are all important; whether the disease will occur or not, as well as the severity of the disease, is greatly influenced by the host mechanisms. In all circumstances, the host's immune system attempts to prevent occurrence of any infection. Any decrease in the host's immune response results in the host's increased susceptibility to infections. These host factors have been largely described as intrinsic factors and extrinsic factors. Intrinsic host factors mainly include extremes of age (32, 81, 122), various comorbidities of the host (DM (123, 124), HIV/AIDS (125, 126), malignancies, transplant history (127–129), chronic obstructive pulmonary disease (COPD) (32)), nutritional status (32, 130), gender (32), race, vaccination or immunization status, presence of distant infection (32), and the psychological state of the host (131). Similarly, various factors extrinsic to the host contribute to occurrence of disease. Indwelling devices are an increasing cause of infections. Indwelling urinary catheters (33), central venous and arterial catheters (57, 64, 132–134), endotracheal tubes, and mechanical ventilators (48) are common causes of HAIs. Any indwelling device will allow potential pathogens to bypass the local defense system of the body. This facilitates the formation of biofilms and allows microorganisms to not only adhere to these biofilms but also resist antimicrobial activity (135). Invasive surgical procedures will transmit pathogens causing infection (51). These agents can be derived from healthcare personnel or may be related to the endogenous colonization of the patient (136–140). Radiation therapy can affect skin integrity and contribute to decreased immunity. Use of antibiotics will alter normal microbial flora of the patient and increase risk of infections (81, 122). These are just a few examples of the numerous mechanisms and changes that occur in the healthcare setting.

To summarize, any factor—intrinsic or extrinsic—that has the propensity to diminish the host's immune response contributes to the complex pathogenicity and interaction with the host causing the disease. For this complex interaction, the various healthcare-related environments provide the appropriate base/platform.

ENVIRONMENT

The healthcare environment has widened in scope over a period of time. In the past, most infections were attributed to the hospital environment; but now, acute and nonacute healthcare settings contribute to spread of infections. Microorganisms are endemic in the healthcare environment and in any healthcare setting; the triad of agent, host, and environment will interact in various ways to cause HAIs.

Acute Healthcare Environment This refers to the hospital setting where acute care is provided to the patients. There are certain environmental factors that are common to all components of the hospital, and there are other unique features associated with specialized forms of healthcare settings.

Adult Care: General Patient Units, Telemetry Units, Step-Down Units, and Intensive Care Units (ICUs) Certain physical factors—heat, cold, humidity, air-conditioning, water reservoirs (water coolers, water tanks)—provide an optimal environment for the agents to replicate in any unit of the hospital. Biological factors include intermediary vectors that contribute to the spread of infections. Examples include insects or snail vectors. Social factors include: methods of food preparation or distribution, medical and surgical waste disposal; room size; and other healthcare amenities. Almost 30% HAIs occur in the ICU (pediatric and adult). Agent, host, and environmental factors play a major role. Patients in the ICU are sicker, with greater comorbidities and risk factors and more likely to be immunocompromised. Endemic microorganisms in the ICU environment such as *P. aeruginosa* (84) and MRSA (95) are provided a greater opportunity to colonize and cause further infections by these host factors. Pediatric and adult ICUs are known to have outbreaks of bacterial, viral, and fungal pathogens secondary to various common sources and person–person contact, both of which are more frequent in the ICU (121, 141–146).

Pediatric Care Care of a pediatric patient poses various challenges different from the adult population. The host in this case has different risk factors for infection; this includes risk factors such as low birth weight and lack of immunization. Environmental factors are different as well. Pediatric populations are prone to contact with sibling visitors who may be responsible for outbreaks in the hospitals especially during seasonal epidemics (147–149). The child play areas provide opportunistic environment for infections. Not only is there more contact among children and person-to-person transmission, toys are known to be major culprits. It is well known that toys harbor pathogenic bacteria (150). A *P. aeruginosa* outbreak in a pediatric oncology unit was attributed to bath toys (151). Also, families and parents spending more time in the patient room—cuddling, feeding, playing, and changing soiled diapers—all provide multiple opportunities for spread of infection between child and family and even child and healthcare workers (122).

Burn Units Burn wound patients are susceptible hosts who are prone to colonization and infection by various nosocomial pathogens and increased morbidity and mortality (152–154). Hydrotherapy equipment is an environmental risk factor that is associated with increased BSI in burn patients with MRSA (155), *A. baumannii* (156), and *P. aeruginosa* (157). Burn wound infections caused by *Aspergillus* spp. and other molds have been implicated to environmental exposure during construction (158, 159).

Nonacute Healthcare Environment Healthcare is being increasingly provided in nonacute settings. Ambulatory care is the most common example. Furthermore, an increasing number of patients are now being managed in long-term care facilities, nursing homes, subacute rehabilitation centers, assisted-living facilities, and hospice. Healthcare is being provided in non-healthcare settings as well. Schools, prisons, military units, and shelters all provide unique environments for spread of infections. Ambulatory care includes outpatient clinics that may be hospital-based or out of the hospital in the form of private physician offices. Ambulatory care also includes urgent care centers, hemodialysis centers, infusion homes for chemotherapy and antibiotics, employee health clinics, public health clinics, and ambulatory surgical centers. Viral infections (hepatitis B, hepatitis C, and rarely HIV) have been reported in ambulatory care setting in association with use of multidose vials, intravenous solutions, and medical devices (160–165). Rubella has been transmitted in outpatient obstetric setting (166). Goodman et al. (167) described multiple cases of infections acquired in the healthcare setting. Cases of contaminated endoscope-related *Salmonella typhimurium* (168), *Mycobacterial* infections causing abscess from contaminated DTP vaccine (169), *S. marcescens*-related septic arthritis from contaminated antiseptic (170) have been documented in ambulatory care setting. Similarly, improper disinfection of ophthalmology equipment has been associated with Adenovirus type 8 epidemic keratoconjunctivitis (171–175).

Healthcare is being increasingly provided at home in the forms of intravenous medication therapy and even in hospice care. Infectious homecare workers and contaminated equipments are risk factors for infections. In prisons and shelters, crowded environment, poor ventilation, and economically disadvantaged individuals with chronic comorbidities such as alcoholism and intravenous drug use (IVDU) can provide a suitable environment for spread of infections including scabies, tuberculosis, hepatitis A virus, and norovirus (176, 177).

To summarize, the hospital and ambulatory care environment provides ample opportunities for pathogens to flourish and cause infections. Appropriate preventive measures and early diagnostic techniques are essential to prevent spread of infection and adverse outcomes in the population.

REFERENCES

1. Garner JS, Bennett JV, Schekler WE, Maki DG, Brachman PS. Surveillance of nosocomial infections. In *Proceedings of the International Conference on Nosocomial Infections,* Atlanta, Center for Disease Control, August 1970. American Hospital Association, Chicago, 1971; pp. 171–181.
2. Center for Disease, Control. National Nosocomial Infection Study site definitions manual (unpublished). Center for Disease Control, Atlanta, 1975.
3. Garner JS, Jarvis WR, Emori TG, Horan TC, Hughes JM. CDC definitions for nosocomial infections, 1988. *Am J Infect Control* 1988;**16**:128–140.
4. Horan TC, Andrus M, Dudeck MA. CDC/NHSN surveillance definition of health care-associated infection and criteria for specific types of infections in the acute care setting. *Am J Infect Control* 2008;**35**:309–332.
5. Klevens RM, Edwards JR, Richards CL, Horan TC, Gaynes RP, Pollack DA, et al. Estimating health care-associated infections and deaths in US hospitals, 2002. *Public Health Rep* 2007;**122**:160–166.
6. Scott RD. II http://www.cdc.gov/ncidod/dhqp/pdf/Scott_CostPaper.pdf.
7. Dembry L, Zervos MJ, and Hierholzer WJ. Nosocomial bacterial infections. In Brachman EA (ed.), *Bacterial Infection in Humans*, 3rd ed. Plenum Publishing Corporation, New York, 1998, pp. 501–528.
8. Haley RW, Culver DH, White JW, Morgan WM, Emori TG. The nationwide nosocomial infection rate: A new need for vital statistics. *Am J Epidemiol* 1985;**121**:159–165.
9. Panlilio A, Culver DH, Gaynes RP, et al. Methicillin-resistant *Staphylococcus aureus* in U.S. hospitals, 1975–1991. *Infect Control Hosp Epidemiol* 1992;**13**:582–586.
10. Archibald L, Phillips L, Monnet D, McGowan JE, Tenover F, Gaynes R. Antimicrobial resistance in isolates from inpatients and outpatients in the United States: Increasing importance of the intensive care unit. *Clin Infect Dis* 1997;**24**:211–215.
11. Barakate MS, Yang YX, Foo SH, Vickery AM, Sharp CA, Fowler LD, Harris JP, West RH, Mcleod C, Benn RA. An epidemiological survey of methicillin-resistant *Staphylococcus aureus* in a tertiary referral hospital. *J Hosp Infect* 2000;**44**:19–26.
12. Rubin RJ, Harrington CA, Poon A, Dietrich K, Greene JA, Moiduddin A. The economic impact of *Staphylococcus aureus* infection in New York City hospitals. *Emerg Infect Dis* 1999;**5**:9–17.
13. Shopsin B, Kreiswirth BN. Molecular epidemiology of methicillin-resistant *Staphylococcus aureus. Emerg Infect Dis* 2001;**7**:323–326.
14. Hidron AI, Edwards JR, Patel J, et al. NHSN annual update: antimicrobial resistant pathogens associated with healthcare-associated infections: Annual summary of data reported to the national healthcare safety network at the centers for disease control and prevention, 2006–2007. *Infect Control Hosp Epidemiol* 2008;**29**:996–1011.

15. Hayden MK, Trenholme GM, Schultz JE, Sahm DF. *In vivo* development of teicoplanin resistance in a *van*B *Enterococcus faecium. J Infect Dis* 1993;**167**:1224–1227.
16. Malani PN, Kauffman CA, Zervos MJ. Enterococcal disease, epidemiology, and treatment. In Malani PN, Kauffman CA, Zervos MJ (eds.), *The Enterococci: Pathogenesis, Molecular Biology, and Antibiotic Resistance.* ASM Press, Washington, DC, 2002; pp. 385–408.
17. Malani PN, Thal LA, Donabedian SM, Robinson-Dunn B, Kauffman CA, Chow JW, Hershberger E, Zervos MJ. Molecular analysis of vancomycin-resistant *Enterococcus faecalis* from Michigan hospitals during a 10-year period. *J Antimicrob Chemother* 2002; **49**:841–843.
18. Moreno F, Grota P, Crisp C, Magnon K, Melcher GP, Jorgensen JH, Evans Patterson J. Clinical and molecular epidemiology of vancomycin-resistant *Enterococcus faecium* during its emergence in a city in southern Texas. *Clin Infect Dis* 1995;**21**:1234–1237.
19. Thal LA, Donabedian SM, Robinson-Dunn B, Chow JW, Dembry LM, Clewell DB, Alshab D, Zervos MJ. Molecular analysis of glycopeptide-resistant *Enterococcus faecium* isolates collected from Michigan hospitals over a 6-year period. *J Clin Microbiol* 1998; **36**:3303–3308.
20. Vergis EN, Hayden MK, Chow JW, Snydman DR, Zervos MJ, Linden PK, Wagener MM, Schmitt B, Muder RR. Determinants of vancomycin resistance and mortality rates in enterococcal bacteremia. *Ann Intern Med* 2001;**135**:484–492.
21. Smith TL, Pearson ML, Wilcox KR, Cruz C, Lancaster MV, Robinson-Dunn B, Tenover FC, Zervos MJ, Band JD, White E, Jarvis WR. Emergence of vancomycin resistance in *Staphylococcus aureus. N Engl J Med* 1999;**340**:493–501.
22. Weber DJ, Rutala WA, Miller MB, Huslage K, Sickbert-Bennett E. Role of hospital surfaces in the transmission of emerging health care-associated pathogens: Norovirus, *Clostridium difficile,* and *Acinetobacter* spp. *Am J Infect Control* 2010;**38**(Suppl): S25–S30.
23. Frédéric Barbut, Anne Richard, Kheira Hamadi, et al. Epidemiology of recurrences or reinfections of *Clostridium difficile*-associated diarrhea. *J Clin Microbiol* 2000;**38**(6): 2386–2388.
24. Barbut F, Corthier G, Charpak Y, Cerf M, Monteil H, Fosse T, Trevoux A, De Barbeyrac B, Boussougant Y, Tigaud S, Tytgat F, Sédallian A, Duborgel S, Collignon A, Le Guern ME, Bernasconi P, Petit JC. Prevalence and pathogenicity of *Clostridium difficile* in hospitalized patients. *Arch Intern Med* 1996;**156**:1449–1454.
25. Bartlett JG. *Clostridium difficile*: History of its role as an enteric pathogen and the current state of knowledge about the organism. *Clin Infect Dis* 1994;**18**:265–272.
26. Kelly CP, Pothoulakis C, LaMont JT. *Clostridium difficile* colitis. *N Eng J Med* 1994;**330**:257–262.
27. McFarland LV, Mulligan ME, Kwok RYY, Stamm WE. Nosocomial acquisition of *Clostridium difficile* infection. *N Engl J Med* 1989;**320**:204–210.
28. Bergogne-Berezin E, Towner KJ, *Acinetobacter* spp. as nosocomial pathogens: Microbiological, clinical, and epidemiological features. *Clin Microbiol Rev* 1996;**9**(2):148–165.
29. Kumarasamy KK, Toleman MA, Walsh TR, et al. Emergence of a new antibiotic resistance mechanism in India, Pakistan, and the UK: A molecular, biological, and epidemiological study. *Lancet Infect Dis* 2010;**10**:597–602.
30. Fridkin SK, Jarvis WR. Epidemiology of nosocomial fungal infections. *Clin Microbiol Rev* 1996;**9**:499–511.
31. Lohr JA, Donowitz LG, Sadler JE III. Hospital-acquired urinary tract infection. *Pediatrics* 1989;**83**:193–199.
32. Emori TG, Gaynes RP. An overview of nosocomial infections, including the role of the microbiology laboratory. *Clin Microbiol Rev* 1993;**6**:428–442.

33. Burke JP, Yeo TW. Nosocomial urinary tract infections In Mayhall CG (ed.), *Hospital Epidemiology and Infection Control,* 3rd ed. Lippincott Williams & Wilkins, Philadelphia, 2004; pp. 267–286.
34. Gardam MA, Amihod B, Orenstein P, et al. Overutilization of indwelling urinary catheters and the development of nosocomial urinary tract infections. *Clin Perform Quality Health Care* 1998;**6**:99–102.
35. Jain P, Parada JP, David A, et al. Overuse of the indwelling urinary tract catheter in hospitalized medical patients. *Arch Intern Med* 1995;**155**:1425–1429.
36. Munasinghe RL, Yazdani H, Siddique M, et al. Appropriateness of use of indwelling urinary catheters in patients admitted to the medical service. *Infect Control Hosp Epidemiol* 2001;**22**:647–649.
37. Bouza E, Rodriquez-Bouze H, Munoz P, et al. Evaluation of indwelling bladder catheterization in a general hospital. *Infect Dis Clin Pract* 1994;**3**:358–362.
38. Saint S, Wiese J, Amory JK, et al. Are physicians aware of which of their patients have indwelling urinary catheters? *Am J Med* 2000;**109**:476–480.
39. Brennan ML, Evans A. Why catheterize?: Audit findings on the use of urinary catheters. *Br J Nurs* 2001;**10**:580–590.
40. Hooton TM, Bradley SF, Cardenas DD, Colgan R, Geerlings SE, Rice JC, Saint S, Schaeffer AJ, Tambayh PA, Tenke P, Nicolle LE. Diagnosis, prevention, and treatment of catheter-associated urinary tract infection in adults: 2009 International Clinical Practice Guidelines from the Infectious Diseases Society of America. *Clin Infect Dis* 2010;**50**(5):625–663.
41. Kappstein I, Schulgen G, Beyes U, et al. Prolongation of hospital stay and extra costs due to ventilator-associated pneumonia in an intensive care unit. *Eur J Clin Microbiol Infect Dis* 1992;**11**:504–508.
42. Niederman MS. Guidelines for the management of respiratory infection: Why do we need them, how should they be developed, and can they be useful? *Curr Opin Pulm Med* 1996;**2**:161–165.
43. Tablan OC, Anderson LJ, Besser R, Bridges C, Hajjeh R. Healthcare Infection Control Practices Advisory Committee, Centers for Disease Control and Prevention. Guidelines for preventing health-care-associated pneumonia, 2003: Recommendations of the CDC and the Healthcare Infection Control Practices Advisory Committee. *MMWR Recomm Rep* 2004; **53**(RR-3):1–36.
44. Craven DE, Kunches LM, Kilinsky V, Lichtenberg DA, Make BJ, McCabe WR. Risk factors for pneumonia and fatality in patients receiving continuous mechanical ventilation. *Am Rev Respir Dis* 1986;**133**:792–796.
45. Hutt E, Kramer AM. Evidence-based guidelines for management of nursing home-acquired pneumonia. *J Fam Pract* 2002;**51**:709–716.
46. Mylotte JM. Nursing-home acquired pneumonia. *Clin Infect Dis* 2002;**35**:1205–1211.
47. Guidelines for the management of adults with hospital-acquired, ventilator-associated, and healthcare-associated pneumonia. *Am J Respir Crit Care Med* 2005;**171**:388–416.
48. Bergmans D, Bonten JM. Nosocomial pneumonia. In Mayhall CG (ed.), *Hospital Epidemiology and Infection Control,* 3rd ed. Lippincott Williams & Wilkins, Philadelphia, 2004; pp. 311–339.
49. Graves EJ. National hospital discharge survey: Annual summary 1987. National Center for health statistics. *Vital Stat* 1989;**13**:11.
50. Cruse P. Wound infection surveillance. *Rev Infect Dis* 1981;**4**:734–737.
51. Wong ES. Surgical site infections. In Mayhall CG (ed.), *Hospital Epidemiology and Infection Control,* 3rd ed. Lippincott Williams & Wilkins, Philadelphia, 2004; pp. 287–310.

52. Cruse PJE, Foord R. The epidemiology of wound infection. A 10-year prospective study of 62,939 wounds. *Surg Clin North Am* 1980;**60**:27–40.
53. Seropian R, Reynolds BM. Wound infections after preoperative depilatory versus razor preparation. *Am J Surg* 1971;**121**:251–254.
54. Tanner J, Woodings D, Moncaster K. Preoperative hair removal to reduce surgical site infection. *Cochrane Database of Systematic Reviews* 2006, Issue 3. Art. No.: CD004122. DOI: 10.1002/14651858.CD004122.pub3.
55. American College of Surgeons Committee on Control of Surgical Infections of the Committee on Pre- and Postoperative, Care. *Manual on Control of Infection in Surgical Patients*, 2nd ed. Lippincott, Philadelphia, 1984.
56. Wenzel RP, Edmond MB. The impact of hospital acquired blood stream infections. *Emerg Infect Dis* 2001;**7**:174–177.
57. Rupp ME, Nosocomial bloodstream infections In Mayhall CG (ed.). *Hospital Epidemiology and Infection Control*, 3rd ed. Lippincott Williams & Wilkins, Philadelphia, 2004; pp. 253–265.
58. Friedman ND, Kaye KS, Stout JE, et al. Health care-associated blood-stream infections in adults: A reason to change the accepted definition of community-acquired infections. *Ann Intern Med* 2002;**137**:791–792.
59. Siegman-Igra Y, Fourer B, Orni-Wasserlauf R, et al. Reappraisal of community-acquired bacteremia: A proposal of a new classifiation for the spectrum of acquisition of bacteremia. *Clin Infect Dis* 2002;**34**:1431–1439.
60. Graham DR, Kelderman MM, Klemm LW, et al. Infectious complications among patients receiving home intravenous therapy with peripheral, central, or peripherally placed central venous catheters. *Am J Med* 1991;**9**:95S–100S.
61. Mimoz O, Karim A, Mercat A, et al. Chlorhexidine compared with povidone-iodine as skin preparation before blood culture. *Ann Intern Med* 1999;**131**:834–837.
62. Maki DG. Nosocomial bacteremia. *Am J Med* 1981;**70**:719–732.
63. Scheckler WE, Scheibel W, Kresge D. Temporal trends in septicemia in a community hospital. *Am J Med* 1991;**91**:90S–94S.
64. Pitter D, Wenzel RP. Nosocomial blood stream infections. *Arch Intern Med* 1995;**155**:1177–1184.
65. Saviteer SM, Samsa GP, Rutala WA. Nosocomial infections in the elderly increased risk per hospital day. *Am J Med* 1988;**84**:661–666.
66. Trilla A, Gatell JM, Mensa J, et al. Risk factors for nosocomial bacteremia in a large Spanish teaching hospital: A case–control study. *Infect Control Hosp Epidemiol* 1991;**12**:150–156.
67. Mylotte JM, Tayara A, Goodnough S. Epidemiology of bloodstream infections in nursing home residents: Evaluation in a large cohort from multiple homes. *Clin Infect Dis* 2002;**35**: 1484–1490.
68. Bodey GP. Infection in cancer patients: A continuing association. *Am J Med* 1986;**81**:11–26.
69. Singer C, Kaplan MH, Armstrong D. Bacteremia and fungemia complicating neoplastic disease: A study of 364 cases. *Am J Med* 1977;**62**:731–742.
70. Mayo JW, Wennzel R. Rates of hospital-acquired bloodstream infection in patients with specific malignancy. *Cancer* 1982;**50**:187–190.
71. Caly WR, Stauss E. A prospective study of bacterial infections in patients with cirrhosis. *J Hepatol* 1993;**18**:353–358.
72. Tokars JI. Bloodstream infections in hemodialysis patients: Getting some deserved attention. *Infect Cont Hosp Epidemiol* 2002;**23**:713–715.
73. Luterman A, Dacso CC, Curreri PW. Infection in burn patients. *Am J Med* 1986;**81**:45–52.
74. Waites KB, Canupp KC, Chen Y, et al. Bacteremia aftr spinal cord injury in initial versus subsequent hospitalizations. *J Spinal Cord Med* 2001;**24**:96–100.

75. Motgomerie JZ, Chan E, Gilmore DS, et al. Low mortality among patients with spinal cord injury and bacteremia. *Rev Infect Dis* 1991;**13**:867–871.
76. Rubin RH. Infectious disease complications of renal transplantation. *Kidney Int* 1993;**44**:221–236.
77. Wenzel RP, hompson RL, Landry SM, et al. Hospital-acquired infection in intensive care unit patients: An overview with emphasis on epidemics. *Infect Control* 1983;**4**:371.
78. Marschall J, Mermel LA, Classen D, et al. SHEA/IDSA practice recommendation: Strategies to prevent central line–associated bloodstream infections in acute care hospitals. *Infect Control Hosp Epidemiol* 2008;**29**:S22–S306.
79. Mausner JS, Kramer S (eds.). *Mausner & Bahn Epidemiology—An Introductory Text.* WB Saunders, Philadelphia, 1985.
80. Fox JP, Elveback L, Gatewood L, et al. Herd immunity. *Am J Epidemiol* 1971;**94**:171–189.
81. Archibald LK, Hierholzer WJ. Principles of infectious disease epidemiology. In Mayhall CG (ed.), *Hospital Epidemiology and Infection Control,* 3rd ed. Philadelphia, Lippincott Williams & Wilkins, 2004; pp. 3–17.
82. Bolyard EA, Tablan OC, Williams WW, Pearson ML, Shapiro CN, Deitchmann SD. Guideline for infection control in healthcare personnel, 1998. Hospital Infection Control Practices Advisory Committee. *Infect Control Hosp Epidemiol* 1998;**19**(6):407–463.
83. Zawacki A, O'Rourke E, Potter-Bynoe G, Macone A, Harbarth S, Goldmann D. An outbreak of *Pseudomonas aeruginosa* pneumonia and bloodstream infection associated with intermittent otitis externa in a healthcare worker. *Infect Control Hosp Epidemiol* 2004;**25**(12):1083–1089.
84. Foca M, Jakob K, Whittier S, et al. Endemic *Pseudomonas aeruginosa* infection in a neonatal intensive care unit. *N Engl J Med* 2000;**343**(10):695–700.
85. Gupta A, Della-Latta P, Todd B, et al. Outbreak of extended-spectrum beta-lactamase-producing *Klebsiella pneumoniae* in a neonatal intensive care unit linked to artificial nails. *Infect Control Hosp Epidemiol* 2004;**25**(3):210–215.
86. Boyce JM, Opal SM, Potter-Bynoe G, Medeiros AA. Spread of methicillin-resistant *Staphylococcus aureus* in a hospital after exposure to a health care worker with chronic sinusitis. *Clin Infect Dis* 1993;**17**(3):496–504.
87. Fliegel PE, Weinstein WM. Rubella outbreak in a prenatal clinic: Management and prevention. *Am J Infect Control* 1982;**10**(1):29–33.
88. Atkinson WL, Markowitz LE, Adams NC, Seastrom GR. Transmission of measles in medical settings—United States, 1985–1989. *Am J Med* 1991;**91**(3B):320S–324S.
89. Carman WF, Elder AG, Wallace LA, et al. Effects of influenza vaccination of health-care workers on mortality of elderly people in long-term care: A randomised controlled trial. *Lancet* 2000;**355**(9198):93–97.
90. CDC., Outbreaks of pertussis associated with hospitals—Kentucky, Pennsylvania, and Oregon, 2003. *MMWR Morb Mortal Wkly Rep* 2005;**54**(3):67–71.
91. Mermel LA, McKay M, Dempsey J, Parenteau S. *Pseudomonas* surgical-site infections linked to a healthcare worker with onychomycosis. *Infect Control Hosp Epidemiol* 2003;**24**(10): 749–752.
92. Barnes GL, Callaghan SL, Kirkwood CD, Bogdanovic-Sakran N, Johnston LJ, Bishop RF. Excretion of serotype G1 rotavirus strains by asymptomatic staff: A possible source of nosocomial infection. *J Pediatr* 2003;**142**(6):722–755.
93. Saiman L, Siegel J. Infection control recommendations for patients with cystic fibrosis: Microbiology, important pathogens, and infection control practices to prevent patient-to-patient transmission. *Infect Control Hosp Epidemiol* 2003;**24**(5 Suppl): S6–S52.

94. Varia M, Wilson S, Sarwal S, et al. Investigation of a nosocomial outbreak of severe acute respiratory syndrome (SARS) in Toronto, *Canada. CMAJ* 2003;**169**(4):285–292.

95. Haley RW, Cushion NB, Tenover FC, et al. Eradication of endemic methicillin-resistant *Staphylococcus aureus* infections from a neonatal intensive care unit. *J Infect Dis* 1995; **171**(3):614–624.

96. Bridges CB, Kuehnert MJ, Hall CB. Transmission of influenza: Implications for control in health care settings. *Clin Infect Dis* 2003;**37**(8):1094–1101.

97. Hall CB. Nosocomial respiratory syncytial virus infections: The "Cold War" has not ended. *Clin Infect Dis* 2000;**31**(2):590–596.

98. Campbell JR, Zaccaria E, Mason EO Jr, Baker CJ. Epidemiological analysis defining concurrent outbreaks of Serratia marcescens and methicillin-resistant Staphylococcus aureus in a neonatal intensive-care unit. *Infect Control Hosp Epidemiol* 1998;**19**(12):924–928.

99. Pena C, Pujol M, Ardanuy C, et al. Epidemiology and successful control of a large outbreak due to *Klebsiella pneumoniae* producing extended-spectrum beta-lactamases. *Antimicrob Agents Chemother* 1998;**42**(1):53–58.

100. Bonten MJ, Slaughter S, Ambergen AW, et al. The role of "colonization pressure" in the spread of vancomycin-resistant enterococci: An important infection control variable. *Arch Intern Med* 1998;**158**(10):1127–1132.

101. Jensenius M, Ringertz SH, Berild D, Bell H, Espinoza R, Grinde B. Prolonged nosocomial outbreak of hepatitis A arising from an alcoholic with pneumonia. *Scand J Infect Dis* 1998; **30**(2):119–123.

102. Valenti WM, Pincus PH, Messner MK. Nosocomial pertussis: Possible spread by a hospital visitor. *Am J Dis Child* 1980;**134**(5):520–521.

103. Christie CD, Glover AM, Willke MJ, Marx ML, Reising SF, Hutchinson NM. Containment of pertussis in the regional pediatric hospital during the Greater Cincinnati epidemic of 1993. *Infect Control Hosp Epidemiol* 1995;**16**(10):556–563.

104. Munoz FM, Ong LT, Seavy D, Medina D, Correa A, Starke Jr., Tuberculosis among adult visitors of children with suspected tuberculosis and employees at a children's hospital. *Infect Control Hosp Epidemiol* 2002;**23**(10):568–572.

105. Garcia R, Raad I, Abi-Said D, et al. Nosocomial respiratory syncytial virus infections: Prevention and control in bone marrow transplant patients. *Infect Control Hosp Epidemiol* 1997; **18**(6):412–416.

106. Whimbey E, Champlin RE, Couch RB, et al. Community respiratory virus infections among hospitalized adult bone marrow transplant recipients. *Clin Infect Dis* 1996;**22**(5):778–782.

107. Saiman L, O'Keefe M, Graham PL, et al. Hospital transmission of community-acquired methicillin-resistant *Staphylococcus aureus* among postpartum women. *Clin Infect Dis* 2003; **37**(10):1313–1319.

108. Wang JT, Chang SC, Ko WJ, et al. A hospital-acquired outbreak of methicillin-resistant *Staphylococcus aureus* infection initiated by a surgeon carrier. *J Hosp Infect* 2001; **47**(2):104–109.

109. Anderson KF, Coulter JR, Keynes DR. Staphylococcal nasal carriage in mothers, babies, and staff in a maternity hospital. *J Hyg* 1961;**59**:15–27.

110. Boyce JM, Potter-Bynoe G, Chenevert C, King T. Environmental contamination due to methicillin-resistant *Staphylococcus aureus*: Possible infection control implications. *Infect Control Hosp Epidemiol* 1997;**18**(9):622–627.

111. Zachary KC, Bayne PS, Morrison VJ, Ford DS, Silver LC, Hooper DC. Contamination of gowns, gloves, and stethoscopes with vancomycin-resistant enterococci. *Infect Control Hosp Epidemiol* 2001;**22**(9):560–564.

112. Perry C, Marshall R, Jones E. Bacterial contamination of uniforms. *J Hosp Infect* 2001; **48**(3):238–241.

113. Morgan DJ, Liang SY, Smith CL, et al. Frequent multidrug-resistant *Acinetobacter baumannii* contamination of gloves, gowns and hands of healthcare workers. *Infect Control Hosp Epidemiol* 2010;**31**:716–721.

114. Bhalla A, Pultz NJ, Gries DM, et al. Acquisition of nosocomial pathogens on hands after contact with environmental surfaces near hospitalized patients. *Infect Control Hosp Epidemiol* 2004; **25**(2):164–167.

115. Duckro AN, Blom DW, Lyle EA, Weinstein RA, Hayden MK. Transfer of vancomycin-resistant enterococci via health care worker hands. *Arch Intern Med* 2005;**165**(3):302–307.

116. Brooks SE, Veal RO, Kramer M, Dore L, Schupf N, Adachi M. Reduction in the incidence of *Clostridium difficile*-associated diarrhea in an acute care hospital and a skilled nursing facility following replacement of electronic thermometers with single-use disposables. *Infect Control Hosp Epidemiol* 1992;**13**(2):98–103.

117. CDC. Nosocomial hepatitis B virus infection associated with reusable fingerstick blood sampling devices—Ohio and New York City, 1996. *MMWR Morb Mortal Wkly Rep* 1997;**46**(10):217–221.

118. Desenclos JC, Bourdiol-Razes M, Rolin B, et al. Hepatitis C in a ward for cystic fibrosis and diabetic patients: Possible transmission by spring-loaded finger-stick devices for self-monitoring of capillary blood glucose. *Infect Control Hosp Epidemiol* 2001;**22**(11):701–707.

119. CDC. Transmission of hepatitis B virus among persons undergoing blood glucose monitoring in long-term-care facilities—Mississippi, North Carolina, and Los Angeles County, California, 2003–2004. *MMWR Morb Mortal Wkly Rep* 2005;**54**(9):220–223.

120. Biddick R, Spilker T, Martin A, LiPuma JJ. Evidence of transmission of *Burkholderia cepacia, Burkholderia multivorans* and *Burkholderia* dolosa among persons with cystic fibrosis. *FEMS Microbiol Lett* 2003;**228**(1):57–62.

121. Griffiths AL, Jamsen K, Carlin JB, et al. Effects of segregation on an epidemic *Pseudomonas aeruginosa* strain in a cystic fibrosis clinic. *Am J Respir Crit Care Med* 2005;**171**(9): 1020–1025.

122. Siegel JD, Rhinehart E, Jackson M, Chiarello L, and the Healthcare Infection Control Practices Advisory Committee, *2007 Guideline for Isolation Precautions: Preventing Transmission of Infectious Agents in Healthcare Settings*. Atlanta, Centers for Disease Control and Prevention. 2007. Available at: http://www.cdc.gov/ncidod/dhqp/pdf/isolation2007.pdf.

123. Thomsen RW, Hundborg HH, Lervang HH, Johnsen SP, Schonheyder HC, Sorensen HT. Risk of community-acquired pneumococcal bacteremia in patients with diabetes: A population-based case–control study. *Diabetes Care* 2004;**27**(5):1143–1147.

124. Carton JA, Maradona JA, Nuno FJ, Fernandez-Alvarez R, Perez-Gonzalez F, Asensi V. Diabetes mellitus and bacteraemia: A comparative study between diabetic and non-diabetic patients. *Eur J Med* 1992;**1**(5):281–287.

125. Hirschtick RE, Glassroth J, Jordan MC, et al. Bacterial pneumonia in persons infected with the human immunodeficiency virus. Pulmonary Complications of HIV Infection Study Group. *N Engl J Med* 1995;**333**(13):845–51.

126. Rosenberg AL, Seneff MG, Atiyeh L, Wagner R, Bojanowski L, Zimmerman JE. The importance of bacterial sepsis in intensive care unit patients with acquired immunodeficiency syndrome: Implications for future care in the age of increasing antiretroviral resistance. *Crit Care Med* 2001;**29**(3):548–556.

127. Malone JL, Ijaz K, Lambert L, et al. Investigation of healthcare-associated transmission of *Mycobacterium tuberculosis* among patients with malignancies at three hospitals and at a residential facility. *Cancer* 2004;**101**(12):2713–2721.

128. Fishman JA, Rubin RH. Infection in organ-transplant recipients. *N Engl J Med* 1998; **338**(24):1741–1751.

129. CDC. Recommendations for preventing transmission of infections among chronic hemodialysis patients. *MMWR Morb Mortal Wkly Rep* 2001;**50**(RR05):1–43.

130. Scrimshaw NS. Malnutrition and nosocomial infection. *Infect Control Hosp Epidemiol* 1989;**10**:191–193.

131. Cohen S, Tyrell AJ, Smith AP. Psychological stress and susceptibility to the common cold. *N Eng J Med* 1991;**325**:606–612.

132. Safdar N, Kluger DM, Maki DG. A review of risk factors for catheter-related bloodstream infection caused by percutaneously inserted, noncuffed central venous catheters: Implications for preventive strategies. *Medicine (Baltimore)* 2002;**81**(6):466–479.

133. Jarvis WR, Robles B. Nosocomial infections in pediatric patients. *Adv Pediatr Infect Dis* 1996;**12**:243–959. (js).

134. Yogaraj JS, Elward AM, Fraser VJ. Rate, risk factors, and outcomes of nosocomial primary bloodstream infection in pediatric intensive care unit patients. *Pediatrics* 2002;**110**(3): 481–485.

135. Donlan RM. Biofilms: Microbial life on surfaces. *Emerg Infect Dis* 2002;**8**(9):881–890.

136. Bonten MJ, Slaughter S, Hayden MK, Nathan C, van Voorhis J, Weinstein RA. External sources of vancomycin-resistant enterococci for intensive care units. *Crit Care Med* 1998;**26**(12): 2001–2004.

137. Flynn DM, Weinstein RA, Nathan C, Gaston MA, Kabins SA. Patients' endogenous flora as the source of "nosocomial" Enterobacter in cardiac surgery. *J Infect Dis* 1987;**156**(2): 363–368.

138. Olson B, Weinstein RA, Nathan C, Chamberlin W, Kabins SA. Epidemiology of endemic *Pseudomonas aeruginosa*: Why infection control efforts have failed. *J Infect Dis* 1984;**150**(6): 808–816.

139. Perl TM, Cullen JJ, Wenzel RP, et al. Intranasal mupirocin to prevent postoperative *Staphylococcus aureus* infections. *N Engl J Med* 2002;**346**(24):1871–1877.

140. Toltzis P, Hoyen C, et al. Factors that predict preexisting colonization with antibiotic-resistant Gram-negative bacilli in patients admitted to a pediatric intensive care unit. *Pediatrics* 1999; **103**(4Pt1):719–723.

141. Villarino ME, Stevens LE, Schable B, et al. Risk factors for epidemic *Xanthomonas maltophilia* infection/colonization in intensive care unit patients. *Infect Control Hosp Epidemiol* 1992; **13**(4):201–206.

142. Sanchez V, Vazquez JA, Barth-Jones D, Dembry L, Sobel JD, Zervos MJ. Nosocomial acquisition of *Candida parapsilosis*: An epidemiologic study. *Am J Med* 1993;**94**(6):577–582.

143. Husni RN, Goldstein LS, Arroliga AC, et al. Risk factors for an outbreak of multi-drug-resistant *Acinetobacter* nosocomial pneumonia among intubated patients. *Chest* 1999;**115**(5): 1378–1382.

144. McDonald LC, Walker M, Carson L, et al. Outbreak of *Acinetobacter* spp. bloodstream infections in a nursery associated with contaminated aerosols and air conditioners. *Pediatr Infect Dis J* 1998;**17**(8):716–722.

145. Trick WE, Kioski CM, Howard KM, et al. Outbreak of *Pseudomonas aeruginosa* ventriculitis among patients in a neurosurgical intensive care unit. *Infect Control Hosp Epidemiol* 2000; **21**(3):204–208.

146. Guidry GG, Black-Payne CA, Payne DK, Jamison RM, George RB, Bocchini JA Jr. Respiratory syncytial virus infection among intubated adults in a university medical intensive care unit. *Chest* 1991;**100**(5):1377–1384.

147. CDC. Outbreaks of pertussis associated with hospitals—Kentucky, Pennsylvania, and Oregon, 2003. *MMWR Morb Mortal Wkly Rep* 2005;**54**(3):67–71.

148. Valenti WM, Pincus PH, Messner MK. Nosocomial pertussis: Possible spread by a hospital visitor. *Am J Dis Child* 1980;**134**(5):520–521.

149. Hatherill M, Levin M, Lawrenson J, Hsiao NY, Reynolds L, Argent A. Evolution of an adenovirus outbreak in a multidisciplinary children's hospital. *J Paediatr Child Health* 2004; **40**(8):449–454.

150. Avila-Aguero ML, German G, Paris MM, Herrera JF. Toys in a pediatric hospital: Are they a bacterial source? *Am J Infect Control* 2004;**32**(5):287–290.

151. Buttery JP, Alabaster SJ, Heine RG, et al. Multiresistant *Pseudomonas aeruginosa* outbreak in a pediatric oncology ward related to bath toys. *Pediatr Infect Dis J* 1998;**17**(6): 509–513.

152. NNIS. National Nosocomial Infections Surveillance (NNIS) System Report, data summary from January 1992 through June 2004, issued October 2004. *Am J Infect Control* 2004; **32**(8):470–485.

153. Wurtz R, Karajovic M, Dacumos E, Jovanovic B, Hanumadass M. Nosocomial infections in a burn intensive care unit. *Burns* 1995;**21**(3):181–184.

154. Rodgers GL, Mortensen J, Fisher MC, Lo A, Cresswell A, Long SS. Predictors of infectious complications after burn injuries in children. *Pediatr Infect Dis J* 2000;**19**(10):990–995.

155. Embil JM, McLeod JA, Al-Barrak AM, et al. An outbreak of methicillin resistant *Staphylococcus aureus* on a burn unit: Potential role of contaminated hydrotherapy equipment. *Burns* 2001; **27**(7):681–688.

156. Wisplinghoff H, Perbix W, Seifert H. Risk factors for nosocomial bloodstream infections due to *Acinetobacter baumannii*: A case–control study of adult burn patients. *Clin Infect Dis* 1999; **28**(1):59–66.

157. Tredget EE, Shankowsky HA, Joffe AM, et al. Epidemiology of infections with *Pseudomonas aeruginosa* in burn patients: The role of hydrotherapy. *Clin Infect Dis* 1992; **15**(6):941–949.

158. Bryce EA, Walker M, Scharf S, et al. An outbreak of cutaneous aspergillosis in a tertiary-care hospital. *Infect Control Hosp Epidemiol* 1996;**17**(3):170–172.

159. Levenson C, Wohlford P, Djou J, Evans S, Zawacki B. Preventing postoperative burn wound aspergillosis. *J Burn Care Rehabil* 1991;**12**(2):132–135.

160. Hlady WG, Hopkins RS, Ogilby TE, Allen ST. Patient-to-patient transmission of hepatitis B in a dermatology practice. *Am J Public Health* 1993;**83**(12):1689–1693.

161. Birnie GG, Quigley EM, Clements GB, Follet EA, Watkinson G. Endoscopic transmission of hepatitis B virus. *Gut* 1983;**24**(2):171–174.

162. Chant K, Lowe D, Rubin G, et al. Patient-to-patient transmission of HIV in private surgical consulting rooms. *Lancet* 1993;**342**(8886–8887):1548–1549.

163. Chant K, Kociuba K, Munro R, et al. Investigation of possible patient-to-patient transmission of hepatitis C in a hospital. *NSW Public Health Bull* 1994;**5**(5):47–51.

164. CDC. Transmission of hepatitis B and C viruses in outpatient settings—New York, Oklahoma, and Nebraska, 2000–2002. *MMWR Morb Mortal Wkly Rep* 2003;**52**(38):901–906.

165. Bronowicki JP, Venard V, Botte C, et al. Patient-to-patient transmission of hepatitis C virus during colonoscopy. *N Engl J Med* 1997;**337**(4):237–240.

166. Fliegel PE, Weinstein WM. Rubella outbreak in a prenatal clinic: Management and prevention. *Am J Infect Control* 1982;**10**(1):29–33.

167. Goodman RA, Solomon SL. Transmission of infectious diseases in outpatient health care settings. *JAMA* 1991;**265**(18):2377–2381.

168. Beecham HJ, Cohen ML, Parkin WE. *Salmonella typhimurium* transmission by fiberoptic upper gastrointestinal endoscopy. *JAMA* 1979;**241**:1013–1015.

169. Borghans JGA, Stanford JL. *Mycobacterium chelonei* in abscesses after injection of diphtheria–pertussis–tetanus–polio vaccine. *Am Rev Respir Dis* 1973;**107**:1–8.

170. Nakashima AK, McCarthy MA, Martone WJ, Anderson RL. Epidemic septic arthritis caused by *Serratia marcescens* and associated with a benzalkonium chloride antiseptic. *J Clin Microbiol* 1987;**25**:1014–1018.

171. Buehler JW, Finton RJ, Goodman RA, et al. Epidemic keratoconjunctivitis: Report of an outbreak in an ophthalmology practice and recommendations for prevention. *Infect Control Hosp Epidemiol* 1984;**5**:390–394.

172. D'Angelo LJ, Hierholzer JC, Holman RC, Smith JD. Epidemic keratoconjunctivitis caused by adenovirus type 8: Epidemiologic and laboratoryaspects of a large outbreak. *Am J Epidemiol* 1981;**113**:44–49.

173. Keenlyside RA, Hierholzer JC, D'Angelo LJ. Keratoconjunctivitis associated with adenovirus type 37: An extended outbreak in an ophthalmologist's office. *J Infect Dis* 1983;**147**:191–198.

174. Koo D, Bouvier B, Wesley M, et al. Epidemic keratoconjunctivitis in a university medical center ophthalmology clinic: Need for re-evaluation of the design and disinfection of instruments. *Infect Control Hosp Epidemiol* 1989;**10**:547–552.

175. Haley CE, McDonald RC, Rossi L, Jones WD Jr, Haley RW, Luby JP. Tuberculosis epidemic among hospital personnel. *Infect Control Hosp Epidemiol* 1989;**10**(5):204–10.

176. CDC. Norovirus outbreak among evacuees from hurricane Katrina—Houston, Texas, September 2005. *MMWR Morb Mortal Wkly Rep* 2005;**54**(40):1016–1018.

177. Cieslak PR, Curtis MB, Coulombier DM, Hathcock AL, Bean NH, Tauxe RV. Preventable disease in correctional facilities. Desmoteric foodborne outbreaks in the United States, 1974–1991. *Arch Intern Med* 1996;**156**(16):1883–1888.

CHAPTER TWO

Pathogen Transmission in the Healthcare Setting

SONJA HANSEN AND RALF-PETER VONBERG

Introduction

Transmission of pathogens has been described in all kinds of healthcare facilities such as a hospital, outpatient care, and long-term care facilities. This chapter will discuss the most frequent reservoirs of pathogens in the healthcare setting as well as the corresponding routes of transmission. Only medical staff that are aware of the basic facts of pathogen transmission will be able to identify (and avoid or properly perform) high-risk medical procedures. The next chapter will then deal with measures to prevent transmission and/or acquisition of nosocomial pathogens (Infection Control Basics).

Epidemiology of Nosocomial Transmissions

ENDOGENOUS INFECTIONS

Pathogens that cause hospital-acquired (nosocomial) infections may derive from the patient's own microbiological flora—for example, from the skin, the respiratory tract, the gastrointestinal tract, or the urogenital tract. These types of infection are called "endogenous nosocomial infections." Some of those are preventable—for example, by the use of appropriate skin disinfection before insertion of a central vascular catheter or by the

Molecular Techniques for the Study of Hospital-Acquired Infection, First Edition. Edited by Steven L. Foley, Anne Y. Chen, Shabbir Simjee, and Marcus J. Zervos.

application of antimicrobial prophylaxis before certain surgical procedures. However, some endogenous nosocomial infections will remain that cannot be prevented. Because it is impossible to totally eradicate a patient's physiological flora there is always some risk of an endogenous nosocomial infection—no matter how much effort in the field of infection control is made.

EXOGENOUS INFECTIONS

The situation is somewhat different for exogenous nosocomial infections. Exogenous nosocomial infections are, by definition, caused by pathogens that were primarily not part of the patient's residential flora. Instead, in some way these pathogens were newly brought to the patient during his or her hospital stay (acquired by transmission). Thus, all exogenous infections are preventable in principle by adherence to infection control recommendations.

INCIDENCE OF NOSOCOMIAL TRANSMISSIONS

The precise incidence of nosocomial transmissions in a hospital can hardly be determined because many transmissions that occur on a ward will remain unnoticed in daily practice. Other factors that may influence the detectable rate of transmission include the pathogen's ability to survive in the environment, the average patient's length of stay on the ward, and the compliance of staff to infection control measures such as hand hygiene, isolation precautions, or the use of protective clothing.

Recent transmission studies came up with an incidence of cross transmission on intensive care units (ICU) between 5.0 (1) and 10.7 (2) per 1.000 patient-days. Another study from a thoracic organ transplant unit reports a transmission rate of 7.8 per 1.000 patient-days as determined by molecular typing of enterococci (3), which served as a marker for the overall transmission rate because of their high prevalence and transmissibility.

RECOGNIZING NOSOCOMIAL TRANSMISSIONS

As mentioned above, nosocomial transmissions usually remain undetected unless specifically searched for. This is especially true for transmissions of common pathogens such as coagulase-negative staphylococci or enterococci. Nosocomial pathogen transmission may also easily be missed if the recipient does not develop a secondary nosocomial infection after transmission.

In contrast, nosocomial transmissions of unusual pathogens or transmissions that lead to a large number of severe or even lethal nosocomial infections are much more likely to be recognized. Thus, the understanding of the mechanism of cross-transmission is absolutely mandatory in the endemic setting, as well as during an obvious nosocomial outbreak.

Nosocomial Pathogens

Since the transmissibility of pathogens varies according to the type of microorganism, the following paragraphs briefly describe the different types of pathogens in the healthcare setting.

BACTERIA

Bacteria are unicellular organisms, about 0.5 to 5 μm in length, and do not possess a nucleus (prokaryotic cells). Most bacteria can rapidly replicate outside the human body (the population usually doubles every 20 minutes) as long as there is a sufficient amount of nutrients around. The genetic information (DNA) of bacteria is coded on a single chromosome that gets copied as the organism divides (vertical transmission). However, some bacteria also hold (up to several hundred) plasmids in addition to their chromosome. Plasmids, too, contain DNA and may encode for virulence factors such as toxin production or antimicrobial resistance. In contrast to the vertical transmission of the chromosome within the species only, plasmids may be exchanged by different species (horizontal transmission during conjugation) via small structures on the bacterial surface (pili). This way, high-level resistance toward beta-lactamasis may rapidly spread in Gram-negative aerobic bacteria such as *Escherichia coli* or *Klebsiella pneumoniae* (4).

A key factor for the nosocomial transmission of bacteria is their ability to survive in the environment remaining infectious (tenacity). The thickness of the peptidoglycan-containing (murein) cell wall of the bacteria affects its tenacity. Bacteria that have a thick cell wall (dark purple in Gram stain indicates Gram-positive) are somewhat protected from drying and thus stay infectious for a much longer time period than bacteria with thin cell walls (red in Gram stain indicates Gram-negative) do. For example, Gram-positive enterococci may survive on cotton gowns, stethoscopes, or other environmental surfaces for as long as three months (5, 6).

Some bacterial species (e.g., *Clostridia* and *Bacilli*) are capable of forming a hypometabolic form called "spores." Bacterial spores are then protected even under extremely disturbing environmental conditions (such as heat, drying, radiation, and chemicals). By this, bacterial spores may survive many years (7). In the microbiological laboratory, bacterial spores are used to check the function of sterilization devices because no other pathogens are as hard to kill as they are. As soon as the environmental conditions improve (e.g., when entering a susceptible host), spores will turn back into the vegetative form of the bacteria and multiplying of the organism begins.

VIRUSES

Viruses are much smaller (about 1% of the size) than bacteria. However, unlike bacteria, viruses cannot multiply in the environment because they need other cells for their own replication.

The structure of the virus determines its likelihood of nosocomial transmission to some extent. All viruses consist of proteins forming a so-call "capsid" that contains the genetic material (either DNA or RNA). Some viruses are moreover surrounded by a lipid membrane bilayer (envelope) that is acquired from the host cell when the virion gets excreted. Those enveloped viruses are quite easy to kill by alcohol-based disinfectants as the disinfecting substance destroys the virus by disrupting this outer membrane. In contrast, some other viruses (e.g., norovirus or adenovirus) lack such a membrane (so-called "naked" viruses). Naked viruses are easier transmitted because much higher concentrations of alcohol (e.g., for the disinfection of hands) are necessary to successfully destroy them (8).

The mutation rate of a viral species may also be epidemiologically relevant. Even though a higher mutation rate does not alter the risk of the transmission of the virus, it still plays a role in the possibility of multiple infections. Viruses that tend to be genetically stable usually lead to a protective immunity after their first course of infection, while genetically variable viruses may cause relapses in one single patient.

FUNGI

Fungi show two major differences compared to bacteria. First, fungi own a nucleus (eukaryotic cells). Second, the cell wall of fungi may contain glucane, mannan, chitin, and/or cellulose, but the bacterial cell wall does not. In terms of transmission, it is important do differentiate between yeasts (e.g., *Candida* spp.) and molds (e.g., *Aspergillus* spp.).

Yeasts replicate by the production of blastoconidia (buds). They are usually transmitted via contact. Small amounts of yeasts are part of the physiological flora of the mucosa. Larger amounts of yeasts on the mucosa grow in immunocompromised patients or are caused by selection under antibacterial therapy (soor).

Molds replicate by the production of spores. Due to their very small size (<5 μm in diameter), airborne transmission of mold spores occurs (9). Molds are never part of the physiologic flora and represent a major health hazard for immunocompromised patients. In contrast to bacterial spores, mold spores are quite easy to inactivate by alcohol.

Sources of Nosocomial Pathogens

Identifying the source of a pathogen is one of the most important measures to prevent further nosocomial transmissions. Especially during nosocomial outbreak situations, knowledge on potential sources for certain pathogens is extremely valuable. In the following, the most important sources of pathogens in the healthcare setting are discussed.

MEDICAL PERSONNEL

Certainly medical staff represents a major source for nosocomial transmission. Personnel may be either constantly colonized (carrier) or even infected themselves by some pathogen. Nevertheless, in most cases pathogens are picked up on the hands of staff when caring for one patient and get easily transferred to another patient. Thus, proper hand hygiene (e.g., using alcohol-based hand disinfection) significantly reduces the likelihood of cross-transmission and subsequent nosocomial infections (10–12).

Sometimes, molecular typing is performed to identify medical personnel that may have caused transmissions of a certain pathogen. The results of such typing should be considered with caution for two reasons: (a) Indistinguishable strains recovered from a patient as well as from staff do not prove the route of transmission (staff to patient vs. patient to staff) (13); and (b) in the case of a low diversity of a particular species, different persons may be colonized by identical strains (e.g., methicillin-resistant *Staphylococcus aureus*) just by chance (14).

PATIENTS AND VISITORS

Individuals in the hospital other than personnel (such as patients or visitors) may also serve as a source for pathogen transmission. There are many outbreaks in the medical literature that began after admission of one single patient (index patient) who spreads an infectious agent all over the entire ward. One way to identify carriers of epidemiologically important pathogens is microbiological diagnostic at the most early time point (screening at admission).

Meanwhile, screening is recommended for methicillin-resistant *Staphylococcus aureus*, vancomycin-resistant enterococci, and *Clostridium difficile* (15, 16). Relatives and friends who suffer from an acute infection themselves at present should not visit patients in a hospital at all.

Sufficient education of patients and visitors about how to perform infection control is one of the most crucial issues in order to avoid pathogen spread from them. Carriers of multidrug-resistant bacteria need to understand that they become isolated in a hospital in a single patient room to protect the more susceptible (e.g., immunocompromised) patients from acquisition of that pathogen. Proper hand hygiene should be taught to both patients and visitors.

ENVIRONMENT

Water Water from the hospital's water supply system may contain pathogens that represent a threat for human health. One of the most important waterborne pathogens are *Legionella*. These bacteria are commonly found in the plumbing system of all kinds of buildings, and they may cause pneumonia (Legionnaires' disease) or a nonpneumonic febrile illness called Pontiac fever (17). Especially severely immunocompromised patients (e.g., with underlying hematological–oncological diseases or transplant patients) are at risk to develop Legionnaires' disease when inhaling contaminated aerosols (e.g., from showers). The exact number of *Legionella* to cause infection is yet unknown. That is why *Legionella*-free water is required for high-risk patient care. Possibilities for the prevention of nosocomial Legionellosis include attempts to either eliminate the bacteria from the plumbing system (e.g., by superheat-and-flush, hyperchlorination, or copper–silver ionization) or to avoid the contact to the bacteria (e.g., by commercially available sterile water, or the use of terminal tap water filters) (18).

Air Some pathogens may be transmitted via air. Please note that airborne transmission should not be mixed up with transmission via droplets (also refer to the next section below). The most important pathogens that cause nosocomial infections after airborne transmission include mould spores (19), *Mycobacterium tuberculosis* (20), and varicella-zoster virus (21). Because these pathogens may be carried in air over long distances and persist for long time periods, special infection control measures are necessary to prevent their transmission. Patients with tuberculosis or varicella should be placed in rooms with negative pressure as long as they shed pathogens, to ensure that those pathogens cannot leave the room when the door gets opened. In contrast, highly susceptible patients without infection should be placed in rooms that are supplied with high-efficacy particulate air (HEPA) filters and that show positive pressure for the protection of the susceptibal individual (for example, from invasive infection by *Aspergillus* spp). Other important measures to prevent an invasive mold infection include the use of N95 face masks for patients when leaving the patient room, wet-cleaning of wards, sealing off areas of demolition and construction, and prospective surveillance of all nosocomial mold infections (22, 23).

FOOD

Drawing an epidemiological curve in the case of an outbreak (by printing the number of newly affected patients over time) may help to identify the underlying mode of transmission.

A sudden onset of the outbreak involving many individuals within a short time (usually two days or less) indicates a newly introduced common source. In contrast, person-to-person transmission often presents with an overall prolonged duration of the outbreak (depending on the incubation period of the specific pathogen) starting from a single index patient before spreading to others. Contaminated food generally affects many patients at the same time. Members of staff, too, can be affected when eating the same food as the patients do.

When dealing with contaminated food it is important to distinguish between infection and intoxication (food poisoning). In the case of a nosocomial infection, patients themselves may become infectious (e.g., for roommates); but when the clinical signs (typically gastronintestinal symptoms such as vomiting, diarrhea, and abdominal cramps) are caused by intoxication, there is no risk for further transmission of the pathogen by the sick individual. This difference has, of course, major implication on the choice of appropriate infection control measures such as isolation in a single room when the patient himself might shed the pathogen.

Frequent mistakes that lead to nosocomial transmission include cooling food too slowly before placing in the refrigerator, undercooking of meat and meat products, not reheating food to temperatures at which food poisoning can be destroyed, preparing food too long in advance, incorrect storage temperature of the food (either cooling or heating), use of contaminated food, cross-contamination between raw and cooked food, infected food handlers, or other breaches of basic hygiene measures during food preparation (24–28).

Typical pathogens from outbreaks that were traced to some kind of malpractice in the hospital's kitchen comprise *Salmonella* spp. (29–31), *Campylobacter* spp. (32, 33), *Bacillus cereus* (34, 35), *Clostridium perfringens* (36, 37), and norovirus (38, 39).

The concept of Hazard Analysis and Critical Control Point (HACCP) may help to prevent diseases derived from contaminated food (40, 41). This concept includes thorough analyis of all potential hazards for the safety of food, the implementation of important check points for the monitoring of food quality, a determination of thresholds that would trigger additional interventions for correction and improvement, and countinuous documentation of all relevant data.

MEDICAL DEVICES

The term "medical device" comprises all kinds of products that get used on patients. Some of those devices are manufactured for single use only, while others may be reprocessed before use or application on a different patient.

Medical devices designed for single use represent a source for HAI only if contaminated during the manufacturing process (intrinsic contamination). This is a rather rare event these days due to rigorous quality management in the industry. However, it still happens once in a while but may then affect very many patients in different locations (42). Especially high risk products in this context are preparations of highly lipid-containing substances such as total parenteral nutrition (43, 44).

Insufficient reprocessing (either disinfection or sterilization, depending on the type of medical device) is much more likely the cause for pathogen transmission and subsequent HAIs. All types of medical devices can be involved in principle—for example, electronic thermometers (45), blood pressure transducers (46), stethoscopes (47), bronchoscopes (48), and cystoscopes (49). In order to avoid an accidental spread of pathogens, the use of "single-use" equipment or devices that are dedicated to a single patient is recommended when caring for patients in single-room isolation.

The third type of unindented contaminated devices are the ones that are manufactured (and sold) for single use only, but still get used multiple times on one or even more than one patient (which then is against the manufacturer's instructions). This is most often the case in so-called "multidose vials" (MDV). MDVs, such as sodium chloride solutions, heparin, or propofol, are provided by the hospital in quite large volumes, but only little amounts are taken out during each single use—still leaving a large volume back in the bottle. Thus, originally sterile products become contaminated, and the introduced pathogens can multiply over time until the next probe of the product gets used (50). Numerous (avoidable) nosocomial outbreaks with all kinds of infections and very many unnecessary deaths are documented in medical literature due to the multiple use of MDVs (51).

Routes of Transmission

There are four main routes of transmission: contact, droplets, airborne transmission, and transmission by vectors. In the following, each route of transmission will be presented in more detail.

TRANSMISSION VIA CONTACT

Contact represents, by far, the most frequent mode of transmission in the healthcare setting. There are two subgroups of contact that deserve distinct discussion: direct contact (skin to skin), and indirect contact (via contaminated devices or pathogens from the environment).

Direct Contact Direct contact transmission requires a direct person-to-person contact, which results in the physical transfer of a pathogen between an infected or colonized person and a susceptible host. Especially in the healthcare setting there are many opportunities for a direct transfer of a microorganism from one person to another such as physical examinations, the drawing of blood samples, patient-care activities, and a large variety of other kinds of medical care. Unprotected contact with infectious agents (e.g., during oral care on patients with herpes simplex virus infection) may lead to transmission (52, 53). Blood samples derived from patients with bloodborne viral infections (e.g., HIV, HBV, or HCV) also represent a risk for healthcare workers when the patient's blood is inoculated accidentally, most likely by needle stick injuries (54).

Direct contact transmission can also occur between patients. There are certain patient populations such as patients in long-term care facilities or board and care facilities in which interpatient spread is extraordinary likely to take place. For example, transmission of norovirus is a well-known problem in these institutions (55, 56) mainly during the winter season. Scabies mites, too, may easily be transferred from an infested patient to others (57, 58).

Indirect Contact Indirect contact transmission involves contact of a susceptible host with contaminated objects (fomites), as, for example, medical devices (59–61) or nursing equipment (62, 63). Fomites are almost anything an infected individual (or reservoir) can touch, and upon which a residue of contagious pathogen can be left. Hands getting in contact with either an infected or colonized body site or with contaminated inanimate objects, subsequently touching another person without performing hand hygiene in between, may also be considered as transmission via indirect contact (64). For additional information on this issue, also refer to the section on nosocomial pathogens.

TRANSMISSION VIA DROPLETS

Droplet transmission is the transfer of respiratory secretions (droplets) containing microorganisms from an infected person to a susceptible host's susceptible mucosal surfaces like conjunctivae, nasal mucosa, or mouth (65). Most infectious agents that spread by droplets are not directly inhaled within the lungs but rather settle on the mucous membranes before. These droplets are larger than 5 μm in size and can be generated by a person primarily during coughing, sneezing, and talking (66, 67), or during the performance of certain procedures, such as bronchoscopy and open suctioning of mechanically ventilated patients (68–70). Droplet transmission requires close contact between the source and the susceptible person since particles may usually travel only about 1 meter (3 feet) or less. Slightly larger distances (up to a total of 2 meters) have been reported from experimental transmission studies or during outbreak investigations of smallpox or SARS (71, 72). The distance a droplet can travel depends upon various factors. These include the absolute number of droplets in the respiratory secretions and the type of mechanism by which the microorganism had been expelled (e.g., sneezing, coughing, or breathing only) (73). Please notice that droplets do not remain suspended in air for a longer time period. That is why there is a difference between so-called "droplet transmission" and true "airborne transmission" (which will be discussed in the following section).

Examples for pathogens that are transmitted by droplets include adenovirus, influenza virus, respiratory syncytial virus (RSV), rhinovirus, SARS-associated coronavirus (SARS-CoV), variola virus (smallpox), group A streptococci (*Streptococcus pyogenes*), *Mycoplasma pneumoniae*, *Neisseria meningitidis*, and *Bordetella pertussis* (74). The use of a surgical face mask is recommended whenever pathogen transmission via droplets is suspected.

There are also some pathogens that are usually not transmitted by droplets but via contact. However, under certain circumstances, they may also be dispersed into the air over short distances; that is why they get mentioned in this section, too. For example, *Staphylococcus aureus* may be dispersed from the nose in the case of the coincidence of viral upper respiratory tract infection (so-called "cloud" phenomenon) (75–77).

AIRBORNE TRANSMISSION

Airborne transmission occurs after the dissemination of small particles (such as droplet nuclei within the respirable size range of <5 μm in diameter) that contain infectious agents. These pathogens then get inhaled by a susceptible host and may even reach the alveoli of the lungs due to the small size of the carrier particle. Notably, droplet nuclei and other small-sized particles may be dispersed for a long time period and over long distances in the air. Thus, it is not necessary for a susceptible person to have "face-to-face contact" with an individual from which these pathogens are spreading in order to also become infected (78–80).

Relevant pathogens that are transmitted by the airborne route are, for example, rubeola virus (measles), varicella-zoster virus (VZV, chickenpox), *Mycobacterium tuberculosis*, and spores of many *Aspergillus* spp. The use of closely fitting face masks (e.g., N95 or FFP-2/-3 masks) is recommended to prevent true airborne transmission. Furthermore, it is important that the building's air supply system maintains a negative pressure in such a patient room compared to surrounding areas. As a result, infectious particles in the air are kept within the patient room when the doors are opened (74).

TRANSMISSION BY VECTORS

In the literature many inanimate contaminated objects (fomites) are described as vectors (81) that cause transmission. These objects are described above as the major element of the indirect transmission. In the following paragraph, animate vectors (usually arthropods such as mosquitos or ticks) will be described since they are able to transfer infectious organisms from one host to another.

Animate vectors may act as either a biological or a mechanical vector. Biological vectors are arthropod vectors in whose bodies the infecting organism develops or multiplies before becoming infective to the recipient individual. Mechanical vectors are arthropod vectors that transmit an infective organism from one host to another but that are not essential to the life cycle of the parasite.

In the healthcare setting, the highest recovery of bacteria were from body surfaces of flies, from German cockroaches, from nonbiting midges (chironomids), and from tenebrionid beetles. In one report, about one-third of all isolates were shown to be resistant to more than three antimicrobials (82). Mechanical transmission of nosocomial infections with multiple antibiotic-resistant bacteria could be shown for houseflies (83, 84). Cockroaches also play an important role as carriers of microorganisms such as bacteria, parasites, and fungi (85–87), and they were especially described as possible vectors of extended spectrum beta-lactamase- (ESBL-) producing *Klebsiella pneumoniae* in a neonatal unit (88).

For mosquito species, evidence was obtained for nosocomial transmission of autochthonous *Plasmodium falciparum* malaria by an indigenous mosquito species (*Anopheles plumbeus*) in Europe (89).

Vectors add an extra dimension to disease transmission since vectors are mobile and therefore increase the transmission range of a disease. Thus, it is important to study their behavior as well as the disease-causing agent in order to implement valuable prevention measures.

Extraordinary Susceptible Patients and High-Risk Areas

The proportion of severely immunocompromised people increases annually in many hospitals worldwide—for example, due to new and improved medical treatment options. However, there are certain patient groups that deserve special mention at this point. Especially patients in intensive care, during hemodialysis treatment, in hematological–oncological wards, or after solid organ transplantation are at an extraordinary risk to develop any kind of nosocomial infection. Besides being more likely to acquire an infection in the first place, these patients will also present with much higher morbidity, mortality, and/or a prolonged hospital stay compared to others. Considering the potential disastrous consequences of HAIs especially in immunocompromised individuals, it seems reasonable to focus on infection control particularly in these patients and to also apply more expensive measures if necessary (e.g., tap water filter for the prevention of nosomial legionellosis or HEPA-filtered air in patient rooms for the prevention of nosocomial aspergillosis).

Several infection control guidelines, such as the "Guidelines for Preventing Opportunistic Infections Among Hematopoietic Stem Cell Transplant Recipients" (23), the "Recommendations for Preventing Transmission of Infections Among Chronic Hemodialysis Patients" (90), and the "Guidelines for the Prevention of Intravascular Catheter-Related Infections" (91), have been published for this purpose. Whenever working in one of the areas mentioned above, medical staff should be aware of this special risk, and strict adherence to the corresponding infection control measures is mandatory at all times.

Financial Impact of Nosocomial Transmissions

As discussed elsewhere in more detail (Chapter 4), HAIs have an enormous impact on the morbidity and mortality of affected patients and lead to very high costs for the healthcare system. The hospital costs of all HAIs (endogenous and exogenous) in the United States have been estimated to exceed $5.9 billion per year (92, 93). The exact costs caused by the transmission of pathogens are difficult to ascertain since the precise incidence of nosocomial transmissions can hardly be determined and not all nosocomial transmissions will eventually lead to a costly infection but instead to colonization. However, the person colonized still may develop an HAI later on during a secondary hospital stay or may become a human source of infectious agents himself, especially if the pathogens persist constantly and the patient becomes a chronic carrier (94–96).

Tremendous problems will emerge from nosocomial outbreaks since affected patients may suffer from possible infections and may require additional treatment in the first place. Secondly, additional (costly) infection control measures will be necessary to stop further spread of pathogens. Almost every nosocomial outbreak will increase the costs for the affected department, especially when a closure of a unit is considered (97). An analysis of an ESBL-producing *Klebsiella pneumoniae* outbreak showed that the largest proportion of costs was related to healthcare worker time providing direct patient care, and approximately one-third of the total outbreak costs could be referred to the lost revenue from blocked patient beds (98). Irrespective of endemically or epidemically occurence of nosocomial transmission—particularly of multidrug-resistant pathogens—additional costs for isolating the patient have also to be considered. These costs may be even higher when single rooms are not available and patients have to be isolated solitarily in multibed rooms (99). A study about the additional costs for preventing the spread of methicillin-resistant *Staphylococcus aureus* on a surgical ward found that the most expensive single measure was blocked beds in multibed rooms which accounted for 82% of the extra costs (100).

Immense costs will also evolve from the prolonged treatment of infected patients. An increased length of stay due to transmission was described for thoracic organ transplantation patients (3), neonatal patients (98), and also for ICU patients in general (101).

To avoid these extra costs and to keep the patients' and personnel's safety, a broad knowledge of the infectious agents' modes of transmission and possible sources is essential for implementing proper infection control measures as far as for a successful outbreak management (102).

REFERENCES

1. Grundmann H, Barwolff S, Tami A, Behnke M, Schwab F, Geffers C. et al. How many infections are caused by patient to-patient transmission in intensive care units? *Crit Care Med* 2005;**33**(5):946–951.
2. Halwani M, Solaymani-Dodaran M, Grundmann H, Coupland C, Slack R. Cross-transmission of nosocomial pathogens in an adult intensive care unit: Incidence and risk factors. *J Hosp Infect* 2006;**63**(1):39–46.

3. Mattner F, Ruden AS, Mattner L, Chaberny IF, Ziesing S, Strueber M. et al. Thoracic organ transplantation may not increase the risk of bacterial transmission in intensive care units. *Int J Hyg Environ Health* 2007;**210**(2):139–145.
4. Gniadkowski M. Evolution and epidemiology of extended-spectrum beta-lactamases (ESBLs and ESBL-producing microorganisms. *Clin Microbiol Infect* 2001;**7**(11):597–608.
5. Zachary KC, Bayne PS, Morrison VJ, Ford DS, Silver LC, Hooper DC. Contamination of gowns, gloves, and stethoscopes with vancomycin-resistant enterococci. *Infect Control Hosp Epidemiol* 2001;**22**(9):560–564.
6. Ray AJ, Hoyen CK, Taub TF, Eckstein EC, Donskey CJ. Nosocomial transmission of vancomycin-resistant enterococci from surfaces. *JAMA* 2002;**287**(11):1400–1401.
7. Setlow P. I will survive: DNA protection in bacterial spores. *Trends Microbiol* 2007; **15**(4):172–180.
8. Weston D. Transmission, management and features of norovirus infection. *Nurs Times* 2005;**101**(5):28–29.
9. Vonberg RP, Gastmeier P. Nosocomial aspergillosis in outbreak settings. *J Hosp Infect* 2006; **63**(3):246–254.
10. Pittet D, Hugonnet S, Harbarth S, Mourouga P, Sauvan V, Touveneau S, et al. Effectiveness of a hospital-wide programme to improve compliance with hand hygiene. Infection Control Programme. *Lancet* 2000;**356**(9238):1307–1312.
11. Kampf G. The six golden rules to improve compliance in hand hygiene. *J Hosp Infect* 2004; **56**(Suppl 2):S3–S5.
12. Gould DJ, Drey NS, Moralejo D, Grimshaw J, Chudleigh J. Interventions to improve hand hygiene compliance in patient care. *J Hosp Infect* 2008;**68**(3):193–202.
13. Vonberg RP, Stamm-Balderjahn S, Hansen S, Zuschneid I, Ruden H, Behnke M, et al. How often do asymptomatic healthcare workers cause methicillin-resistant *Staphylococcus aureus* outbreaks? A systematic evaluation. *Infect Control Hosp Epidemiol* 2006;**27**(10):1123–1127.
14. Kreiswirth B, Kornblum J, Arbeit RD, Eisner W, Maslow JN, McGeer A, et al. Evidence for a clonal origin of methicillin resistance in *Staphylococcus aureus*. *Science* 1993;**259**(5092):227–230.
15. Muto CA, Jernigan JA, Ostrowsky BE, Richet HM, Jarvis WR, Boyce JM, et al. SHEA guideline for preventing nosocomial transmission of multidrug-resistant strains of *Staphylococcus aureus* and enterococcus. *Infect Control Hosp Epidemiol* 2003;**24**(5):362–386.
16. Vonberg RP, Kuijper E, Wilcox M, Barbut F, Tull P, Gastmeier P, et al. Infection control measures to limit the spread of *Clostridium difficile*. *Clin Microbiol Infect* 2008;**14**(Suppl. 5):2–20.
17. Diederen BM. *Legionella* spp. and Legionnaires' disease. *J Infect* 2008;**56**(1):1–12.
18. Chaberny IF, Ziesing S, Gastmeier P. Legionella prevention in intensive care units. *Anasthesiol Intensivmed Notfallmed Schmerzther* 2004;**39**(3):127–131.
19. Lutz BD, Jin J, Rinaldi MG, Wickes BL, Huycke MM. Outbreak of invasive *Aspergillus* infection in surgical patients, associated with a contaminated air-handling system. *Clin Infect Dis* 2003;**37**(6):786–793.
20. Narvskaya O, Otten T, Limeschenko E, Sapozhnikova N, Graschenkova O, Steklova L, et al. Nosocomial outbreak of multidrug-resistant tuberculosis caused by a strain of *Mycobacterium tuberculosis* W-Beijing family in St. Petersburg, Russia. *Eur J Clin Microbiol Infect Dis* 2002; **21**(8):596–602.
21. Gustafson TL, Lavely GB, Brawner ER Jr., Hutcheson RH Jr., Wright PF, Schaffner W. An outbreak of airborne nosocomial varicella. *Pediatrics* 1982;**70**(4):550–556.
22. Centers for Disease Control and Prevention (CDC). Guidelines for prevention of nosocomial pneumonia. Centers for Disease Control and Prevention. *MMWR Recomm Rep* 1997;**46** (RR-1):1–79.

23. Centers for Disease Control and Prevention (CDC). Guidelines for preventing opportunistic infections among hematopoietic stem cell transplant recipients. *MMWR Recomm Rep* 2000; **49**(RR-10):1–7.
24. Wilkinson PJ, Dart SP, Hadlington CJ. Cook–chill, cook–freeze, cook–hold, sous vide: Risks for hospital patients? *J Hosp Infect* 1991;**18**(Suppl A): 222–229.
25. Regan CM, Syed Q, Tunstall PJ. A hospital outbreak of *Clostridium perfringens* food poisoning—Implications for food hygiene review in hospitals. *J Hosp Infect* 1995;**29**(1):69–73.
26. Barrie D. The provision of food and catering services in hospital. *J Hosp Infect* 1996; **33**(1):13–33.
27. Todd EC, Greig JD, Bartleson CA, Michaels BS. Outbreaks where food workers have been implicated in the spread of foodborne disease. Part 3. Factors contributing to outbreaks and description of outbreak categories. *J Food Prot* 2007;**70**(9):2199–2217.
28. Jones SL, Parry SM, O'Brien SJ, Palmer Sr., Operational practices associated with foodborne disease outbreaks in the catering industry in England and Wales. *J Food Prot* 2008; **71**(8):1659–1665.
29. Kistemann T, Dangendorf F, Krizek L, Sahl HG, Engelhart S, Exner M. GIS-supported investigation of a nosocomial Salmonella outbreak. *Int J Hyg Environ Health* 2000; **203**(2):117–126.
30. Sion C, Garrino MG, Glupczynski Y, Avesani V, Delmee M. Nosocomial outbreak of *Salmonella enteritidis* in a university hospital. *Infect Control Hosp Epidemiol* 2000;**21**(3):182–183.
31. Frank C, Buchholz U, Maass M, Schroder A, Bracht KH, Domke PG, et al. Protracted outbreak of *S. enteritidis* PT 21c in a large Hamburg nursing home. *BMC Public Health* 2007;**7**:243.
32. Yoda K, Uchimura M. An outbreak of *Campylobacter jejuni* food poisoning caused by secondary contamination in cooking practice at a high school. *Jpn J Infect Dis* 2006;**59**(6):408–409.
33. Jelovcan S, Schmid D, Lederer I, Hell M, Rehberger K, Arnhold D, et al. Cluster of nosocomial campylobacteriosis, Austria 2006. *J Hosp Infect* 2008;**69**(1):97–98.
34. Ghelardi E, Celandroni F, Salvetti S, Barsotti C, Baggiani A, Senesi S. Identification and characterization of toxigenic *Bacillus cereus* isolates responsible for two food-poisoning outbreaks. *FEMS Microbiol Lett* 2002;**208**(1):129–134.
35. McIntyre L, Bernard K, Beniac D, Isaac-Renton JL, Naseby DC. Identification of *Bacillus cereus* group species associated with food poisoning outbreaks in British Columbia, Canada. *Appl Environ Microbiol* 2008;**74**(23):7451–7453.
36. Yamagishi T, Sakamoto K, Sakurai S, Konishi K, Daimon Y, Matsuda M, et al. A nosocomial outbreak of food poisoning caused by enterotoxigenic *Clostridium* perfringens. *Microbiol Immunol* 1983;**27**(3):291–296.
37. Wada A, Masuda Y, Fukayama M, Hatakeyama T, Yanagawa Y, Watanabe H, et al. Nosocomial diarrhoea in the elderly due to enterotoxigenic *Clostridium perfringens*. *Microbiol Immunol* 1996;**40**(10):767–771.
38. Oogane T, Hirata A, Funatogawa K, Kobayashi K, Sato T, Kimura H. Food poisoning outbreak caused by norovirus GII/4 in school lunch, Tochigi prefecture, Japan. *Jpn J Infect Dis* 2008; **61**(5):423–424.
39. Martinez A, Dominguez A, Torner N, Ruiz L, Camps N, Barrabeig I, et al. Epidemiology of foodborne norovirus outbreaks in Catalonia, Spain. *BMC Infect Dis* 2008;**8**:47.
40. Bobeng BJ, David BD. HACCP models for quality control of entree production in hospital foodservice systems. I. Development of hazard analysis critical control point models. *J Am Diet Assoc* 1978;**73**(5):524–529.
41. Worsfold D. A guide to HACCP and function catering. *J R Soc Health* 2001;**121**(4):224–229.

42. Centers for Disease Control and Prevention (CDC). Epidemiologic notes and reports. Nosocomial bacteremias associated with intravenous fluid therapy—USA. 1971. *MMWR Morb Mortal Wkly Rep* 1997;**46**(51):1227–1233.

43. Centers for Disease Control and Prevention (CDC). Clinical sepsis and death in a newborn nursery associated with contaminated parenteral medications—Brazil, 1996. *MMWR Morb Mortal Wkly Rep* 1998;**47**(29):610–612.

44. Tresoldi AT, Padoveze MC, Trabasso P, Veiga JF, Marba ST, von Nowakonski A, et al. *Enterobacter cloacae* sepsis outbreak in a newborn unit caused by contaminated total parenteral nutrition solution. *Am J Infect Control* 2000;**28**(3):258–261.

45. Livornese LL Jr, Dias S, Samel C, Romanowski B, Taylor S, May P, et al. Hospital-acquired infection with vancomycin-resistant *Enterococcus faecium* transmitted by electronic thermometers. *Ann Intern Med* 1992;**117**(2):112–116.

46. Aduan RP, Iannini PB, Salaki J. Nosocomial bacteremia associated with contaminated blood pressure transducers: Report of an outbreak and a review of the literature. *Am J Infect Control* 1980;**8**(2):33–40.

47. Youngster I, Berkovitch M, Heyman E, Lazarovitch Z, Goldman M. The stethoscope as a vector of infectious diseases in the paediatric division. *Acta Paediatr* 2008;**97**(9):1253–1255.

48. Kirschke DL, Jones TF, Craig AS, Chu PS, Mayernick GG, Patel JA, et al. *Pseudomonas aeruginosa* and *Serratia marcescens* contamination associated with a manufacturing defect in bronchoscopes. *N Engl J Med* 2003;**348**(3):214–220.

49. Wendelboe AM, Baumbach J, Blossom DB, Frank P, Srinivasan A, Sewell CM. Outbreak of cystoscopy related infections with *Pseudomonas aeruginosa*: New Mexico, 2007. *J Urol* 2008; **180**(2):588–592.

50. Mattner F, Gastmeier P. Bacterial contamination of multiple-dose vials: A prevalence study. *Am J Infect Control* 2004;**32**(1):12–16.

51. Vonberg RP, Gastmeier P. Hospital-acquired infections related to contaminated substances. *J Hosp Infect* 2007;**65**(1):15–23.

52. Spruance SL. Pathogenesis of herpes simplex labialis: Excretion of virus in the oral cavity. *J Clin Microbiol* 1984;**19**(5):675–679.

53. Adler SP. Herpes simplex virus. In Mayhall CG (ed.), *Hospital Epidemiology and Infection Control*. Lippincott Williams & Wilkins, Philadelphia, 2004;733–736.

54. FitzSimons D, Francois G, De Carli G, Shouval D, Pruss-Ustun A, Puro V, et al. Hepatitis B virus, hepatitis C virus and other blood-borne infections in healthcare workers: Guidelines for prevention and management in industrialised countries. *Occup Environ Med* 2008;**65**(7): 446–451.

55. Schmid D, Lederer I, Pichler AM, Berghold C, Schreier E, Allerberger F. An outbreak of norovirus infection affecting an Austrian nursing home and a hospital. *Wien Klin Wochenschr* 2005;**117**(23–24):802–808.

56. Grmek KI, Peternelj B, Pohar M, Kraigher A. Outbreak of norovirus infection in a nursing home in northern Slovenia, July 2007. *Euro Surveill* 2007;**12**(10):E071011.

57. Koene RP, Tjioe M, Hoondert K, van d, V, Olde Rikkert MG, Wulfen M, et al. Scabies outbreak in a hospital and in 8 health-care institutions caused by an elderly patient with scabies crustosa. *Ned Tijdschr Geneeskd* 2006;**150**(16):918–923.

58. Tjioe M, Vissers WH. Scabies outbreaks in nursing homes for the elderly: Recognition, treatment options and control of reinfestation. *Drugs Aging* 2008;**25**(4):299–306.

59. Polish LB, Shapiro CN, Bauer F, Klotz P, Ginier P, Roberto RR, et al. Nosocomial transmission of hepatitis B virus associated with the use of a spring-loaded finger-stick device. *N Engl J Med* 1992;**326**(11):721–725.

60. Ransjo U, Good Z, Jalakas K, Kuhn I, Siggelkow I, Aberg B, et al. An outbreak of *Klebsiella oxytoca* septicemias associated with the use of invasive blood pressure monitoring equipment. *Acta Anaesthesiol Scand* 1992;**36**(3):289–291.
61. McDonald LC, Banerjee SN, Jarvis WR. Line-associated bloodstream infections in pediatric intensive-care-unit patients associated with a needleless device and intermittent intravenous therapy. *Infect Control Hosp Epidemiol* 1998;**19**(10):772–777.
62. Sherertz RJ, Sullivan ML. An outbreak of infections with *Acinetobacter calcoaceticus* in burn patients: Contamination of patients' mattresses. *J Infect Dis* 1985;**151**(2):252–258.
63. Patterson JE, Vecchio J, Pantelick EL, Farrel P, Mazon D, Zervos MJ, et al. Association of contaminated gloves with transmission of *Acinetobacter calcoaceticus* var. *anitratus* in an intensive care unit. *Am J Med* 1991;**91**(5):479–483.
64. Pittet D, Allegranzi B, Sax H, Dharan S, Pessoa-Silva CL, Donaldson L, et al. Evidence-based model for hand transmission during patient care and the role of improved practices. *Lancet Infect Dis* 2006;**6**(10):641–652.
65. Hall CB, Douglas RG Jr, Schnabel KC, Geiman JM. Infectivity of respiratory syncytial virus by various routes of inoculation. *Infect Immun* 1981;**33**(3):779–783.
66. Wells WF. On airborne infection: Study II. Droplets and droplet nuclei. *Am J Hygiene* 1934;**20**:611–618.
67. Papineni RS, Rosenthal FS. The size distribution of droplets in the exhaled breath of healthy human subjects. *J Aerosol Med* 1997;**10**(2):105–116.
68. Christian MD, Loutfy M, McDonald LC, Martinez KF, Ofner M, Wong T, et al. Possible SARS coronavirus transmission during cardiopulmonary resuscitation. *Emerg Infect Dis* 2004; **10**(2):287–293.
69. Fowler RA, Guest CB, Lapinsky SE, Sibbald WJ, Louie M, Tang P, et al. Transmission of severe acute respiratory syndrome during intubation and mechanical ventilation. *Am J Respir Crit Care Med* 2004;**169**(11):1198–1202.
70. Muller MP, McGeer A. Febrile respiratory illness in the intensive care unit setting: an infection control perspective. *Curr Opin Crit Care* 2006;**12**(1):37–42.
71. Downie AW, Meiklejohn M, St Vincent L, Rao AR, Sundara Babu BV, Kempe CH. The recovery of smallpox virus from patients and their environment in a smallpox hospital. *Bull World Health Organ* 1965;**33**(5):615–622.
72. Wong TW, Lee CK, Tam W, Lau JT, Yu TS, Lui SF, et al. Cluster of SARS among medical students exposed to single patient, Hong Kong. *Emerg Infect Dis* 2004;**10**(2):269–276.
73. Xie X, Li Y, Chwang AT, Ho PL, Seto WH. How far droplets can move in indoor environments—Revisiting the Wells evaporation-falling curve. *Indoor Air* 2007;**17**(3): 211–225.
74. Siegel D, Rhinehart E, Jackson M, Chiarello L, the Healthcare Infection Control Practices Advisory Committee. Guideline for isolation precautions: Preventing transmission of infectious agents in healthcare settings 2007. http://www.cdcgov/ncidod/dhqp/pdf/guidelines/ Isolation2007pdf 2007.
75. Eichenwald HF, Kotsevalov O, Fasso LA. The "cloud baby": An example of bacterial-viral interaction. *Am J Dis Child* 1960;**100**:161–173.
76. Sheretz RJ, Reagan DR, Hampton KD, Robertson KL, Streed SA, Hoen HM, et al. A cloud adult: The *Staphylococcus aureus*–virus interaction revisited. *Ann Intern Med* 1996;**124**(6): 539–547.
77. Bassetti S, Bischoff WE, Walter M, Bassetti-Wyss BA, Mason L, Reboussin BA, et al. Dispersal of *Staphylococcus aureus* into the air associated with a rhinovirus infection. *Infect Control Hosp Epidemiol* 2005;**26**(2):196–203.

78. Bloch AB, Orenstein WA, Ewing WM, Spain WH, Mallison GF, Herrmann KL et al. Measles outbreak in a pediatric practice: Airborne transmission in an office setting. *Pediatrics* 1985; **75**(4):676–683.

79. Iwen PC, Davis JC, Reed EC, Winfield BA, Hinrichs SH. Airborne fungal spore monitoring in a protective environment during hospital construction, and correlation with an outbreak of invasive aspergillosis. *Infect Control Hosp Epidemiol* 1994;**15**(5):303–306.

80. Pegues DA, Lasker BA, McNeil MM, Hamm PM, Lundal JL, Kubak BM. Cluster of cases of invasive aspergillosis in a transplant intensive care unit: Evidence of person-to-person airborne transmission. *Clin Infect Dis* 2002;**34**(3):412–416.

81. Burdge DR, Nakielna EM, Noble MA. Case-control and vector studies of nosocomial acquisition of *Pseudomonas cepacia* in adult patients with cystic fibrosis. *Infect Control Hosp Epidemiol* 1993;**14**(3):127–130.

82. Sramova H, Daniel M, Absolonova V, Dedicova D, Jedlickova Z, Lhotova H, et al. Epidemiological role of arthropods detectable in health facilities. *J Hosp Infect* 1992;**20**(4): 281–292.

83. Fotedar R, Banerjee U, Samantray JC, Shriniwas. Vector potential of hospital houseflies with special reference to *Klebsiella* species. *Epidemiol Infect* 1992;**109**(1):143–147.

84. Graczyk TK, Knight R, Gilman RH, Cranfield MR. The role of non-biting flies in the epidemiology of human infectious diseases. *Microbes Infect* 2001;**3**(3):231–235.

85. Fotedar R, Shriniwas UB, Verma A. Cockroaches (*Blattella germanica*) as carriers of micro-organisms of medical importance in hospitals. *Epidemiol Infect* 1991;**107**(1):181–187.

86. Baumholtz MA, Parish LC, Witkowski JA, Nutting WB. The medical importance of cockroaches. *Int J Dermatol* 1997;**36**(2):90–96.

87. Pai HH, Chen WC, Peng CF. Cockroaches as potential vectors of nosocomial infections. *Infect Control Hosp Epidemiol* 2004;**25**(11):979–984.

88. Cotton MF, Wasserman E, Pieper CH, Theron DC, van Tubbergh D, Campbell G, et al. Invasive disease due to extended spectrum beta-lactamase-producing *Klebsiella pneumoniae* in a neonatal unit: The possible role of cockroaches. *J Hosp Infect* 2000;**44**(1):13–17.

89. Kruger A, Rech A, Su XZ, Tannich E. Two cases of autochthonous *Plasmodium falciparum* malaria in Germany with evidence for local transmission by indigenous *Anopheles plumbeus*. *Trop Med Int Health* 2001;**6**(12):983–985.

90. Centers for Disease Control and Prevention (CDC). Recommendations for preventing transmission of infections among chronic hemodialysis patients. *MMWR Recomm Rep* 2001;**50**(RR-5):1–43.

91. O'Grady NP, Alexander M, Dellinger EP, Gerberding JL, Heard SO, Maki DG, et al. Guidelines for the prevention of intravascular catheter-related infections. Centers for Disease Control and Prevention. *MMWR Recomm Rep* 2002;**51**(RR-10):1–29.

92. Jarvis WR. Selected aspects of the socioeconomic impact of nosocomial infections: Morbidity, mortality, cost, and prevention. *Infect Control Hosp Epidemiol* 1996;**17**(8):552–557.

93. Centers for Disease Control and Prevention (CDC). Monitoring hospital-acquired infections to promote patient safety—United States, 1990–1999. *MMWR Morb Mortal Wkly Rep* 2000; **49**(8):149–153.

94. Massari M, Petrosillo N, Ippolito G, Solforosi L, Bonazzi L, Clementi M, et al. Transmission of hepatitis C virus in a gynecological surgery setting. *J Clin Microbiol* 2001;**39**(8): 2860–2863.

95. Lagging LM, Aneman C, Nenonen N, Brandberg A, Grip L, Norkrans G, et al. Nosocomial transmission of HCV in a cardiology ward during the window phase of infection: An epidemiological and molecular investigation. *Scand J Infect Dis* 2002;**34**(8):580–582.

96. Kondili LA, Genovese D, Argentini C, Chionne P, Toscani P, Fabro R, et al. Nosocomial transmission in simultaneous outbreaks of hepatitis C and B virus infections in a hemodialysis center. *Eur J Clin Microbiol Infect Dis* 2006;**25**(8):527–531.
97. Hansen S, Stamm-Balderjahn S, Zuschneid I, Behnke M, Ruden H, Vonberg RP, et al. Closure of medical departments during nosocomial outbreaks: Data from a systematic analysis of the literature. *J Hosp Infect* 2007;**65**(4):348–353.
98. Stone PW, Gupta A, Loughrey M, Della-Latta P, Cimiotti J, Larson E, et al. Attributable costs and length of stay of an extended-spectrum beta-lactamase-producing *Klebsiella pneumoniae* outbreak in a neonatal intensive care unit. *Infect Control Hosp Epidemiol* 2003;**24**(8):601–606.
99. Gastmeier P, Schwab F, Geffers C, Ruden H. To isolate or not to isolate? Analysis of data from the German Nosocomial Infection Surveillance System regarding the placement of patients with methicillin-resistant *Staphylococcus aureus* in private rooms in intensive care units. *Infect Control Hosp Epidemiol* 2004;**25**(2):109–113.
100. Herr CE, Heckrodt TH, Hofmann FA, Schnettler R, Eikmann TF. Additional costs for preventing the spread of methicillin-resistant *Staphylococcus aureus* and a strategy for reducing these costs on a surgical ward. *Infect Control Hosp Epidemiol* 2003;**24**(9):673–678.
101. Beyersmann J, Gastmeier P, Grundmann H, Barwolff S, Geffers C, Behnke M, et al. Transmission-associated nosocomial infections: Prolongation of intensive care unit stay and risk factor analysis using multistate models. *Am J Infect Control* 2008;**36**(2):98–103.
102. Gastmeier P, Stamm-Balderjahn S, Hansen S, Nitzschke-Tiemann F, Zuschneid I, Groneberg K, et al. How outbreaks can contribute to prevention of nosocomial infection: Analysis of 1,022 outbreaks. *Infect Control Hosp Epidemiol* 2005;**26**(4):357–361.

CHAPTER THREE

Infection Control Basics

LOUISE-MARIE DEMBRY AND CARLOS TORRES-VIERA

Introduction

Healthcare-associated infection refers to any infection caused by any infectious agent acquired as a consequence of a person's treatment for other conditions within the healthcare setting or which is acquired by a healthcare worker in the course of their healthcare duties.

Healthcare-associated infections (HAIs) are recognized as a significant cause of morbidity and mortality. It is considered that about 1.7 million people develop an HAI every year in the United States, and this is associated with approximately 99,000 deaths per year (1). HAIs are not only a problem for the developed world where between 5% and 10% of people admitted to a hospital will develop an HAI, but it is an even more serious problem for developing countries where the risk of infection can exceed 25% (2). The cost of HAIs in the United States has been estimated to be $4.5–5.7 billion per year (3).

Although the major infection control movement started in the 1970s, the demonstration of the effect of infection control programs in the reduction of HAIs only came with the publication of the landmark "Study on the Efficacy of Nosocomial Infection Control" (SENIC). This study showed a 32% reduction in hospital-associated infection in those hospitals with a surveillance and control component (4). Eighty percent of all HAIs can be accounted for by four pathologies: urinary tract infections, bloodstream infections, pneumonia, and surgical-site infections (5). This chapter provides information regarding the basics of infection prevention and control in acute healthcare settings.

Molecular Techniques for the Study of Hospital-Acquired Infection, First Edition. Edited by Steven L. Foley, Anne Y. Chen, Shabbir Simjee, and Marcus J. Zervos.

HAND HYGIENE

Human skin is normally colonized with bacteria; bacterial counts vary in different areas of the body, with the perineal, inguinal areas, and axilla being the most heavily colonized. Total counts of bacteria on the hands of healthcare personnel vary between 3.9×10^4 and 4.6×10^6, and the number increases with length of clinical activities (6).

These bacteria are divided into two principal types of flora:

1. *Resident flora*, which are permanent inhabitants of the skin. They are located either on the surface or under the superficial layers of the stratum corneum and have a protective role by preventing the colonization of the skin with resistant bacteria. The most common microorganism in this group is coagulase-negative staphylococci. They are not pathogens in intact skin but can cause infections in nonintact skin, eyes, or foreign bodies.
2. *Transient flora*, which consist of bacteria, fungi, and viruses that are only found on the skin for relatively short periods of time. They are able to be transmitted to other individuals and play an important role in healthcare-associated transmission of resistant microorganisms (7). Gram-positive and Gram-negative organisms such as *Staphylococcus aureus*, vancomycin-resistant enterococci (VRE), *Pseudomonas aeruginosa*, and *Escherichia coli* are representative of this transient flora.

Since nearly 10^6 skin squames containing microorganisms are shed daily by individuals, it is expected that the environment around patients (gowns, linen, furniture, etc.) can become heavily contaminated with patients' skin flora (8).

When taking care of patients, significant contamination of hands can occur. Colonization of healthcare workers' hands has been described in diverse studies and involves different microorganisms such as *Staphylococcus aureus* (10.5–78.3%), vancomycin-resistant enterococci (41%), *Pseudomonas* spp. (1.3–25%), and *Clostridium difficile* (14–59%), just to name a few (6, 9–12). Cross-transmission of pathogens can be achieved provided that the organism is capable of surviving first on the patient's skin or nearby environment and then survive for at least several minutes on healthcare workers' hands, that deficient or no hand hygiene is performed and finally that the contaminated hands of the healthcare worker come into direct contact with another patient's skin or environment with which the patient can come in direct contact (13). Hands are considered the main method of cross-transmission of microorganisms in healthcare settings and hand hygiene continues to be the simplest, most important and effective way of reducing the spread of antimicrobial-resistant pathogens in healthcare institutions.

Hand hygiene is a term that applies to hand washing (washing hands with non-antimicrobial soap and water), antiseptic hand wash or rub (washing hands with water and soap or other detergent or with a rub containing an antiseptic), or surgical hand antisepsis (a process that uses an antimicrobial agent to remove and/or kill transient flora and reduce resident flora in preparation for invasive procedures) (7). Antimicrobial agents used for hand hygiene have varying characteristics (e.g., persistence, residual activity) and tendency to irritate skin.

Evidence of the role of contaminated hands in the cross-transmission of pathogens in the healthcare setting comes from different types of sources, including experimental models, mathematical models, outbreak investigations, and hospital-based studies in which a temporal association between improvement in hand hygiene compliance and a decrease in the rate of infection has been observed (14–16). The role of hand hygiene in reducing healthcare-associated infections was clearly demonstrated by Ignatz Semmelweis in 1861. After implementing a hand hygiene method that consisted of soaking physicians' hands in a chlorinated solution, there was a significant reduction in maternal puerperal sepsis from 18% to 4% (14). A more recent example is the campaign developed at the University of Geneva Hospitals, where improvement with hand hygiene compliance was associated with a reduction in HAIs and methicillin-resistant *Staphylococcus aureus* (MRSA) transmission (17).

Despite the large body of literature evidencing the benefits of hand hygiene in preventing HAIs and the publication of specific guidelines, compliance with hand hygiene in healthcare settings continues to be disappointingly low. There are various explanations for this, including: the perception of higher compliance with hand hygiene by healthcare personnel as compared to actual compliance; misperception of the opportunities to transmit microorganisms; lack of time; lack of resources; and so on.

Several strategies have been implemented (alone or in combination) to improve compliance with hand hygiene; they include educational activities, incentive programs, system changes, and so on, but the fact is that promotion of hand hygiene compliance continues to be a challenging task.

The Environment and Infections

Nowadays nobody argues that the environment does not play any role in the transmission of organisms but there is no agreement about the magnitude of that role specifically in the setting of healthcare-associated infections. What does seem to be clear is that the significance of that role is different, depending on the particular organism.

In 1991 Rhame (18) suggested six levels of proof, ordered by the rigor with which they could potentially help to establish the causative role of inanimate objects in causation of human diseases:

1. The organism can survive after inoculation onto fomites.
2. The pathogen can be cultured from in-use fomites.
3. The pathogen can proliferate in the fomites.
4. Some fraction of acquisition cannot be accounted for by other recognized methods of transmission.
5. Retrospective case–control studies show an association between exposure to the fomite(s) and infection.
6. Prospective studies allocating exposure to the fomite to a subset of patients show an association between the exposure and infection.

In addition to these six levels, Weber and Rutala (19) have suggested two more: (1) Molecular analysis of isolates recovered from patients and the environment are similar and (2) reduction or elimination of disease transmission after decontamination of the fomite or elimination of the source. Microorganisms can be transmitted from the inanimate environment to patients by different routes that include surfaces, air, and water.

SURFACES

Multiple studies have shown that pathogenic organisms (including antibiotic resistant strains) such as *Staphylococcus aureus* (MRSA and MSSA), vancomycin-resistant enterococci

(VRE), *Clostridium difficile*, Gram-negative organisms like *Acinetobacter* spp., and viruses such as respiratory syncytial virus (RSV) and norovirus can extensively contaminate surfaces and remain viable not only inside the patient's room but outside their room as well including nursing stations and other common areas. VRE, for example, has been recovered in up to 46% of environmental cultures obtained in rooms of VRE patients with diarrhea and on 15% of surfaces cultured in the rooms of patients without diarrhea (20). VRE is able to colonize skin, and there is evidence that the degree of contamination of the environment increases with the number of body sites colonized. One study has shown that when three to four body sites are colonized with VRE, the frequency of environmental contamination can be as high as 60–70% (21). The degree of contamination is not only high but also prolonged, and it has been demonstrated that this microorganism can remain viable from several days to up to 58 days depending on the characteristics of the contaminated surface (e.g., countertop, polyvinyl, cloth, or plastic surfaces) (22–24). In the case of MRSA, the amount of contamination seems to be less extensive, but it is still significant with a proportion of hospital surfaces contaminated that ranges from 1% to 64% (19, 25–32). As is the case with VRE, MRSA can remain viable for periods of time that range from a few days to two weeks on formica surfaces and up to 9 weeks on cotton blankets (31, 32).

Acinetobacter baumannii is a Gram-negative organism that is found in soil and water and can also extensively contaminate the environment for prolonged periods of time (up to 33 days on plastic laminated surfaces) (31, 33–35). As a final example, *Clostridium difficile* has been shown to contaminate inanimate surfaces in hospitals (27%), and its active spores have been recovered for up to 5 months on hospital floors (31, 36–37). It continues to be a matter of debate as to what is the real contribution of environmental contamination in the transmission of pathogenic microorganisms from patient to patient in the healthcare setting. Although some studies suggest that there is a real role for this type of transmission, most of the studies lack a high level of scientific precision given the lack of a molecular epidemiology component to establish the link between the environmental strain to patients' strains and the less rigorous quasi-experimental design of the studies. However, studies have shown that VRE can be transmitted from the environment to hands or gloves and from there to other surfaces (38). Similarly, there is documentation of transfer of VRE from medical equipment to patients particulary in outbreak settings (39, 40). Although less well documented, there is also evidence of such transmission in the case of MRSA (26, 41). Studies have shown that by eliminating the contaminated environmental source of VRE, MRSA, *Clostridium difficile*, or *Acinetobacter* spp., there was a reduction and/or elimination of outbreaks (42–49). It is true that in most of these studies the environmental cleaning intervention was associated with other infection control interventions; nonetheless, this constitutes another type of evidence that supports the concept of transmission of pathogenic organisms from the environment to patients.

AIR

Many infectious diseases are transmitted via air such as *Mycobacterium tuberculosis*, *Brucella* spp., *Coxiella burnetii*, *Aspergillus* spp., and other filamentous fungi, measles, varicella, and so on. Many of the infectious diseases transmitted by air in healthcare settings have humans as the source and get transmitted via either airborne or droplet mechanisms (or potentially, depending on the circumstances, by both). However, the inanimate environment can itself be a source of infectious particles transmitted via air as is clearly the case with aspergillosis.

WATER

The capacity of some microorganisms to survive and multiply in water has been recognized for many years and described in numerous studies (50–70). Exposure to waterborne microorganisms in hospitals occurs when patients shower, bathe, or drink water, but it also occurs through contact with contaminated medical equipment (e.g., dialysis) and when tap water is used to rinse medical equipment after disinfection (e.g., endoscopes, nebulizers, etc.) or to dilute medications. Water quality in hospitals is primarily impacted by biofilm formation and corrosion of pipes and water tanks which occur naturally over time. Biofilms are complex ecosystems composed of communities of microorganisms adhering in a slimy matrix to a surface. Removal of biofilms is difficult because their slimy matrix protects the bacteria from disinfectants and antibiotics (54).

Organisms where water constitutes a source for HAI include *Legionella pneumophila* (52–54). *Legionella* is commonly present in hospital water systems and is able to multiply in this environment. Several factors contribute to this amplification, including obstruction and stagnation of water, water temperatures between 25°C and 45°C, and the presence of biofilms in the pipe system (54). It is also recognized that *Legionella* can survive inside free-living amoebae that provide a safe environment against disinfectants (55). *Legionella* can be transmitted by inhalation of contaminated aerosolized fluids or microaspiration. Healthcare-associated infections where other Gram-negative organisms have been implicated include *Pseudomonas aeruginosa* (58–60), *Stenotrophomonas maltophilia* (61), *Acinetobacter* spp (62, 63), *Aeromonas* (64, 65) and atypical mycobacteria (66–68). These microorganisms are well adapted to proliferate in water. More recently it has also been suggested that infections with *Aspergillus*, whose main mechanism of transmission is via the airborne route from air loaded with *Aspergillus* spores, may also be transmitted via the waterborne route when water is aerosolized (71).

STERILIZATION AND DISINFECTION

Inadequate cleaning, disinfection, or sterilization of medical equipment has resulted in the transmission of organisms such as hepatitis B (72–74) and hepatitis C (73, 75–77), bacteria such as *Pseudomonas aeruginosa* (78, 79), and atypical mycobacteria (80, 81). Not all patient-care items need to be sterilized; the need for disinfection or sterilization depends on the intended use of the item.

Cleaning is the process of removing all foreign material from objects by using water and detergent or soap to wash and scrub the objects. This process reduces the burden of microorganisms from the object. Disinfection is the process that eliminates most or all pathogenic microorganisms except spores using either heat/steam (thermal) or chemicals.

There are three levels of disinfection:

1. Low-level disinfection kills some viruses and most bacteria and some fungi but does not kill some more resistant organisms such as *Mycobacterium tuberculosis* or bacterial spores.
2. Intermediate-level disinfection inactivates most viruses, bacteria (including *Mycobacterium tuberculosis*), and fungi but does not kill bacterial spores.
3. High-level disinfection kills all microorganisms except high numbers of the most resistant bacterial spores.

Sterilization is a process that renders an item or product free of all forms of viable microorganisms, including spores. This process can be carried out by means such as dry heat, steam under pressure, ethylene oxide, and other gases or by prolonged soaking times in chemical disinfectants.

In 1968 Spaulding suggested an approach to disinfection and sterilization that continues to be useful today (82). The scheme is based on the risk of infection associated with the intended use of the item. Accordingly, items are classified as follows:

1. *Critical*: Items that enter sterile body compartments (e.g., vascular system, urinary systems) and, if contaminated, carry a high risk of infection. These items should be sterilized before use.
2. *Semicritical*: Items that come in contact with mucosal surfaces or nonintact skin. These items should be free of bacteria but not necessarily all bacterial spores; thus they should be subjected to high-level disinfection. Examples of items in this group are colonoscopes, bronchoscopes, laryngeal blades, and so on.
3. *Noncritical*: Items that come in contact with intact skin. Because intact skin constitutes a very good barrier against microorganisms, these items require only low-level disinfection. Examples of items included in this group are patient beds, stretchers, blood-pressure cuffs, and so on.

It is important to keep in mind that in order to carry out an effective process of disinfection and sterilization, the first step must be cleaning of the object.

Transmission of Microorganisms

In order for infections to occur, there are a series of conditions that have to be met. These conditions constitute the chain of infection (or organism) transmission. First, there must be an infectious agent such as a virus, bacteria, protozoa, fungus, or infectious protein particle known as a prion. Second, a reservoir must exist for the infectious agent which is a place where the microorganism maintains its presence and replicates. The organism must be able to exit its reservoir and gain access to a susceptible individual through one or more mechanisms of transmission which depends on the characteristics of the specific microorganism. Some microorganisms may have more than one mode of transmission but are predominately transmitted by one mechanism. For example, influenza is predominantly transmitted by respiratory droplets, but in some circumstances it can be also transmitted by airborne or contact. Interrupting the chain of transmission in the healthcare setting in order to prevent infections is the main objective of infection prevention and control programs.

The modes of transmission are classified into three principal routes: contact (direct or indirect), droplet, and airborne.

CONTACT TRANSMISSION

Contact transmission implies the transfer of an infectious agent from an infected or colonized person to a susceptible individual via direct contact (direct contact transmission) or indirectly via a contaminated intermediate object (patient device, instrument, environment, etc.) or person. Contact transmission is the most common means of transmission, and examples of microorganisms transmitted this way include bacteria such as methicillin-sensitive and methicillin-resistant *Staphylococcus aureus*, vancomycin-susceptible and vancomycin-resistant enterococci, and viruses such as RSV or parainfluenza virus.

DROPLET AND AIRBORNE TRANSMISSION

Droplet transmission implies the transmission of infectious agents from a reservoir to a susceptible host by infected respiratory droplets produced by the source individual when coughing, sneezing, talking, and so on. Droplets are usually defined as having a size >5 μm and, once expelled by the respiratory mucosa of the source, are able to travel only short distances before falling to the ground. This short distance has been traditionally defined as ≤3 feet, although investigations during the outbreak of SARS in 2003 suggest that persons located at a further distance (within 10 feet from the source) could be affected (83). Examples of microorganisms transmitted by this route are influenza virus and *Neisseria meningitidis*.

Tuberculosis, aspergillosis, and viruses such as measles, smallpox, and so on, are airborne transmitted. This refers to the transmission of infectious particles from the source to susceptible individuals by way of small-particle aerosols. Aerosols are the suspension of solid or liquid particles in gas. As mentioned before, when people cough or sneeze, thousands of droplets are expelled into the air. Most of these droplets are >5 μm in size and tend to fall to the ground rapidly. However those of smaller size tend to become even smaller by rapid evaporation from their surface and are converted into small droplet nuclei (usually ≤5 μm in size). These small particles can remain suspended for long periods of time (e.g., a 2-μm droplet nucleus can take 4.2 hours to fall a distance of 2 meters in a room with no air disturbances) and travel long distances by convection currents, and thus they may be widely disseminated before settling on or entering a susceptible host's airway. Because of their small size and aerodynamic characteristics, they easily reach the lower respiratory tract and initiate infection. It is important to understand that the definition of droplet versus airborne transmission is operatively useful, but its limits are less clear than originally thought because the range of sizes of droplets produced by a source and their aerodynamic characteristics may be modified by elements such as evaporation, temperature, humidity, and so on. Droplets of 10 μm in size may rapidly change size into small droplet nuclei by rapid evaporation (84–88).

Although in hospitals most airborne microorganisms are generated within the building itself by patients and/or infected personnel, not all airborne-transmitted organisms have individuals as their source and some of them will become aerosolized from the environment (e.g., *Aspergillus*). Not all aerosolized organisms from an individual source will come from the respiratory tract either, because skin squamae can also be aerosolized (89). Some Gram-positive bacteria such as *Staphylococcus aureus* and some Gram-negative bacteria (e.g., *Acinetobacter* spp or *Legionella* spp.) can be dispersed and occasionally transmitted by aerosolization.

PRECAUTIONS TO PREVENT TRANSMISSION OF INFECTIOUS AGENTS IN HEALTHCARE SETTINGS

The main role of infection prevention and control is to prevent the transmission of infectious agents by breaking the chain of transmission. Over time, improvements in the understanding of organisms' modes of transmission have led to more evidence-based and easier-to-understand-and-apply approaches to infection prevention and control. One fundamental concept in infection prevention is isolation precautions. Patients who are infected or colonized by pathogenic organisms may need to have precautions applied to prevent transmission to other individuals. In the past, different types of isolation systems were developed based on specific categories such as mechanism of transmission or specific diseases or diagnosis.

In the 1980s with the advent of the human immunodeficiency virus/acquired immunodeficiency syndrome (HIV/AIDS) epidemic, it became necessary to implement a new strategy to protect the healthcare worker from bloodborne pathogens (HIV, hepatitis B, etc.) by preventing contact with blood and some other body fluids. This gave rise to the concept of Universal Precautions, which was based on the concept that it was not always possible to identify people who are infectious or to distinguish them from those who are not infectious. This shifted the focus to routine use of blood and bloody substance precautions regardless of known or presumed bloodborne pathogen infectious status. Universal Precautions included: Handle all bloody body fluids as potentially infectious, use barrier precautions (gloves, gowns, etc.) when contact with these bloody fluids was anticipated, and wash hands immediately after removing gloves or if one was directly exposed to blood or bloody fluids without barrier protection.

A second important change came in the late 1980s with the introduction of body substance isolation, which considered all body fluids except sweat as potentially infectious. This new classification was aimed not only to protect the healthcare worker but also to protect patients.

Finally, the Centers for Disease Control and Prevention (CDC) and the Hospital Infection Control Practices Advisory Committee implemented in 1996 (and updated in 2007) a new system of isolation that not only acknowledged the goals of the previous two systems but also recognized the importance of healthcare workers' hands in the transmission of organisms and that some pathogens require additional control measures to prevent spread, depending on their mechanism of transmission (90).

There are two tiers to the new system:

1. *Standard Precautions.* It is the primary approach to preventing the transmission of organisms and it is based on the principle that all body fluids except sweat can carry pathogenic organisms and thus are potentially infectious. These precautions apply to all patients regardless of their known or suspected infectious status. Its components include hand hygiene and use of gloves, gown, mask, and eye protection or face shields, depending on the expected contact with body fluids, mucous membranes, or nonintact skin. In the new revised *Guideline for Isolation Precautions: Preventing Transmission of Infectious Agents in Healthcare Settings* released in 2007, three new elements were added: First is *respiratory hygiene/cough etiquette*, which is aimed at patients and persons accompanying them to a healthcare facility who might have an undiagnosed transmissible respiratory disease and who are symptomatic (e.g., cough, increased respiratory secretions, rhinorrhea, etc.). Its main elements are source control measures (covering mouth/nose when coughing or sneezing), hand hygiene after contact with respiratory secretions, and spatial separation (>3 feet) of symptomatic persons in common waiting areas. Second is *safe injection practices*, which include the use of sterile single-use, disposable needles and syringes, single-dose vials of medications whenever possible, proper disposal of sharps, and so on.

Third is the *use of masks* for insertion of catheters or injection of material into spinal or epidural spaces via lumbar puncture procedures.

2. *Transmission-Based Precautions*. These precautions apply to patients with known or suspected infectious diseases, and they are based on the major modes of transmission of organisms described earlier: contact, droplet, and airborne. It recommends the use of personal protective equipment (gloves, gowns, mask, respirator) and in some cases special rooms or special ventilation. Because some infectious agents have the potential to be transmitted by more than one mechanism, a combination of these precautions may need to be applied. It is important to remember that the use of transmission-based precautions is in addition to standard precautions and not a substitute for them.

CONTACT PRECAUTIONS

These precautions are aimed at preventing transmission of microorganisms that spread by direct (skin-to-skin) or indirect (through contact with the environment, fomites, etc.) contact. It suggests the placement of the patient infected or colonized with an organism whose mode of transmission is through contact in a single room or cohorting with another patient (s) infected or colonized with the same organism. Gloves and gown should be donned before entering the room and disposed of before exiting the room, hand hygiene should be performed before donning and after removal of personal protective equipment, and dedicated medical equipment should be used, followed by cleaning and low-level disinfection before being used on other patients. Mobilization and transport of patients outside their rooms should also be discouraged. Contact precautions are required for patients colonized or infected with VRE or MRSA, those with diarrhea due to *Clostridium difficile*, and patients with RSV or norovirus infection, to name just a few examples.

DROPLET PRECAUTIONS

These precautions are indicated for patients with infections caused by organisms transmitted by droplets such as influenza, *Neisseria meningitides*, *Mycoplasma pneumoniae*, *Bordetella pertussis*, and so on. Patients should be placed in a private room; if a private room is not available, patients may be cohorted with another patient infected with the same microorganism. A mask should be worn by healthcare personnel and visitors when coming within 3 feet of the patient. Patients should wear a mask if they need to leave their room for diagnostic testing.

AIRBORNE PRECAUTIONS

These precautions are indicated for patients with infections caused by organisms transmitted by droplet nuclei that can remain suspended in the air and travel long distances such as *Mycobacterium tuberculosis*, measles, varicella-zoster, smallpox, and so on. When admitted to the healthcare facility, these patients should be placed in a private room with negative air pressure relative to the surrounding areas, 6–12 air exchanges per hour, and air exhausted directly to the outside or passed through a high-efficiency particulate air (HEPA) filter if recirculated through the general ventilation system. These rooms are referred to as airborne infection isolation rooms (AIIRs). The minimum negative pressure in the room should be

>0.01 inch of water gauge or >2.5 pascals as compared to the surrounding areas. HEPA filters are able to trap at least 99.97% of particles of 0.3 microns in size or larger and thus can efficiently remove droplet nuclei. The door of the room should remain closed at all times to maintain the negative pressure differential. Airborne precautions also consist of healthcare personnel and visitors who enter the room wearing a respirator (e.g., N-95) that meets the following National Institute for Occupational Safety and Health (NIOSH) requirements: (a) the ability to filter particles 1 micron in size with a filter efficiency of ≥95%, (b) availability in different sizes to fit different facial characteristics and (c) the ability to be fit-tested. The patient should leave the room only for essential medical tests and should wear a surgical mask when outside the AIIR.

PROTECTIVE ENVIRONMENT

When patients who are undergoing, or have recently received, an allogeneic stem cell transplant are admitted to a hospital, it is recommended to place them in a protective environment room (also referred to as a positive-pressure room). The goal of this type of isolation is to reduce the risk of infection with environmental invasive fungal pathogens, such as *Aspergillus* spp., for which these patients are at high risk because of their high level of immunosuppression. The requirements for this type of isolation room include: HEPA filtration of incoming air, ≥12 air changes per hour, positive pressure in relation to the corridor, minimization of dust, and prohibition of dried and fresh flowers in the room.

SURVEILLANCE

Surveillance can be defined as the systematic recording, counting, and analysis of the occurrence and distribution of diseases. The objective of surveillance is not only to know the extent of a problem in terms of the burden of disease, trends, and epidemiological features but in some cases also to identify the risks that may act to increase or decrease the incidence or prevalence of disease. The optimal goal of surveillance in infection prevention is to serve as a tool to decrease HAIs and their associated morbidity and mortality.

Surveillance can be hospital-wide or targeted. In the first case all clinical areas are surveyed, and in the second case only some predetermined areas or type of infections are surveyed for HAIs. Hospital-wide surveillance has disadvantages such as it is very time and resource intensive. An example of hospital wide surveillance is the identification of antibiotic-resistant organisms. This surveillance can be accomplished by evaluating the clinical culture reports from the microbiology laboratory. In targeted surveillance, the focus is on a specific area of the hospital, population or specific infections.

Whatever the surveillance program in mind, there are multiple elements to be considered before its implementation, such as the type and size of the hospital, the proper definition of the outcome to measure and intervening variables as well as the population at risk, the characteristics of the data source and the data itself, the availability of resources to implement surveillance effectively, the potential impact of the information obtained through surveillance in helping to reduce the healthcare-associated infections, and so on.

WASTE MANAGEMENT

Ever since the beach wash-ups of medical waste close to part of the New Jersey coastline in 1987, the issue of medical waste disposal has been a major concern and subject to regulation due to the potential for infectious diseases transmission via medical waste. This has led to an increase in the volume of hospital-associated waste identified as regulated medical waste (potentially infectious) and a decrease in the options for treatment and disposal of this waste (91). Part of the problem comes from the lack of uniform definitions as to what is medical waste and infectious waste. According to the Medical Waste Tracking Act of 1988, medical waste is defined as "any waste that is generated in the diagnosis, treatment, or immunization of human beings or animals, in research pertaining thereto, or in the production or testing of biologicals." This definition includes, but is not limited to:

- Blood-soaked bandages
- Culture dishes and other glassware
- Discarded surgical gloves
- Discarded surgical instruments
- Discarded needles used to give injections or draw blood
- Cultures, stocks, swabs used to inoculate cultures
- Removed body organs
- Discarded lancets

Infectious waste would be the part of hospital waste that could potentially transmit infectious diseases. However, there is no epidemiologic evidence to suggest that most waste generated in healthcare facilities is any more infectious than household waste (although there is a greater number of bacterial species association with such waste). Similarly, there is no evidence to suggest that traditional waste disposal from healthcare facilities, with the exception of sharps leading to injuries, have transmitted infectious diseases (92).

Although there is no general concensus about what should be designated as infectious waste that requires special handling, the CDC considers the following types of medical waste as potentially infectious and thus subject to special handling: microbiological waste, human blood and blood products, pathological waste of human origin, contaminated animal waste, and sharps regardless of whether they are contaminated or not. The Environmental Protection Agency (EPA) also adds isolation waste to this list.

It is estimated that around 2 million tons of hospital waste are generated annually in the United States. This represents about 1% of the total national waste output (93). Most estimates are that 10–15% of medical waste generated by hospitals is infectious and that, given the lack of uniform definitions, this percentage varies depending on the generator's definition. Regulated medical waste can be treated by diverse methods that can be divided into four groups: thermal (incineration, steam sterilization, etc), mechanical/chemical (maceration and disinfection), irradiative (cobalt, gamma radiation, ultraviolet, etc.) or biological methods (enzymes).

Summary

Healthcare-associated infections represent common and costly events in healthcare settings. Although it is unreasonable to think that all of these events would be preventable with the current state of science and technology, the fact is that a significant proportion of them can be prevented. Well-structured infection prevention and control programs are fundamental to reaching the goal of reducing the rate of healthcare-associated infections. It is believed that the majority of instances of healthcare-associated colonization and/or infection of patients in healthcare settings occur as a result of patient-to-patient tranmission via the hands of healthcare personnel. Other mechanisms of transmission include contact with contaminated environment(s), surfaces or fomites, and airborne or droplet exposures. The chain of transmision of infectious agents in healthcare settings can be broken by following standard precautions for all patient interactions and by the implementation of transmission-based precautions if needed, given the characteristic mode of transmission of a specific diagnosed or suspected microorganism.

REFERENCES

1. Monina R, Edwards JR, Richard CL, et al. Estimating health care-associated infections and deaths in U.S. hospitals, 2002. *Public Health Rep* 2007;**122**:160–166.
2. Allegrazi B, Pittet D. Healthcare-associated infection in developing countries: Simple solutions to meet complex challenges. *Infect Control Hosp Epidemiol* 2007;**28**:1323–1327.
3. Burke J. Infection control—A problem for patient safety. *N Engl J Med* 2003;**348**:651–656.
4. Haley RW, Culver DH, White JW, et al. The efficacy of infection surveillance and control programs in preventing nosocomial infections in U.S. hospitals. *Am J Epidemiol* 1985; **121**:182–205.
5. Haley RW, Culver DH, White JW, et al. The nationwide nosocomial infection rate: A new need for vital statistics. *Am J Epidemiol* 1985;**121**:159–167.
6. Kampf G, Kramer A. Epidemiologic background of hand hygiene and evaluation of the most important agents for scrub and rubs. *Clin Microbiol Rev* 2004;**17**:863–893.
7. Boyce JM, Pittet D. Guidelines for hand hygiene in health-care settings. Recommendations of the Healthcare Infection Control Practices Advisory Committee and the HICPAC/SHEA/APIC/IDSA Hand Hygiene Task Force. *Am J Infect Control* 2002;**30**:S1–S46.
8. Noble WC. Dispersal of skin microorganisms. *Br J Dermatol* 1975;**93**:477–485.
9. Hayden MK. Insights into the epidemiology and control of infection with vancomycin-resistant enterococci. *Clin Infect Dis* 2000;**31**:1058–1065.
10. Mcfarland LV, Mulligan ME, Kwok RY, et al. Nosocomial acquisition of *Clostridium difficile* infection. *N Engl J Med* 1989;**320**:204–210.
11. Bertrand X, Bailly P, Blasco G, et al. Large outbreak in a surgical intensive care unit of colonizatioin and infection with *Pseudomonas aeruginosa* that overexpressed an active efflux pump. *Clin Infect Dis* 2000;**31**:e9-14.
12. Foca M, Jakob K, Whittier S, et al. Endemic *Pseudomonas aeruginosa* infection in a neonatal intensive care unit. *N Engl J Med* 2000;**343**:695–700.
13. Pittet D, Allegranzi B, Sax H, et al. Evidence-based model for hand transmission during patient care and the role of improved practices. *Lancet Inf Dis* 2006;**6**:641–652.
14. Nuland SB. *The Doctor's Plague: Germs, Childbed Fever, and the Strange Story of Ignac Semmelweis*, 1st ed. W.W. Norton & Company, New York, 2003.
15. Larson E. A causal link between handwashing and risk of infection? Examination of the evidence. *Infect Control Hosp Epidemiol* 1988;**9**:28–36.
16. Cooper BS, Medley GF, Scott GM. Preliminary analysis of the transmission dynamics of nosocomial infections. Stochastic and management effects. *J Hospital Infect* 1999;**43**:131–147.
17. Pittet D, Hugonnet S, Harbarth S, et al. Effectiveness of a hospital-wide programme to improve compliance with hand hygiene. *Lancet* 2000;**356**:1307–1312.

18. Rhame FS. The inanimate environment. In Bennett JV, Brachman PS (eds.), *Hospital Infections*, 3rd ed. Little, Brown and Company, Boston, 1998, pp. 299–278.
19. Weber DJ, Rutala WA. The environment as a source of nosocomial infections. In Wenzel RP (ed.), *Prevention and Control of Nosocomial Infections*, 4th ed. Lippincott Williams & Wilkins, Philadelphia, 2003, pp. 575–597.
20. Boyce JM, Opal SM, Chow JW, et al. Outbreak of multidrug-resistant *Enterococcus faecium* with transferable *vanB* class vancomcyin resistance. *J Clin Microbiol* 1994;**32**:1148–1153.
21. Bonten MJ, Hayden MK, Nathan C, et al. Epidemiology of colonization of patients and environment with vancomycin-resistant enterococci. *Lancet* 1996;**348**:1615–1619.
22. Bala H. Contamination, disinfection, and cross-colonization: Are hospital surfaces reservoirs for nosocomial infections? *Clin Infect Dis* 2004;**39**:1182–1189.
23. Noskin GA, Stosor V, Cooper I, et al. Recovery of vancomycin-resistant enterococci on fingertips and environmental surfaces. *Infect Control Hosp Epidemiol* 1996;**17**:770–771.
24. Bonilla HF, Zervos MJ, Kauffman CA. Long-term survival of vancomycin-resistant *Enterococcus faecium* on a contaminated surface. *Infect Control Hosp Epidemiol* 1996;**17**:770–772.
25. Boyce JM, White RL, Causey WA, et al. Burn units as a source of methicillin-resistant *Staphylococcus aureus* infections. *JAMA* 1983;**249**:2803–2807.
26. Boyce JM, Potter-Bynoe G, Chenevert C, et al. Enironmental contamination due to methicillin-resistant *Staphylococcus aureus*; Possible infection control implications. *Infect Control Hosp Epidemiol* 1997;**18**:622–627.
27. Duckworth GJ, Jordens JZ. Adherence and survival properties of an epidemic methicillin-resistant strain of *Staphylococcus aureus* compared with those of methicillin-sensitive strains. *J Med Microbiol* 1990;**32**:195–200.
28. Boyce JM, Havill NL, Otter JA, et al. Widespread environmental contamination associated with patients with diarrhea and methicillin-resistant *Staphylococcus aureus* colonization of the gastrointestinal tract. *Infect Control Hosp Epidemiol* 2007;**28**:1142–1147.
29. Neely AN, Maley MP. Survival of enteroccci and staphylococci on hospital fabric and plastic. *J Clin Microbiol* 2000;**38**:724–726.
30. Wagenvoort JH, Slujsman W, Penders RJ. Better environmental survival of outbreak vs. sporadic MRSA isolates. *J Hosp Infect* 2000;**45**:231–234.
31. Kramer A, Schwebke I, Kampf G. How long do nosocomial pathogens persist on inanimate surfaces? A systematic review. *BMC Infect Dis* 2006;**6**:130–138.
32. Beard-Pegler MA, Stubbs E, Vickery AM. Observations on the resistance to drying of staphylococcal strain. *J Med Microbiol* 1990;**32**:195–200.
33. Wendt C, Dietze B, Dietz E, et al. Survival of *Acinetobacter baumanii* on dry surfaces. *J Clin Microbiol* 1997;**35**:1394–1397.
34. Jawad A, Seifert H, Snelling AM, et al. Survival of *Acinetobacter baumanii* on dry surfaces: Comparison of outbreak and sporadic isolates. *J Clin Microbiol* 1998;**36**:1938–1941.
35. Webster C, Towner KJ, Humphreys H. Survival of *Acinetobacter* on three clinically related inanimate surfaces. *Infect Control Hosp Epidemiol* 2000;**21**:246.
36. Samore MH, Venkataram L, DeGirolami PC, et al. Clinical and molecular epidemiology of sporadic and clustered cases of nosocomial *Clostridium difficile* diarrhea. *Am J Med* 1996;**100**:32–40.
37. Kim KH, Fekety R, Batts DH, et al. isolation of *Clostridium difficile* from the environment and contacts of patients with antibiotic-associated colitis. *J Infect Dis* 1981;**143**:42–50.
38. Grabsch EA, Burell LJ, Padiglione A, et al. Risk of environmental and healthcare worker contamination with vancomycin-resistant enterococci during outpatient procedures and hemodialysis. *Infect Control Hosp Epidemiol* 2006;**27**:287–293.

39. Ray AJ, Hoyen CK, Taub TF, et al. Nosocomial transmission of vancomycin-resitant enterococci from surfaces. *JAMA* 2002;**287**:1400–1401.
40. Duckro AN, Blom DW, Lyle EA, et al. Transfer of vancomycin-resitant enterococci via health care workers hands. *Arch Intern Med* 2005;**165**:302–307.
41. Bhalla A, Pultz NJ, Gries DM, et al. Acquisitions of nosocomial pathogens on hands after contact with environmental surfaces near hospitalized patients. *Infect Control Hosp Epidemiol* 2004;**25**:164–167.
42. Huang SS, Datta R, Platt R. Risk of acquiring antibiotic-resistant bacteria from prior room occupants. *Arch Intern Med* 2006;**166**:1945–1951.
43. Hayden MK, Bonten MJ, Blom DW, et al. Reduction in acquisition of vancomycin-resistant enterococcus after enforcement of routine environmental cleaning measures. *Clin Infect Dis* 2006;**42**:1552–1560.
44. Dress M, Snydman D, Schmid CH, et al. Prior environmental contamination increases risk for acquisition of vancomycin-resistant enterococci. *Clin Infect Dis* 2008;**46**:678–685.
45. Mahamat A, MacKenzie FM, Brooker K, et al. Impact of infection control interventions and antibiotic use on hospital MRSA: A multivariate interrupted time-series analysis. *Int J Antimicrob Agents* 2007;**30**:169–176.
46. Rampling A, Wiseman S, Davis L, et al. Evidence that hospital hygiene is important in the control of methicilline-resistant *Staphylococcus aureus*. *J Hosp Infect* 2001;**49**:109–116.
47. Wilcox MH, Fawley WN, Wigglesworth N, et al. Comparison of the effect of detergent vs. hypochlorite cleaning on environmental contamination and incidence of *Clostridium difficile* infection. *J Hosp Infect* 2003;**54**:109–114.
48. Apisarnthanarak A, Zack JE, Mayfield JL, et al. Effectiveness of environmental and infection control programs to reduce transmission of *Clostridium difficile*. *Clin Infect Dis* 2004; **39**:601–602.
49. Martin AJ, Collins CJ, Ruddy R. Simultaneous control of norovirus and *Clostridium difficile* outbreaks due to enhanced infection prevention and control measures. *J Hosp Infect* 2008;**68**:180–181.
50. Moffet HL, Williams T. Bacteria recovered from distilled water and inhalation therapy equipment. *AJDC* 1967;**114**:7–12.
51. Anaissie EJ, Penzak SR, Dignani C. The hospital water supply as a source of nosocomial infections. A plea for action. *Arch Intern Med* 2002;**162**:1483–1492.
52. Kool JL, Bermgmire-Sweat D, Buttler JL, et al. Hospital characteristics associated with colonization of water systems by *Legionella* and risk of nosocomial Legionaires disease: A cohort study of 15 hospitals. *Infect Control Hosp Epidemiol* 1999;**20**:798–805.
53. Stout Je, Yu V. *Legionella* in the hospital water supply: A plea for decision making based on evidence-based medicine. *Infect Control Hosp Epidemiol* 2001;**22**:670–672.
54. Yu V, Liu Z, Stout JE, et al. *Legionella* disinfection of water distribution systems; Principles, problems, and practice. *Infect Control Hosp Epidemiol* 1993;**14**:571–575.
55. Berger P, Papazian L, Drancourt M, et al. Ameba-associated microorganisms and diagnosis of nosocomial pneumonia. *Emerg Infect Dis* 2006;**12**:248–255.
56. Jennigan DB, Hofman J, Cetron MS, et al. Outbreak of Legionnaires disease among cruise ship passengers exposed to a contaminated whirlpool spa. *Lancet* 1996;**347**:494–499.
57. Blatt SP, Parkinson MD, Pace E, et al. Nosocomial Legionnaires disease: Aspiration as a primary mode of transmission. *Am J Med* 1993;**95**:16–22.
58. Muscarella L. Contribution of tap water and environmental surfaces to nosocomial transmission of antibiotic-resistant *Pseudomonas aeruginosa*. *Infect Control Hosp Epidemiol* 2004; **25**:342–345.

59. Berrouane YF, McNutt LA, Buschelman BJ, et al. Outbreak of severe *Pseudomonas aeruginosa* infections caused by a contaminated drain in a whirlpool bathtub. *Clin Infect Dis* 2000;**31**:1331–1337.
60. Rudnick J, Beck-Sague CM, Anderson RL, et al. Gram-negative bacteremia in open-heart surgery patients traced to potable tap water contamination of pressure-monitoring equipment. *Infect Control Hosp Epidemiol* 1996;**17**:281–285.
61. Verweij PE, Meis JF, Christmann V, et al. Nosocomial outbreak of colonization and infection with *Stenothrophomonas maltophilia* in preterm infants associated with contaminated tap water. *Epidemiol Infect* 1998;**120**:251–256.
62. Villegas MV, Hartstein AI. *Acinetobacter* outbreaks, 1977–2000. *Infect Control Hosp Epidemiol* 2003;**24**:284–295.
63. Maragakis LL, Cosgrove SE, Song X, et al. An outbreak of multidrug-resistant *Acinetobacter baumannii* associated with pulsatile lavage wound treatment. *JAMA* 2004;**292**:3006–3011.
64. Picard B, Goullet P. Epidemiological complexity of hospital *Aeromonas* infections revealed by electrophoretic typing of esterases. *Epidemiol Infect* 1987;**98**:5–14.
65. Sartor C, Limouzin-Perotti F, Legre R, et al. Nosocomial infections with *Aeromonas hydrophila* from leeches. *Clin Infect Dis* 2002;**35**:e1–e5.
66. Vaerewicjck MJ, Huys G, Palomino JC, et al. Mycobateria in drinking water distribution systems: Ecology and significance for human health. *FEMS Microbiol Rev* 2005;**29**:911–934.
67. Wallace RJ Jr, Brown BA, Griffith DE. Nosocomial outbreaks/pseudo-outbreaks caused by nontuberculous mycobacteria. *Annu Rev Microbiol.* 1998;**52**:453–490.
68. Phillips MS, Von Reyn CF. Nosocomial infections due to nontuberculous mycobacteria. *Clin Infect Dis* 2001;**33**:1363–1374.
69. Nasser R, Rahi A, Haddad M, et al. Outbreak of *Burkholderia cepacia* bacteremia traced to contaminated hospital water used for dilution of an alcohol skin antiseptic. *Infect Control Hosp Epidemiol* 2004;**25**:231–239.
70. Gorbushinna AA. Life on the rocks. *Environ Microbiol* 2007;**7**:1613–1731.
71. Anaissie EJ, Costa SF. Nosocomial aspergillosis is waterborne. *Clin Infect Dis* 2001;**33**: 1546–1548.
72. Birnie GG, Quingley EM, Clements GB, et al. Endoscopic transmission of hepatitis B. *Gut* 1983;**24**:171–174.
73. Morris J, Duckworth GJ, Ridgway GL. Gastrointestinal endocopy decontamination failure and the risk of transmission of blood-borne viruses: A review. *J Hosp Infect* 2006;**63**:1–13.
74. Spach DH, Silverstein FE, Stamm WE. Transmission of infection by gastroeintestinal endocoscopy and bronchoscopy. *Ann. Intern Med* 1993;**118**:117–128.
75. Bronowicki JP, Venard V, Botte C, et al. patient-to-patient transmission of hepatitis C virus during colonoscopy. *N Engl J Med* 1997;**337**:237–240.
76. Delwaide J, Gerard C, Vaira D, et al. Hepatitis C virus transmission following invasive medical procedures. *J Intern Med* 1999;**245**:107–108.
77. Nelson DB, Muscarella LF. Current issues in endoscope reprocessing and infection control during gastrointestinal endoscopy. *World J Gastroenterol* 2006;**12**:3953–3964.
78. Kayabas U, Bayraktar M, Otlu B, et al. An outbreak of *Pseudomonas aeruginosa* because of inadequate disinfection procedures in a urology unit: A pulsed-field gel electrophoresis-based epidemiologic study. *Am J Infect Control* 2008;**36**:33–38.
79. Gillespie JL, Arnold KE, Noble-Wang J, et al. Outbreak of *Pseudomonas aerugionsa* infections after transrectal ultrasound-guided prostate biopsy. *Urology* 2007;**69**:912–914.
80. Meyers H, Brown-Elliot BA, Moore D, et al. An outbreak of *Mycobacterium chelonae* infection following liposuction. *Clin Infect Dis* 2002;**34**:1500–1507.

81. Murillo J, Torres J, Bofill L, et al. Skin and wound infection by rapidly growing mycobacteria: An unexpected complication of liposuction and liposculpture. *Arch Dermatol* 2000;**136**:1347–1352.
82. Rutala WA, Weber DJ. Disinfection and sterilization in health care facilities: What clinitians need to know. *Clin Infect Dis* 2004;**39**:702–709.
83. Wong TW, Lee CK, Tam W, et al. Cluster of SARS among medical students exposed to a single patient, Hong Kong. *Emerg Infect Dis* 2004;**10**:269–276.
84. Xie X, Li Y, Chwang ATY, et al. How far droplets can move in indoor environments-revisiting the Wells evaporation-falling curve. *Indoor Air* 2007;**17**:211–225.
85. Nicas M, Nazaroff WW, Hubbard A. Toward understanding the risk of secondary airborne infection: Emissin of respirable pathogens. *J Occup Environ Hyg* 2005;**2**:143–154.
86. Beggs CB. The airborne transmission of infection in hospital buildings: Fact or fiction? *Indoor Built Environ* 2003;**12**:9–18.
87. Noakes CJ, Beggs CB, Sleigh PA, et al. Modelling the transmission of airborne infections in enclosed spaces. *Epidemiol Infect* 2006;**134**:1082–1091.
88. Ly Y, Leung GM, Tang JW, et al. Role of ventilation in airborne transmission of infectious agents in the built environment—A multidisciplinary systematic review. *Indoor Air* 2007;**17**:2–18.
89. Spendlove JC, Fannin KF. Source, significance, and control of indoor microbial aerosols: human health aspects. *Public Health Rep* 1983;**98**:229–244.
90. Siegel JD, Rhinehart E, Jackson M, and the Healthcare Infection Control Practices Advisory Committee. *2007 Guideline for Isolation Precautions: Preventing Transmission Agents in Healthcare Settings*, June 2007.
91. US Environmental Protection Agency. Standards for the tracking and management of medical waste; interim final rule and request for comments. *Fed Regist* 1989;**54**:12326–12395.
92. Rutala WA, Mayhall CG. Medical waste. *Infect Control Hosp Epidemiol* 1992;**13**:38–48.
93. Rutala WA, Odette RL, Samsa GP. Management of infectious waste by US hospitals. *JAMA* 1989;**262**:1635–1640.

CHAPTER FOUR

Cost Effectiveness of Infection Control Program

MARC-OLIVER WRIGHT AND ELI N. PERENCEVICH

Introduction

Estimates of healthcare-associated infections and their resultant costs vary widely, but the summary data paint a rather bleak picture. There are more than 2 million hospital admissions in the United States each year, and approximately 4.5% of these patients will die (30,000 direct and 70,000 indirect deaths); this is the sixth overall leading cause of death, with an associated cost nearing $6.7 billion per year (2002 US dollars) (1–4). Thus, it may seem that committing financial investment in infection control programs is an intuitive remedy and one that healthcare organizations should readily embrace. However, such programs are often viewed as "cost centers" in that direct operating costs are not offset by revenue generated for the organization. A review of 28 regional healthcare facilities in the southeastern United States found that the attributable costs of healthcare-associated infections exceeded the allotted budget for infection control programs by factor of 4.6 (5). Although it cannot be expected that professionals in healthcare epidemiology develop the in-depth expertise of a health economist, a general understanding of cost justification can be an invaluable asset in seeking and justifying existing or additional needed resources.

This chapter will introduce healthcare costs and reimbursement, indicate how to quantify attributable costs related to infections, and outline basic financial analyses with an emphasis on making a business case for quality improvement. The chapter will provide a practical example for a creating a business proposal to request additional full-time equivalent

Molecular Techniques for the Study of Hospital-Acquired Infection, First Edition. Edited by Steven L. Foley, Anne Y. Chen, Shabbir Simjee, and Marcus J. Zervos.

employees (FTEs). Lastly, a published case study describing the successful expansion of an infection control program will be summarized.

Healthcare Costs and Reimbursement

Healthcare organizations function to serve their patient population, but must do so in a manner that either neutralizes expenditures (nonprofit organizations) or perhaps generates a return on investment (for profit). Failure to do so, particularly over a prolonged period of time, is likely to result in the organization closing its doors or, at best, merging and streamlining its resources with a more financially stable partner.

Total costs of programs may be either fixed or variable. Fixed costs include contractual obligations such as utility costs, facility maintenance, and others that are neither dependent on patient volume nor easily modified or exchanged for cash in the short term. For example, a hospital cannot build a new inpatient wing or intensive care unit overnight to meet increased admissions or length of stay. Variable costs are usually related to patient care such as pharmaceuticals, consumables, or laboratory tests and can increase or decrease dramatically and relatively quickly (open or close a new unit or service) (3). Employee salaries are commonly considered fixed in the short term because they are usually tied with job security (e.g., severance) (6). The vast majority (84–90%) of hospital costs are fixed (7). The sum of fixed and variable costs equals an organization's total operating expenses and must be offset by incoming revenue from reimbursed patient care and (to a small extent) supplemental income-generating activities (e.g., leased real estate, third-party buy-back of devices for reprocessing, etc.). Reimbursed patient care is the amount that is *paid* by the patient and/or third-party payer (e.g., private insurance, Medicare, Medicaid) to the healthcare organization. Large third-party payers receive discounts off of the charges (total amount on a patient's bill) because such charges are inflated with fees greater than the actual cost of the care provided in order to ensure that all costs are reimbursed to the point of solvency (8). This intentional adjustment to cost can be of the magnitude of 60–80%; and if actual cost data are unavailable, hospital charges can be adjusted back to actual costs by using a cost-to-charge ratio, determined annually by CMS (9, 10).

Healthcare facilities have never been directly reimbursed for maintaining an infection control program. Until recently, it was possible for an organization to be reimbursed for the care provided to a patient following a "reasonably preventable" adverse event such as catheter-associated urinary tract infections, central venous catheter bloodstream infections, and some surgical site infections following clean procedures such as cardiac surgery. This came to an end October 1, 2008 as part of an implementation of the Federal Deficit Reduction Act 2006 (10). Patients identified as experiencing "reasonably preventable" events including some infections during their hospitalization are no longer reimbursable if that event results in the assignment of a higher-cost diagnosis-related group (DRG). The following example from CMS concerns a patient admitted for an intracranial hemorrhage (ICH) and the reasonably preventable event of a fall resulting in a dislocated patella. The 2008 average payment for a principal diagnosis of an ICH is $5347.98. If the patient dislocated their patella at home and arrived at the hospital with the ICH and dislocation (present on admission as a secondary diagnosis), the average payment for this higher-cost DRG would be $6177.43. If, however, the same fall occurs following admission to the neurosurgery intensive care unit (ICU), the payment reverts to $5347.98 (10). The cost incurred by the organization for treating the dislocated patella is likely similar, but the reimbursement of such treatment is only received if the fall occurred prior to admission and not as a result of care received. The same scenario applies to the healthcare-associated infections described above, each of which are intended to reduce the federal budget deficit as well as incentivize healthcare organizations to reduce these preventable events. However, the potential for unintended consequences is present and their occurrence and extent are unknown. Furthermore, if these indirect incentives are to be successful in prevention, these events must be measurable, unambiguous, and truly preventable (11). While ventilator-associated pneumonia is an adverse outcome capable of significant morbidity and mortality, its identification is highly subjective and difficult to measure and its degree of preventability is subject to interpretation. These characteristics suggest that VAP is a poor choice for quality metrics or benchmarking and as such may be a poor choice for inclusion as part of the nonreimbursable CMS events (12). There is every reason to believe that the list of healthcare-associated infections deemed reasonably preventable (and thereby no longer reimbursable) will likely expand in the coming years.

Costs of Healthcare-Associated Infections

Quantifying healthcare-associated infections and other complications in terms of dollars saved or lost can be difficult. If the intended analysis is from the organization's point of view (e.g., justifying the need for an additional position), administrators will likely prefer that the source of the cost data used in the analysis be specific to the organization (8). Micro-costing refers to costs obtained at the individual level and specific to the care provided. It is commonly extracted from a hospital cost-accounting system and is especially useful for assessing incremental cost of new technologies. Micro-costing may also include time and motion studies with appropriated hourly salaries. This allows cost estimates to include how long a particular intervention increases or decreases expenditures through the change in workflow requirement on the part of the employee (13). Although ideal for internal purposes, it is not recommended for comparing across institutions without a thorough price comparison and may be improved with the aforementioned cost-to-charge ratio to better represent true costs. In calculating the cost of adverse outcomes, such as healthcare-associated infections, it is important to include only those costs that are not recouped as part of the reimbursement process (3). Costs from patients with healthcare-associated infections are compared to a reference group of patients who did not acquire the infection. Ideally, these case and reference groups are similar to one another (matched) with respect to factors that would contribute to costs aside from the adverse event such as severity of illness or comorbid conditions and length of stay prior to the onset of infection (3, 8). Of note, when examining antimicrobial-resistant organisms in the context of a financial analysis, a reference group selection is especially important (14). Reference groups with an infection due to the antibiotic-susceptible strain addresses the incremental cost associated with resistance, rather than the infection itself, and may underestimate the true financial benefit of prevention. Reference groups for analyzing outcomes associated with infections due to antimicrobial-resistant organisms should include both (a) patients with an infection due to a susceptible strain and (b) those patients who never acquired an infection to more closely approximate the costs. Importantly, for any type of infection, only outcomes (length of stay or costs) that occur after the infection appears should be counted. This is important since preinfection length of stay (and thus costs) can be quite long, but this time period is a risk factor for infection and cannot be attributed to the infection itself (15).

If internal patient-level data are not available, the costs of many healthcare-associated infections can be found in the literature. There are a number of downsides to using such reported figures. Costs (and charges) can differ greatly across institutions, regions of the same country, or internationally (9). Using data from published reports subjects the analysis to the same strengths and limitations of the original author's study. Two recent systematic reviews of published studies focusing on economic analyses of healthcare-associated infections concluded that not only do the estimates of these costs vary widely, but so do the methods utilized and quality of the reports (2, 16). For example, while the cost of a surgical site infection reported by Stone and colleagues was $25,546, the eight point estimates reviewed ranged from $1783 to $134,602 in excess costs. Bloodstream infections costs ranged from $1822 to $107,156 with an average of $36,441 (2). If published data are to be used, the methods and setting of the published report should be carefully considered and selected to most closely resemble the setting in which the analysis is being conducted.

COST ADJUSTMENT

Whether an analysis includes internal cost estimates or published data expressed in prior year's dollars, it is necessary to convert these estimates to current year dollar values. This can be done using the medical services component of the Consumer Price Index (17). Adjusting for inflation is especially important if the estimates are from more than a single year. Similarly, if benefits to an intervention are expected to be realized in future years, these values should be discounted to reflected their current market value. As described by Perencevich et al. (17), this discounting process accounts for anticipated inflation and is calculated as follows: Estimated savings/$[1 + (0.3)^n]$, where n is number of years ahead in time when the benefit is expected to occur (17). If an MRSA screening program prevents a case of MRSA 2 years from the initial screen and the savings of prevention is $23,000, the current value of this savings would be $21,679.71 $(23{,}000/(1.03)^2)$.

COSTS BEYOND THE WALLS

With internal and literature cost estimates alike, the perspective of loss or gain is on the part of the organization while the societal costs are often ignored (18). Societal costs may include mortality, disability and quality of life for the patient or increased antimicrobial resistance in the environment. The decision of whether or not to include these costs may be best answered both in terms of feasibility and, perhaps more importantly, from the perspective of the decision-maker. If the decision to commit institutional resources to a particular intervention is exclusively on the part of organizational leadership, then perhaps societal costs can be excluded from the analysis or serve as supporting evidence in an addendum. Most internal cost estimates should similarly be restricted to costs incurred at the hospital during the index hospitalization. Subsequent readmissions following discharge or treatment provided in the outpatient setting are often not included but may be useful if readily available (19). Lastly, there is the increasing tendency of affected patients and families to initiate litigation procedures against the facilities in which they acquired their infections. A recent survey in Philadelphia found that 44% of cases are resolved in favor of the plaintiff, the verdicts are often in excess of a million dollars, and the most common healthcare-associated infections being litigated come from postoperative surgical site infections and outcomes caused by MRSA (20).

Direct cost estimates are sufficient if the economic analysis is narrow in focus and not compared to disparate initiatives. If, for example, the decision to be made is whether or not to screen patients for colonization with an antibiotic-resistant organism, such as methicillin-resistant *Staphylococcus aureus* (MRSA), a direct cost analysis between the options to screen or not screen patients is appropriate. Comparing competing infection control initiatives aimed at the same outcome may also be appropriately analyzed by cost metrics alone, and models aimed at doing such have been previously described (21). If, however, the decision to be made is between an infection control initiative and an enhanced cancer-screening program, direct cost comparisons are insufficient (3). To make such a comparison would be analogous to comparing apples to oranges. A more equitable approach to comparing disparate initiatives requires comparing the costs of each with respect to gained quality-adjusted life-years (QALYs). QALYs are the additional years gained by an initiative adjusted by a utility weight ranging from 0 (death) to full-functional wellness (1.0) (3, 21). In doing so, the analysis places a value on not only life itself, but the quality of life. For example, discharge to a skilled nursing facility for an infection would have a lower weight (e.g., 0.6) than discharge to home (1.0) and a higher score than death (0.0) due to the same infection. The costs of each intervention are then expressed with regard to dollars per QALY. Using the previously mentioned example, if an MRSA infection is avoided (by screening and appropriate isolation of colonized patients) and the (now) noninfected patient is discharged to home with a utility weight of 0.9 (minimal comorbid conditions unrelated to MRSA) to survive an additional 10 years, their QALYs gained by the intervention are 9.0 (10 years $\times$ 0.9 QALYs/year = 9.0 QALYs). If the cost of the intervention is \$100,000, the cost per QALY for the MRSA screening program is \$11,111.11 per QALY (\$100,000/9.0) if the intervention only prevents infection in this one single patient.

This same method can be applied to competing interventions to assess their respective cost per QALY, and informed decision-making with regard to appropriate resource allocation can be made in an unbiased fashion. When Fraser and Olsen (1) compared the cost effectiveness of an infection control program against screening programs for heart disease, cervical and breast cancer programs in terms of estimated costs per QALY infection programs were 2.5 to 80 times more cost effective (1). Interventions are generally considered fiscally suitable for implementation if their cost per QALY is \$50,000 or less, though the exact limit is a matter of continuous debate (22). Of note, QALY-based cost-utility analysis is not typically utilized by hospitals in business-cases analyses, but is more often thought of as the research standard for completing cost-effectiveness analysis at the societal or large institutional (e.g., Veterans Administration) level (23).

ANALYSIS

Having identified sources of cost data, adjusting these values to current value, and potentially examining them in terms of their respective cost per QALY gained, the infection control program leaders are now faced with the tough decision of how to best analyze and present the results to decision-makers. In this section, different methods of analysis are introduced, with an emphasis on cost-effective analysis.

There are four basic types of economic analysis used with regards to hospital epidemiology programs; cost minimization, cost benefit, cost utility, and cost effectiveness (3). A subtype of economic analysis most commonly used in healthcare is the business-case analysis. These analyses are useful for either helping to decide whether to implement a given intervention or program (as opposed to no change compared to baseline) or deciding which of several potential interventions to implement.

Cost minimization is the most basic, in which two equally effective options are weighed solely on the basis of cost alone (3). With respect to infection control programs, this type of analysis is most commonly seen in product selection or cost-reduction committees where the purchasing department explores options for reducing hospital expenditures. If hospital-grade disinfectant X costs $43.65 per unit and hospital-grade disinfectant Y has the same active ingredients and FDA approval for use but costs $32.67 per unit, the decision is relatively easy. This method of analysis is only appropriate when the two or more options are of equal utility. If disinfectant Y causes allergic reactions in environmental services staff, it is not reasonable to assume the two products are equal in effectiveness, regardless of their comparability with regard to active ingredients.

In cost–benefit analysis all elements regarding the intervention and subsequent outcomes are expressed in monetary units. If death is a potentially averted outcome as a result of the intervention, then a cost–benefit analysis of the intervention must include the appropriated cost of a human life. Similarly, quality of life must also be delineated in terms of dollars. Failing to account for these costs or benefits and describing the analysis as a cost–benefit analysis is a misclassification (17). After the costs of the intervention and potential cost savings are fully calculated, the two costs are compared. If the intervention is cost-neutral or profitable with respect to the costs, the intervention is considered worth implementing.

A cost–utility analysis compares benefits of intervention with respect to the aforementioned QALYs. By doing so, it accounts for mortality and quality of life measures in a manner that allows for different programs of unequal scope and costs to be compared with one another (3, 24). It most closely resembles cost-effectiveness analysis (described below). Zanetti et al. (25) illustrated a cost–utility analysis when they examined the costs and benefits of antibiotic prophylaxis for coronary artery bypass graft surgery by comparing vancomycin, cefazolin, or no prophylaxis at all. Though cefazolin was superior with respect to the absence of antibiotic prophylaxis, vancomycin was superior to cefazolin in terms of cost and QALYs (25).

COST EFFECTIVENESS

The most common form of evaluating the economics of infection control in the literature to date focuses on the cost of infection alone ("how much do surgical site infections cost?"). In evaluating the effectiveness of intervention with respect to these costs, cost effectiveness predominates the published reports (2). In its simplest form, cost effectiveness examines the relationship between two or more opportunities in terms of the increase in expenditures necessary to modify the probability of an event and the improved outcomes of that modified probability (3, 24).

Before beginning a cost-effectiveness analysis, it may be helpful to determine if one is actually necessary. For example, when considering an intervention to reduce catheter-associated urinary tract infection, Foley catheter A costs $6 per unit and is a standard urinary catheter and Foley catheter B costs $5 per unit but has antimicrobial properties that have demonstrated reduced rates of infection compared to Foley A (or other similarly comparable Foley); a cost-effectiveness analysis is not necessary. Foley B is both less expensive and comes with a decreased probability for infection. When one option is less expensive and more effective (or, alternatively, more expensive and less effective) at achieving desired results, a formal analysis is unnecessary. This becomes essentially the aforementioned cost-minimization analysis with the added benefit of improved outcomes. Unfortunately, these cut-and-dried scenarios are less common than their more complicated counterparts, namely when Option A is more expensive but more effective than Option B (24). Cost-effectiveness analyses evaluates the costs of a particular intervention or opportunity with respect to the most natural unit of comparison such as infections prevented and is expressed in terms of dollars per unit (e.g., $5000 per avoided surgical site infection) (3).

Cost-effectiveness analysis becomes increasingly complex when there are more options to choose from. If instead of Option A (standard practice) and Option B (intervention) there are five different options to choose from (A–E), each addressing the same outcome, a cost-effectiveness ratio may help simplify the decision-making. Beginning with A and B, an incremental cost-effectiveness ratio (ICER) is calculated as $(\text{Costs}_A - \text{Costs}_B)/(\text{Outcomes}_A - \text{Outcomes}_B)$, where option B may be either an alternate intervention or baseline practice (21, 24). ICERs are calculated with respect to each other. If one option is more costly but slightly more effective than another, a true cost per additional outcome can be generated. This allows the decision-maker to fully evaluate which is worth the necessary investment. In a setting of limited resources, lower ICERs generally suggest better value for the investment (21). A limitation to this approach is that all options (A–E) evaluated must address the same outcome (e.g., surgical site infection). One option cannot be focused on MRSA infection reduction while another targets urinary tract infections.

Similar interventions aimed at reducing healthcare-associated infections may be different with respect to cost-effectiveness in different settings. Settings where the outcome has a greater likelihood of occurring (sans intervention) will have a higher return on investment than the same program where the risk is not as great. Dr. Matthew Davis highlights this phenomenon with regard to an intervention aimed at improving pneumococcal vaccination during hospitalization (26). According to this law of diminishing returns, the degree of cost-effectiveness is determined, in part, by how "big" the problem is. The same intervention aimed at reducing the incidence of MRSA infections will be more cost effective in an endemic setting compared to settings where MRSA infections are a rare event. This highlights the need to perform economic analyses individually rather than relying exclusively on results of similar interventions reported in the literature.

BUSINESS-CASE ANALYSIS

Most economic analyses for hospital epidemiology programs exclude some patient outcomes such as mortality. The audience for such analyses (e.g., hospital administration) may be more focused on cost and investment return for the organization alone, rather than for the society as a whole. As such, program justification and interventions aimed at quality improvement usually address investment and return for the organization and fail to include investment and outcomes external to the organization. Whether by design or due to a lack of available data, failing to account for all potential outcomes renders the analysis to being a business-case analysis rather than cost effectiveness (17). A business-case analysis adopts the framework of cost effectiveness, but only includes variables directly related to cost or profit of the investing entity (e.g., hospital) (see Figure 4.1). Thus while cost-effectiveness studies are the most commonly cited form of economic analysis in the infection control literature, they are predominately misclassified business-case analyses (17). A successful business case "exists if the entity that invests in the intervention realizes a financial return on its investment in a reasonable time frame" (27).

1. Identity and describe the problem and potential solution
2. Meet with administration
3. Calculate costs of the intervention
4. Calculate the potential impact of the intervention
5. Calculate the cost of the problem
6. Calculate the difference between Step 3 and estimated cost savings [Step 3 – (Step 5 X incremental reduction from Step 4)]
7. Assess the potential for unintended consequences
8. Build support, gain approval and implement
9. Prospectively collect data post implementation and provide feedback

FIGURE 4.1 Essential steps to completing a business case analysis for an infection control program. Adapted from Perencevich et al. (17).

A common type of business-case analysis comes in the form of program justification in which an infection control department may be in the position of needing to justify existing resources in the face of proposed budget cuts. The lessons described by the BJC Healthcare System later in this chapter came as a result of such an opportunity. Rather than undergo a reduction in resources, they were able to propose and attain additional resources, resulting in a near tripling their number of FTEs over a few short years (28). Importantly, the methods for economic analysis in the setting of resource justification are much the same. Rather than adding resources to the program and anticipating benefits, justification begins with an existing program, calculating the cost savings of diminished resources and describing the effects of such cuts in terms of services no longer able to be provided. A business-case analysis makes sense in this setting because it may be difficult to project what, if any, increase in adverse patient outcomes may occur as a result of such cuts (17).

Examples of Cost-Effectiveness Studies

To further illustrate the utility of cost-effectiveness analyses with regard to infection control programs, this section will highlight examples reported in the literature. Strengths and limitations of these examples will be described because not all reports adhere to the principles of such analysis described above.

Muto et al. (29) evaluated the cost effectiveness of performing active surveillance cultures for vancomycin-resistant *Enterococcus* (VRE) in two large medical facilities: In one of these, surveillance was performed on high-risk admissions, while the other served as the control facility in which no such surveillance occurred. Attributable costs of the intervention described in the study included (a) personnel costs for obtaining the specimens, laboratory supplies, and technician time and (b) costs for the personal protective equipment used for patients identified as positive that were placed on contact isolation and totaled $253,099 over 2 years. The cost of the adverse outcome (bacteremia due to VRE infection) was approximated from recent estimates in the literature ($27,190 per episode). They found that the surveillance program had a positive impact on patient outcomes compared to the control facility (1 VRE bacteremia versus 29 infections at the control facility during the same time period) and that the intervention was of financial benefit to the intervening facility, with an average net annual cost savings of $254,110.50. The bacteremia cost data were extracted from the literature; however, the study from which this figure was obtained derived the cost of bacteremia due to VRE compared to patients with bacteremia due to the susceptible strain. Despite this limitation, the authors were thorough in the assessment of the costs of the intervention, including not only the cost of the test itself but also the hourly salary of persons obtaining and testing the specimen as well as the resultant contact isolation materials utilized for colonized patients. The authors do not state whether any of the costs were adjusted for inflation over the two-year study (29).

Chaiyakunapruk et al. (30) showcase a more complex example by evaluating the cost-effectiveness of chlorhexidine gluconate (CHG) versus povidone iodine for central venous catheter site care. They performed a systematic review to identify randomized controlled clinical trials in which the two antiseptic agents were evaluated. They pooled the data of these eight individual studies to form a mathematical model with probabilities for each of the respective outcomes (line infection, site infection, and survival/death). Costs were ascertained from micro-cost data of the authors' organization and applied to the model. Costs of the outcome included laboratory tests, pharmaceuticals, and increased hospital stay, with an average for central line-associated bloodstream infections of $7113 per episode. The results of this study demonstrated that selectively using CHG resulted in better patient outcomes and at a cost savings compared with the less expensive povidone iodine (30).

Practical Examples for Infection Control

One of the most common requests for additional resources in hospital epidemiology programs is the need for additional FTEs. Salary and benefits compensation also make the business case one of the more expensive and therefore difficult to successfully achieve. This section outlines the basic steps involved in seeking additional personnel resources. A condensed version of a mock proposal is shown in Figure 4.2.

Following a modified approach to the steps outlined in Figure 4.1, begin by outlining in writing what needs are currently not being met due insufficient personnel resources. Be specific and, if possible, approximate the amount of time necessary to complete each task in a given time period (e.g., "Perform central-line-associated bloodstream infection surveillance in cardiac care unit: 2.5 hours per week."). Add to this list known or anticipated expectations that will require an investment of resources. For example, if the next year's National Patient Safety Goals are available, identify which tasks will require the department's involvement and approximate the amount of time that will need to be committed. Lastly, add specific and measurable opportunities for improvement in which the addition of personnel may impact upon. An example would be if central-line-associated bloodstream infections are unacceptably high (compared to baseline, external benchmarks, or institutional goals) and the Institute for Healthcare Improvement (IHI) "central-line bundle" has not yet been implemented. For each of the above tasks, reference external benchmarks or requirements as able (the IHI bundle is a 2008 National Patient Safety Goal, for example). Sum the above time commitments to a uniform time interval (e.g., 60 hours per week) and calculate the number of needed FTEs (60 hours per week = 1.5 FTE). Use the above problem list to frame ideal and suitable candidate profiles and meet with a human resources (HR) representative to present these profiles and establish an approximate cost to fulfill the position. If additional nonpersonnel resources are needed (e.g., computer), approximate these costs as well and sum with the salary and benefits cost from HR. This initial figure is the upfront investment, and subsequent years may need to be calculated but will mostly consist of the compensation plus an average merit increase.

UTI REDUCTION INITIATIVE PROPOSAL

Rationale

Catheter-associated urinary tract infections are the most common healthcare-associated infection. Recent estimates suggest that Institution X has an unacceptably high rate of infection compared with national benchmarks. Beginning in October 2008, CMS will no longer reimburse higher diagnosis-related groups assigned to persons with these infections.

The Infection Control Department does not currently have the personnel resources available to dedicate sufficiently to this effort. By focusing surveillance and prevention strategies in this area, Institution X will be able to greatly reduce the rate of infection, resulting in a net cost savings to the institution.

Specific Daily Tasks and Approximate Time Requirements

1. Assess all Foley-catheterized inpatients for appropriate use and maintenance (15–30 minutes per patient per day, totaling 3 hours per day).
2. Assess insertion and maintenance activities of clinical staff (1 hour per day).
3. Conduct catheter-associated UTI surveillance, collate and present results (2 hours per day).
4. Educate direct care providers regarding appropriate utilization, insertion practice, and maintenance of Foley catheters (1 hour per week).
5. Observe and collect hand hygiene data as part of routine assessments (1 hour per day).
6. Serve on Nursing Quality Improvement Council (0.5 hours per week).

Total required: 40.5 hours per week. 1.0 FTE: RN required (involves direct patient care), IC experience and MSN in education a plus.

FIGURE 4.2 Mock proposal of requesting an additional FTE for an infection control program. The aim of this hypothetical program is specifically targeted toward a reduction of Foley-catheter-associated urinary tract infections (UTIs).

Return to the task list described above; and for each task in which there is a measurable opportunity for improvement by (in part) dedicating additional personnel, approximate the potential level of improvement. These goals must be achievable; utilize published reports of successful targeted interventions as well as internal or external benchmarks. If the intensive care unit had 10 central-line-associated bloodstream infections in the preceding year and 2300 line days, the rate is 4.35 per 1000 central-line days, more than double the external benchmark published by the CDC and certainly more than the increasingly common reports of attaining zero infections (31). In this example a 50% reduction would reduce the number of infections by five. Identify the attributable cost for each outcome variable for which a goal has been identified as described in the prior section describing costs of healthcare-associated infections. Multiply this cost by the number of adverse outcomes to be avoided for an estimated cost savings. Then calculate the difference between the potential cost savings and projected resource investment to determine a net return on investment. Ideally, this final figure is either cost neutral or preferably of projected financial benefit to the organization. Develop a basic implementation plan with timeline and benchmarks for success.

Before bringing this proposal to the final decision-makers, meet with multidisciplinary leadership to seek and gain their support. Seek and respond to feedback and modify the proposal as appropriate. It is more difficult to decline a request when there is widespread endorsement. Physician support can be especially helpful in a setting where their services are an anchor to revenue-generating activities (17). If the key decision-maker(s) reject the proposal, seek feedback with regard to what elements could be modified in order to attain approval, but don't overestimate performance with fewer resources or add objectives that cannot be reasonably achieved. Once approved, prospectively monitor outcome measures and assess the financial impact of successes with feedback to appropriate stakeholders and decision-maker(s). Success breeds success, and subsequent proposals will likely find an easier path to being approved.

Surveillance Technology

Hospital epidemiology programs have reported enhanced surveillance capabilities with the advent of surveillance technology programs (32). However, to date, no reports have assessed whether adopting these programs resulted in improved patient outcomes (33). Most commercially available programs are subscription-based with substantial capital investment required, though these costs are not publicly reported. Marketing materials from one commercial entity offers annual financial analysis on the cost of healthcare-associated infections (34). In-house developed systems are costly to develop, with one published report of an in-house clinical data warehouse for infection control requiring upwards of 4000 person-hours for development alone (35).

If a traditional cost-effective analysis is not feasible because a financial return on investment cannot be approximated from improved patient outcomes, a more creative approach may be suitable, likely in the framework of a business-case analysis. Many of the commercial entities may be start-up companies seeking to acquire new and preferably high-profile organizations to use as marketing for seeking additional clients. They may alternatively be partnered with a major distributor of medical or pharmaceutical supplies which may, in turn, have an existing relationship with the healthcare organization. They may be interested in pursuing research opportunities resulting in peer-reviewed publications highlighting the utility of their product. Each of the above leverages the healthcare organization to pursue competitive pricing with the hopes of reducing the upfront investment. Initiatives aimed at public reporting of healthcare-associated infections lead to a partnership between the state hospital association, a major healthcare insurance company, and a surveillance technology company in Alabama and reported a 13% reduction in infections during the first year of the program (36). In-house development of surveillance technology programs may be more difficult. They require institutional commitment of resources not in the context of a contractual agreement as with a commercial entity, but more often in the form of capital investment in dedicated hardware and software and the expertise of trained personnel. Furthermore, the return on investment in the form of a functioning system may be protracted compared with the packaged products offered commercially. Additional financial support may be available via research grants, but this too requires dedicated investment with regard to proposal development, submission, and deliverables.

A business case for surveillance technology can be made, though perhaps not in the traditional sense outlined in this chapter. The strengths of the proposal may include a reduction of projected upfront costs through competitive pricing and resources outside of the institution. Its necessity can be outlined through reports of increased demands for meaningful data, enhanced surveillance capabilities, a reduction in time spent performing surveillance, and a redistribution of these assets away from data collection and toward implementing change to reduce adverse outcomes. By prospectively monitoring via time-motion studies, quality improvement efforts, and healthcare-associated infections following implementation, a retrospective cost justification may ensure continued support in the long term.

BJC CASE STUDY

Following a series of mergers in the 1990s, the infection control program at BJC Healthcare underwent dramatic revisions to their department with respect to services provided and resource allocation. Denise Murphy described these events in great detail in a published report, a summary of which follows here (28).

Mergers often involve aligning resources from the previously distinct entities and eliminating duplicate work. In healthcare, it is not uncommon for this to result in fewer, not more, FTEs, particularly in areas not involved in direct patient care (e.g., administration, infection control). When BJC underwent a series of mergers, the 18 existing ICPs harnessed this anxiety to formulate a "survival plan." Their plan evolved from one of survival to expansion and success (see Figure 4.3).

They began by evaluating their existing infrastructure primarily from the point of view of being a corporate division, rather than multiple distinct entities or departments. Policies were reviewed and inconsistent practices were standardized in accordance with best practice recommendations. The collection and storage of surveillance data was evaluated with regard to several aspects. The BJC group elected to adopt the NHSN surveillance definitions to introduce uniformity in surveillance practices. They developed a central database for the storage of surveillance data and reports.

During this initial phase, they developed a long-term vision of what the department needed to successfully address the needs of the organization. They develop a 5-year plan and a mission statement that reflected these needs, emphasizing their role throughout the "continuum of care" and openly addressing the fact that their services must be provided in a "cost-effective manner." With this, they began a comprehensive review of their existing practice with regard to this long-term vision and identified where further effort was required and what resources were needed to successfully bridge the gap from where they were to where they wanted to be.

Throughout this process they maintained open dialogues with both their supporting infection control committee and senior executive leadership, including the organization's business leaders, and sought their approval and appropriate feedback. They note that by including such variables as the attributable cost of healthcare-associated infections in their analyses, the infection control group was able to communicate the financial implications of failing to act on potential performance improvement activities. After identifying high-risk, high-volume procedures for which infection rates were unacceptably high compared to external benchmarks, they proposed an initiative aimed at reducing these infections, outlined necessary resources along with an implementation plan, and presented said proposal, with potential for cost savings, to executive leadership. Following implementation, they prospectively monitored outcomes and calculated the attributable cost savings associated with reduced adverse outcomes. In one initiative alone, the net cost savings approached \$103,000 in one year, with the costs of the intervention including not only time and materials on behalf of the department, but also the time requirements for the direct care providers in receipt of the intervention (needs assessment, education, and follow-up).

Of important note, the BJC group coupled this business-sense-based approach with a change in philosophy regarding how infection control programs and personnel should work. They invested heavily in efforts aimed at efficiency by leveraging information technology tools (e.g., PDAs) to encourage and empower ICPs to be a more visible and available resource in the patient care areas and by removing data collection that did not

1. Infrastructure
    a. Streamline practice
        i. Corporate structure
        ii. Leadership
        iii. Policies
    b. Information technology
        i. Uniform data collection (same surveillance definitions)
        ii. Uniform data storage (central database)
        iii. Needs assessment for hardware, software and user training
2. Gaining direction and building the case
    a. Complete evaluation of current practice
    b. Develop a long-term plan
    c. Complete gap analysis between long-term plan and current practice
    d. Develop the business case
        i. How to get "there" from "here"
        ii. Identify needed resources and the projected costs (bad outcomes) of continuing with established practice
        iii. Meet with keystakeholders (e.g. customers and administration) and gain their support
3. Implementation and evaluation
    a. Personnel
        i. Close knowledge and training gaps
        ii. Provide the necessary resources
        iii. Raise expectations, continue to build support for change
    b. Change practice
        i. Data collection must be "value-added" (discontinue otherwise)
        ii. Focus the deliverables to the needs of the customer
        iii. Leverage IT for increased efficiency
        iv. Divide and conquer
            1. Dedicated expert resources for emergent issues
            2. Focus teams for targeted projects
    c. Evaluation
        i. Prospectively collect and report outcomes
        ii. Evaluate successes in terms of cost

FIGURE 4.3 Outline describing the successful enhancement in both resource allocation and practice of the infection control program at BJC Healthcare following a series of corporate mergers. Adapted from Murphy (28).

meet specific criteria (reliable, measurable, and value added). They fostered an environment internally that encouraged adaptability and change on the part of the ICPs, increased expectations on behalf of the staff and provided the resources to help personnel achieve these new goals.

Between 1996 and 2001 the newly renamed Infection Control and Healthcare Epidemiology Consortium at BJC increased their allocated FTEs from 10.6 to 27.7, reduced healthcare-associated infections in targeted high-risk areas by as much as 68%, and evolved from being enclaves of data collectors to a unified corporate entity with a long-term vision focused on implementing change to drive quality improvement, receiving increased resources and proactively demonstrating the return on investment to executive leadership (28).

Conclusions

In order to demonstrate the cost effectiveness or return on investment of an intervention, an additional resource request, or an entire program, hospital epidemiology personnel must understand where costs are accrued and how adverse outcomes lead to attributable costs.

They must be able to quantify these costs and adjust them accordingly via inflation or discounting. To address the problem, they must form hypotheses about how such outcomes may be reduced or even eliminated. The actionable items of the hypothesis that require resource allocation must then be quantified in terms of cost and compared with the potential return on investment. The results of this analysis may then be used as part of a program proposal or justification. Once approved, prospective monitoring with regard to patient outcomes, attributable cost savings, and return on investment should be collected and communicated to decision-makers as appropriate.

Healthcare expenditures are projected to reach 18.4% of the Untied States gross domestic product by 2013 (37). Small and large healthcare organizations alike are struggling to avoid financial losses, and infection control programs are unlikely to detach their reputation as non-revenue-generating cost centers. The cloud of mandatory reporting and other legislative effort towards healthcare-associated infections does have silver lining; it has elevated the profile of hospital epidemiology programs in the eyes of the public. This provides such programs with the opportunity to leverage such heightened awareness with administration to seek and obtain the needed resources to prevent adverse patient outcomes. However, healthcare administrators are unlikely to allocate additional resources indiscriminately. Approaching the need for additional resources with a business frame of mind allows hospital epidemiology personnel to frame their requests in a manner that can be more easily interpreted and accepted by a wider audience including healthcare administration.

REFERENCES

1. Fraser VJ, Olsen MA. The business of health care epidemiology: Creating a vision for service excellence. *Am J Infect Control.* 2002;**30**(2):77–85.
2. Stone PW, Braccia D, Larson E. Systematic review of economic analyses of health care-associated infections. *Am J Infect Control.* 2005;**33**(9):501–509.
3. Cosgrove SE, Perencevich EN. Economic evaluation of healthcare-associated infections and infection control interventions. In, *Bennet and Brachman's Hospital Infections*, 5th ed. Bennet JV, Jarvis WR, Brachman PS. (eds.), Lippincott and Williams, Philadelphia, 2007.
4. Jarvis W. Infection control and changing healthcare delivery systems, *Emerg Infect Dis* 2001;**7**:170–173.
5. Anderson DJ, Kirkland KB, Kaye KS, Thacker PA 2nd, Kanafani ZA, Auten G, Sexton DJ. Underresourced hospital infection control and prevention programs: Penny wise, pound foolish? *Infect Control Hosp Epidemiol* 2007;**28**(7):767–773.
6. Graves N, McGowan JE, Jr. Nosocomial infection, the Deficit Reduction Act, and incentives for hospitals. *JAMA* 2008;**300**(13):1577–1579.
7. Graves N. Economics and preventing hospital-acquired infection. *Emerg Infect Dis* 2004; **10**(4):561–566.
8. Finkler SA. The distinction between cost and charges. *Ann Intern Med* 1982;**96**(1):102–109.
9. Howard D, Cordell R, McGowan JE Jr, Packard RM, Scott RD, Solomon SL. Workshop Group. Measuring the economic costs of antimicrobial resistance in hospital settings: Summary of the Centers for Disease Control and Prevention—Emory Workshop. *Clin Infect Dis* 2001; **33**(9):1573–1578.
10. Center for Medicare and Medicaid Services web site: http://www.cms.hhs.gov. Accessed November 2, 2008.

11. Pronovost PJ, Goeschel CA, Wachter RM. The wisdom and justice of not paying for "preventable complications". *JAMA* 2008;**299**(18):2197–2199.
12. Klompas M, Platt R. Ventilator-associated pneumonia—The wrong quality measure for benchmarking. *Ann Intern Med* 2007;**147**(11):803–805.
13. Frick KD.Microcosting presented at Health Care Costs: Standardized Methods & Estimates for Research & Policy Applications Workshop, December 6–7 2007, Rockville, MD. Slides available at http://healthservices.cancer.gov/publications/workshops/hcc/cost_ws_frick.pdf.
14. Harris AD, Samore MH, Lipsitch M, Kaye KS, Perencevich EN, Carmeli Y. Control-group selection importance in studies of antimicrobial resistance: Examples applied to *Pseudomonas aeruginosa,* enterococci, and *Escherichia coli. Clin Infect Dis* 2002;**34**(12):1558–1563.
15. Perencevich EN, Thom KA. Commentary: Preventing *Clostridium difficile*-associated disease: Is it time to pay the piper? *Infect Control Hosp Epidemiol* 2008;**29**(9):829–831.
16. Halton K, Graves N. Economic evaluation and catheter-related bloodstream infections. *Emerg Infect Dis* 2007;**13**(6):815–823.
17. Perencevich EN, Stone PW, Wright SB, Carmeli Y, Fisman DN, Cosgrove SE. Society for Healthcare Epidemiology of America. Raising standards while watching the bottom line: making a business case for infection control. *Infect Control Hosp Epidemiol* 2007; **28**(10):1121–1133.
18. Cosgrove SE, Carmeli Y. The impact of antimicrobial resistance on health and economic outcomes. *Clin Infect Dis* 2003;**36**(11):1433–1437.
19. Perencevich EN, Sands KE, Cosgrove SE, Guadagnoli E, Meara E, Platt R. Health and economic impact of surgical site infections diagnosed after hospital discharge. *Emerg Infect Dis* 2003;**9**(2):196–203.
20. Guinan JL, McGuckin M, Shubin A, Tighe J. A descriptive review of malpractice claims for health care-acquired infections in Philadelphia. *Am J Infect Control* 2005;**33**(5):310–312.
21. Graves N, Halton K, Lairson D. Economics and preventing hospital-acquired infection: Broadening the perspective. *Infect Control Hosp Epidemiol* 2007;**28**(2):178–184.
22. Bell CM, Urbach DR, Ray JG, Bayoumi A, Rosen AB, Greenberg D, Neumann PJ. Bias in published cost effectiveness studies: Systematic review. *BMJ* 2006;**332**(7543):699–703.
23. Gold MR, Siegel JE, Russell LB, Weinstein MC. *Cost-Effectiveness in Health and Medicine*, 1st ed. Oxford University Press, New York, 1996.
24. Saint S, Chenoweth C, Fendrick AM. The role of economic evaluation in infection control. *Am J Infect Control* 2001;**29**(5):338–344.
25. Zanetti G, Goldie SJ, Platt R. Clinical consequences and cost of limiting use of vancomycin for perioperative prophylaxis: Example of coronary artery bypass surgery. *Emerg Infect Dis* 2001; **(5)**:820–827.
26. Davis MM. Challenges in cost-effectiveness analyses of hospital interventions to improve quality. *Infect Control Hosp Epidemiol* 2008;**29**(5):395–397.
27. Leatherman S, Berwick D, Iles D, Lewin LS, Davidoff F, Nolan T, Bisognano M. The business case for quality: Case studies and an anlysis. *Health Aff (Millwood)* 2003;**22**:17–30.
28. Murphy DA. From expert data collectors to interventionists: Changing the focus for infection control professionals. *Am J Infect Control* 2002;**30**(2):120–132.
29. Muto CA, Giannetta ET, Durbin LJ, Simonton BM, Farr BM. Cost-effectiveness of perirectal surveillance cultures for controlling vancomycin-resistant *Enterococcus. Infect Control Hosp Epidemiol* 2002;**23**(8):429–435.
30. Chaiyakunapruk N, Veenstra DL, Lipsky BA, Sullivan SD, Saint S. Vascular catheter site care: The clinical and economic benefits of chlorhexidine gluconate compared with povidone iodine. *Clin Infect Dis* 2003;**37**(6):764–771.

31. Richards C. Getting to zero: An emerging policy framework for the elimination of hospital-associated infections. *Infect Control Hosp Epidemiol* 2009;**30**(1):71–73.
32. Wright MO. Automated surveillance and infection control: Towards a better tomorrow. *Am J Infect Control* 2008;**36**(3):S1–S6.
33. Furuno JP, Schweizer ML, McGregor JC, Perencevich EN. Economics of infection control surveillance technology: Cost-effective or just cost? *Am J Infect Control* 2008;**36**(3 Suppl): S12–S17.
34. Cardinal Health MedMined Services web site: http://cardinalhealth.com/medmined/services/index.asp. Accessed December 3, 2008.
35. Wisniewski MF, Kieszkowski P, Zagorski BM, Trick WE, Sommers M, Weinstein RA. Development of a clinical data warehouse for hospital infection control. *J Am Med Inform Assoc* 2003;**10**(5):454–462.
36. Alabama Hospital Quality Initiative web site: http://www.ahqi.org/index.cfm. Accessed December 15, 2008.
37. Stone PW, Hedblom EC, Murphy DM, Miller SB. The economic impact of infection control: making the business case for increased infection control resources. *Am J Infect Control* 2005; **33**(9):542–547.

CHAPTER FIVE

Outbreak Investigations (Importance of the Healthcare Epidemiologist)

FAIQA ALAM CHEEMA AND MARCUS J. ZERVOS

Introduction

Healthcare epidemiology has been practiced since the mid-1800s. Nightingale, Semmelweis, Lister, and Holmes all made significant contributions to the field. The term "hospital epidemiologist" was first used in an article published in 1940 that described measures to prevent outbreak of diarrhea (1). Healthcare epidemiologist refers to anyone who concerns themselves with the determinants of hospital-acquired disease or injuries; such efforts are usually undertaken with prevention in mind. Traditionally, hospital epidemiology has been referred to as infection control but is increasingly being applied to clinical performance and quality management.

Nosocomial infections are an important source of morbidity and mortality in hospital settings, afflicting an estimated 2 million patients in the United States each year (2). Early information has shown that this number represents approximately 5% of hospitalized patients and result in 88,000 deaths and 4.5 billion in healthcare cost (3–6). The new goal is to have zero infection rates.

Bloodstream infections are one of the most serious complications of hospitalization (7–10). In a recent matched cohort study of intensive care unit (ICU) patients, the

Molecular Techniques for the Study of Hospital-Acquired Infection, First Edition. Edited by Steven L. Foley, Anne Y. Chen, Shabbir Simjee, and Marcus J. Zervos.

length of stay among survivors for primary bloodstream infection was increased by a median of 8.5 days and cost was increased to a median of $34,000 (11). Cost of surgical site infection is estimated to 3 billion per year. A recent matched cohort study of wound infections in a community hospital was associated with $3089 in excess cost, 6.5 extra days of inpatient stay, and an attributable mortality rate of 4.3% (12). In nosocomial pneumonias, VAP results in 4–5 days of excess ICU stay in survivors (13, 14). The cost per case has been estimated to range from $10,000 to $29,000. Each symptomatic urinary tract infection adds approximately $700 to the cost of hospitalization, a figure that quadruples if bacteremia develops (15, 16).

Increasingly, hospital-acquired infections are multidrug-resistant pathogens. The presence of underlying conditions (such as diabetes, renal failure, or malignancies), long hospitalizations, surgical procedures, indwelling catheters, and discriminate use of broad spectrum antibiotics has been cited as risk factors for acquiring infections. The majority of instances of antimicrobial resistance are associated with Gram-positive nosocomial pathogens, which include methicillin-resistnt *Staphylococcus aureus* (MRSA) (17–20) and vancomycin-resitant *Enterococcus* (VRE) (21–26).

MRSA infections alone increase LOS for nosocomial infections 12 days for MRSA versus 4 days for MSSA. The median length of stay for surgical site MRSA infection is 23 days versus 14 days for MSSA. Direct hospital cost from nosocomial MRSA bacteremia is 2.8 times more than that for MSSA bacteremia. Nosocomial MRSA infections are associated with higher mortality versus MSSA (21% versus 8%). MRSA SSTI (skin soft tissue infection) is associated with a higher 90-day mortality rate (20.7% for MRSA versus 6.7% for MSSA) (27, 28). Among the Gram-negative bacilli, extended-spectrum beta-lactamase-producing strains of *Escheria coli* and *Kliebsiella pnuemonia* have been of emerging concern.

Infectious disease clinicians, hospital epidemiologists, and infection prevention specialists may frequently encounter outbreak scenarios in which patients are likely to be infected with genetically similar organisms. Although many of these outbreaks are due to a common source (e.g., because they are limited to a specific time and place), the source of other outbreaks is not so visible (29). Therefore, understanding pathogen distribution and relatedness is essential for determining the epidemiology of nosocomial infections and aiding in the design of rationale pathogen control methods (2).

In the past, a number of methods have been used to study the epidemiology of hospital infections, including observational analyses, biochemical tests, nutritional requirements, antibiograms, immunological testing, serogrouping, and bacteriphage. Over the past two decades, newer technologies are based on DNA, or molecular analysis. These DNA-based molecular methodologies, including PFGE, restriction-based methods, and PCR-based typing methods are used (see corresponding chapters in the Part II of this book).

Molecular typing methods have become powerful tools for epidemiologic investigations of healthcare-associated infections (2, 30–32). When used appropriately as a part of an epidemiological investigation, strain typing facilitates the job of a healthcare epidemiologist. Practioners in this field must be familiar with the available methods and must understand their limitations, their cost, and the applicability of the various techniques in order to choose the most appropriate method for a given purpose. Results of molecular typing should not be used alone and strain typing data should be included as a part of complete, well-designed epidemiological investigations.

Also establishing clonality of pathogens can aid in the identification of source (environmental or personnel) of organism, distinguish infections from noninfectious strains, and distinguish relapse from reinfections. If an infection is due to relapse, this may be an indication that an initial treatment regimen was not effective and that alternative therapy must be required (2).

Investigating Nosocomial Infections

A number of nosocomial infections are endemic infections and are defined as sporadic infections that constitute the background rate of infections at the healthcare facility; the rate of such infections fluctuates from month to month but overall is not statistically different from the background rate of these infections. Of all nosocomial infections, endemic infections account for the majority of the infections and are the focus of almost all infections control activities. Epidemic infections are defined as the occurrence of infections at a rate statistically more significant than the background rate; these infection clusters are often unexpected and involve either an unusual organism or an organism with an unusual susceptibility pattern. There are a number of key factors that are essential in conduction a successful epidemiological investigation. Surveillance is the cornerstone for rapid recognition of endemic or epidemiological nosocomial infections, including the recognition that a problem exists, establishing a case-controlled definition, confirmation of cases and completion of case finding. The investigation is typically multifaceted involving an infection control specialist, an infectious disease physician, a laboratory personnel, and often a pharmacist (33).

Once an aberration is detected, an investigation can be initiated. The first step in any investigation is to ensure that critically important data (isolates/materials) that may be associated with the outbreak are saved. Identification of affected personnel, and a review of the characteristics of the representative case patients in relation to time, person, and place are essential in the early stages of the investigation. In the case–control portion of the investigation, characteristic of affected persons are compared with those of a similar but unaffected person.

Laboratory personnel should also be alerted that any of the infecting organisms from current and past possible "cases" should be saved, and it is important to keep any subsequent isolates of the outbreak strain that may be recovered during the investigation. The pathogen associated with outbreak is characterized using molecular typing methods to assist in the clinical epidemiological assessment. Also included in investigative steps include asking an important question: "Is this unusual?" An equally important measure is to calculate attack rate and compare with baseline rate to correctly identify it as an epidemic. Laboratory participation would assist by providing archival data on occurrence.

A hypothesis about causation is then generated about the epidemiology of infection, including mode of spread, reservoirs, and vectors and specific control measures initiated. Ongoing and follow-up surveillance is necessary to ensure that control measures are effective and to determine efficacy of treatment regimen.

General Concepts for Strain Typing

Three assumptions are generally made in using molecular typing for the purpose of epidemiological studies or microorganisms: First, are the isolates responsible for the outbreak the recent progeny of a common ancestor? Second, do these isolates have the same genotype? Third, do these epidemiologically unrelated strains have different genotypes? The concept of "clonality" is a fundamental principle in strain typing; microbial isolates recovered from different sources are considered to be clones if they have identical phenotypic and genetic traits. This idea clonality is based on the belief that isolates from common origins will share common phenotypes and genotypes. Therefore, the determination of clonality cannot be made with absolute certainty, but instead represents a statistical likelihood of identity amongst a group of independently isolated organism. The better the discriminatory power of the technique used to identify the isolate, the more likely the clonality of isolate can be accurately determined.

The most useful typing methods fulfill three criteria in that they have typeability, which is the ability to give an unambiguous result for each isolate; they have reproducibility, which is the capacity to give same result on repeat testing; and they have discriminatory power, which is the ability to differentiate among epidemiologically unrelated strains. Choosing a typing method depends not only on the strength of the particular method in each of the above-mentioned areas but also on the organism in question. Both the ease of performance (which is the technical complexity of the technique) and the ease of interpretation are important criteria for choosing a typing system (31, 34, 35). Although phenotyping methods have been successfully been used for epidemiologic purposes, they have largely been replaced by molecular methods. Phenotyping methods for typing include biotyping, serotyping, bacteriophage susceptibility testing, antimicrobial susceptibility testing, and bacteriocin-producing testing. Phenotypic methods involve cost in labor and material and are restricted to a few species; for example, anti-sera for *Salmonella* serotyping will not work to type Gram-positive organism. Hence they are limited in their discriminatory power and reproducibility.

Genetic methods for delineation of strain relatedness include PFGE, restriction fragment-length polymorphism (e.g. RFLP), DNA probes, ribotyping, electrophoretic karyotyping, PCR application, multilocus enzyme electrophoresis, and nucleated sequence. Genotypic methods involve direct DNA analysis of chromosomal or extra-chromosomal genetic elements. These techniques, although costly, are relatively easy to learn and are applicable to a variety of species. These techniques have improved typeability, reproducibility, and discriminatory power compared to phenotypic techniques. Genotypic methods are also less affected by natural variation in a population, although changes such as insertion of DNA or deletion of DNA from chromosome, the gain or loss of extra-chromosomal DNA, or random mutation may lead to difficulty in interpretations (2).

PULSE FIELD GEL ELECTROPHORESIS (PFGE)

Chromosomal DNA is the fundamental component of identity of the cell and therefore represents a preferred measure for assessing strain interrelatedness. DNA is digested with restriction enzymes, resulting in a series of fragments of different sizes that form different patterns when analyzed by agarose gel electrophoresis. Differences in these patterns are referred to as restriction fragment-length polymorphism (RFLPs). Enzymes used to cleave DNA often recognize numerous sites within the bacterial chromosome, resulting in too many band fragments to efficiently and accurately compare following conventional agarose gel electrophoresis. The resulting DNA fragments are too large to be separated by conventional agarose gel electrophoresis. A number of alternative methods, generally classified as PFGE, are capable of separating these large DNA fragments (36–41). To interpret DNA fragment pattern generated by PFGE and transform them into epidemiologically useful information for typing nosocomial pathogens, the clinical microbiologist must understand how to compare PFGE patterns and how random genetic events can alter these patterns. Banding patterns from large chromosomal fragments can be compared by visual inspection for a small number of isolates. Isolates that differ by less than or equal to three bands are related strains and represent a single genetic event. PFGE patterns can be digitalized in a TIFF format, with patterns normalized; comparing large numbers of isolates also generate dandrogramic analysis. Major limitations of PFGE include (a) the need for technical expertise and (b) the initial cost of equipment, although many laboratories are skilled in this technique.

PLASMID ANALYSIS

Plasmid (extra-chromosomal DNA is present in most bacteria). Plasmid typing was the first molecular method to be used as a bacterial typing tool (42–47). In plasmid typing, plasmid DNA is extracted and subjected to restriction-enzyme digestion. Some bacteria have large plasmids in the range 100–150 kb, making their separation difficult. For these strains, a restriction endonuclease digestion step following plasmid isolation will aid in typing. Evaluation of plasmid content is not useful in delineation of clonal relationships. An exception may be when isolates from a suspected nosocomial outbreak have three or more plasmids in common. Plasmid analysis has been applied in clinical situations to determine the evolution and spread of antibiotic resistance among isolates with different PFGE profiles or among different species of organism within a hospital (25, 48, 49). Plasmids are not generally helpful for differentiation between endemic and epidemic strains, because plasmids are often mobile extra-chromosomal DNA fragments that can be acquired and deleted. A consequence of the plasmid mobility is that epidemiologically related isolates can exhibit different plasmid profiles. Many plasmids carry antibiotic resistance determinants that are contained within mobile genetic elements (transposons) that can move in or out of plasmids and the chromosomes, allowing the DNA component of plasmid protein to change rapidly.

TYPING METHOD USING PCR

PCR is a powerful molecular method that has been adapted for use as a typing tool for epidemiological investigation (50, 51). It permits the synthesis of large quantities of a targeted nucleic acid sequence (52). It amplifies minute quantities of microbial DNA component, present in a sample, which allows for detection and identification of microbes and can generate a "molecular fingerprint" for each organism based on its unique sequence of DNA or RNA. Compared with other methods, PCR offers the advantage of speed (results obtained in minutes to hours) and is unrivaled in sensitivity. PCR can also be extremely specific, depending on choice of primers. A growing number of organisms have been studied using this approach (53–62). The high sensitivity of PCR can lead to its greatest limitations leading to false-positive result due to amplification of contaminated DNA present in a sample. Therefore, PCR should be performed by personnel trained in these techniques in a laboratory specifically set up for these procedures.

Multiplex PCR In order to increase efficiency of PCR typing and reduce reagent costs, multiple sets of primers can be included in a single reaction tube in a process termed multiplex PCR (63, 64).

Nested PCR Nested PCR can be carried out when there is an extreme need for sensitivity and specificity. It involves the sequential use of two PCR primer sets.

Arbitrarily Primed PCR Arbitrarily primed PCR (AP-PCR) and the similar randomly amplified polymorphic DNA assay are variations of the PCR technique in which a random primer, which is not targeted to amplify any specific bacterial DNA sequence, is used for amplification (65–67). AP-PCR has several advantages: It is widely applicable to many bacterial species and is rapid and fairly easy to perform, compared to other typing systems. A disadvantage of AP-PCR is the difficulty standardization; small changes in reaction may give variability in banding pattern resulting in low reproducibility.

SOUTHERN BLOT ANALAYSIS: RIBOTYPING

In this method, the restriction fragment separated by agarose gel electrophoresis is transferred onto nitrocellulose or nylon membrane, and a chemically or radioactive labeled fragment of DNA or RNA is used as a probe to detect fragments that contain sequences homologous to a probe. One of the most commonly used targets for Southern blotting is the gene for rRNA, and targeting of the rRNA gene is referred as ribotyping. The discriminatory power of ribotyping has been shown to be less than that of the PFGE or PCR method. A benefit of ribotyping is that it is highly automated, reducing the amount of human capital needed to perform the technique and limiting user variability (68).

AMPLIFIED FRAGMENT-LENGTH POLYMORPHISM (AFLP) ANALYSIS

In AFLP analysis, chromosomal DNA is digested with a restriction endonuclease, generating a large number of fragments. In order to make the interpretation of result more feasible, only a specific subset is used for isolation comparison. PCR primers are designed to hybridize to the adapter sequence, the remaining restriction site sequence, and an additional one or two nucleotides of the unknown template sequence. Following PCR, the reaction products are separated by gel electrophoresis and their banding patterns are resolved.

COMPARISON AND SELECTION OF TECHNIQUE

In the analysis of nosocomial infection, detective-like solving problem skills are often required. There should always be a clear objective for use of a particular strain type, and should limit strain typing to only the isolates needed to define the clinical or epidemiological entity. The choice of a strain method will depend on the medical capability and expertise of the laboratory that serves the hospital, but one should first decide whether there is a real need to use a molecular epidemiological approach to study the situation in question. The choice of a test will also depend on the cost and the performance characteristic of the method (discriminatory power, reproducibility, and the availability of a relevant database). The molecular characterization can assist in separating relapse from reinfection; or, in the case of bacteremia, it can determine whether the organism is from the infection or contamination. In a group of isolates, the characterization of isolate by a method such as PFGE can assist in establishment of clonal relationships that help in assessing the question of patient-to-patient spread of an organism. Plasmid or transposon analysis of strain is used when there is a suspicion of dissemination of a particular resistance gene or set of genes. Repetitive typing or use of a second method does not significantly alter the epidemiological assessment, provided that the isolates are typeable and appropriate controls are used in the analysis.

When comparing the different molecular methods, it is important to consider what each method is actually assessing. Additionally, there is a need to have an understanding of the underlying genetic diversity of the species of microorganism being typed to have a more full understanding of the typing result. In some instances, minor genetic differences may be of epidemiological significance in more clonal organism that, by definition, has low degree of genetic variability. A key way to accomplish understanding of diversity is through development of a large isolate database. CDC has begun to develop a national database for MRSA isolates and has set up a naming scheme for a number of MRSA isolates.

SINGLE LOCUS SEQUENCE TYPING (SLST) AND MULTILOCUS SEQUENCE TYPING (MLST)

At present, the SLST approach with the most promise involves analysis of a particular region of staphylococcal protein A gene (*spa*) which is polymorphic. Multilocus sequence typing is based on the sequencing of multiple housekeeping genes and is the genetic equivalent of multilocus enzyme electrophoresis. The sequences of these genes are determined by routine DNA sequencing, after which they are analyzed by a publicly available database. MLST was originally employed to identify hypervirulent lineages of *Nisseria meningitides*. However, this approach has now been applied to a variety of other pathogens, including *S. aureus* (49, 69–73) and *Enterococcus spp.* (74, 75) for the assignment of *Staphylococcus* pneumonia strains to major hypervirulent, penicillin-resistant, and multiple-antibiotic-resitant clones and to a large number of other organisms.

Conclusions

The evaluation of hospital-acquired infection will continue to rely on clinical infection surveillance as the first step to understanding disease epidemiology and management of infections (2). Additionally, the tests chosen should be rapid and cost effective and facilitate in reduction of nosocomial infections. Molecular testing will continue to be an essential tool for rapid and cost-effective means of detecting epidemiologically significant organisms.

In the future, concerns about the emergence of nosocomial infections, increasing antimicrobial resistance, and increase in morbidity, mortality, and costs associated with hospital-acquired infections will drive the need for refinement of molecular approaches to aid in epidemiological analyses and diagnosis of nosocomial infections.

REFERENCES

1. Felson J, Wolarsky W. The hospital epidemiologist. *Hospitals* 1940;**14**:41.
2. Singh A, Goering RV, Simjee S, Foley SL, Zervos MJ. The application of molecular techniques to the study of hospital infection. *Clin Microbiol Rev* 2006;**19**:512–530.
3. Centers for Disease Control and Prevention. *Addressing Emerging Infectious Disease Threats; A Preventive Strategy for the United States*. Centers for Disease Control and Prevention, Atlanta, 1994.
4. Dembry L, Zervos MJ, Hierholzer WJ. Nosocomial Bacterial Infections, 3rd ed., In Brachman EA, (ed.), *Bacterial Infections in Humans*. Plenum Publishing Corporation, New York, pp. 501–528.
5. Jarvis WR. Usefulness of molecular epidemiology for outbreak investigations. *Infect Control Hosp Epidemiol* 1994;**15**:500–503.

6. McGowan JE Jr. Economic impact of antimicrobial resistance. *Emerg Infect Dis* 2001; **7**:286–292.
7. Pittet D, Wenzel RP. Nosocomial bloodstream infections. Secular trends in rates, mortality, and contribution to total hospital deaths. *Arch Intern Med* 1995;**155**:1177–1184.
8. Renaud B, Brun-Buisson C. Outcomes of primary and catheter related bacteremia. A cohort and case–control study critically ill patients. *Am J Respir Crit Care Med* 2001;**163**:1584–1590.
9. Wenzel R, Edmond M. The impact of hospital acquired blood stream infections. *Emerg Infect Dis* 2001;**7**:174–177.
10. Pittet D, Tarara D, Wenzel RP. Nosocomial bloodstream infections in critically ill patients: excess length of stay, extra costs and attributable mortality. *JAMA* 1994;**271**:1598–1601.
11. DiGiovinie B, Chenoweth C, Watts C, et al. The attributable mortality and cost of primary nosocomial blood stream infections in the intensive care unit. *Am J Respir Crit Care Med* 1999;**160**:976–981.
12. Kirkland KB, Briggs JP, Trivett SL, et al. The impact of surgical infections in the 1990s: Attributable mortality, excess length of hospitalization and extra costs. *Infect Control Hosp Epidemiol* 1999;**20**:725–730.
13. Heyland DK, Cook DJ, Griffith L, et al. and the Canadian Critical Care Trial Group. The attributable morality of ventilator-associated pneumonia in the critically ill patient. The Canadian Critical Trials Group. *Am J Respir Crit Care Med* 1999;**159**:1249–1256.
14. Papzaian L, Bregeon F, Thirion X, et al. Effect of ventilator associated pneumonia on mortality and morbidity. *Am J Respir Crit Care Med* 1996;**154**:91–97.
15. Saint S. Clinical and economic consequence of nosocomial catheter-related bacteriuria. *Am J Infect Control* 2000;**28**:68–75.
16. Maki D, Tambyah P. Engineering out the risk of infection with urinary catheters. *Emerg Infect Dis* 2001;**7**:1–6.
17. Barakate, MS, Yang YX, Foo SH, Vickery AM, Sharon CA, Fowler LD, Harris JP, West RH, Mcleod C, Benn RA. An epidemiological survey of methicillin-resistant *Staphylococcus aureus* in a tertiary referral hospital. *J Hosp Infect* 2000;**44**:19–26.
18. Rubin R, Harrington CA, Poon A, Dietrich K, Greene JA, Moiduddin A. The economic impact of *Stapylococcus aureus* infections in New York City hospitals. *Emerg Infect Dis* 1999;**5**:9–17.
19. Shopsin B, Kreiswirth BN. Molecular epeidemiology of methicillin-resistant *Staphylococcus aureus. Emerg Infect. Dis* 2001;**7**:323–326.
20. Smith TL, Pearson ML, Wilcox KR, Cruz C, Lancaster MV, Robinson-Dunn B, Tenover FC, Zervos MJ, Band JD, White E, Jarvis WR. Emergence of vancomycin resistance in *Staphylococcus aureus. N Engl J Med* 1999;**340**:493–501.
21. Hayden MK, Trenholm GM, Schultz JE, Sahm DF. *In vivo* development of teicoplanin resistance in a van B *Enterococcus faecium. J Infect Dis* 1993;**167**:1224–1227.
22. Malani PN, Kauffman CA, Zervos MJ. *Enterococcal Disease, Epidemiology, and Treatment.* ASM Press, Washington, DC, 2002, pp. 385–408.
23. Malani PN, Thal LA, Donabedian SM, Robinson-Dunn B, Kauffmann CA, Chow JW, Zervos MJ. Molecular analysis of vancomycin-resistant *Enterococcus fecalis* from Michigan hospitals during a 10-year period. *J Antimicrob Chemother* 2002;**49**:841–843.
24. Moreno F, Grota P, Crisp C, Magnon K, Melcher GP, Jorgensen JH, Evans Patterson J. Clinical and molecular epidemiology of vancomycin-resistant *Enterococcus faecium* during its emergence in a city in southern Texas, *Clin Infect Dis* 1995;**21**:1234–1237.
25. Thal LA, Donabedian SM, Robinsun-Dunn B, Chow JW, Dumbry LM, Clewell DB, Alishab D, Zervos MJ. Molecular analysis of glycopeptide-resistant *Enterococcus faecium* isolates collected from Michigan hospitals over a 6-year period. *J Clin Microbiol* 1998;**36**:3303–3308.

26. Vergis EN, Hayden MK, Chow JW, Snydmen DR, Zervos MJ, Linden PK, Wagener MM, Schmitt B. Determinants of vancomycin resistance and mortality rates in eneterococcal bacteremia. *Ann Intern Med* 2001;**135**:484–492.
27. Abramson MA, Sexton DJ. Nosocomial methicillin-resistant and methicillin-susceptible *Staphylococcus aureus* primary bacteremia: At what costs? *Infect Control Hosp Epidemiol* 1999;**20**: 408–411.
28. Engemann JJ, Carmeli Y, Cosgrove SE, Fowler VG, Bronstein MZ, Trivette SL, Briggs JP, Sexton DJ, Kaye KS. Adverse clinical and economic outcomes attributable to methicillin resistance among patients with *Staphylococcus aureus* surgical site infection. *Clin Infect Dis* 2003;**36**: 592–598.
29. Hafkin J, Chandler L, Maslow J. *Practical Health care Epidemiology,* 3rd ed. University of Chicao Press, Chicago, 2010.
30. Fey PD, Rupp ME. Molecular epidemiology in the public health and hospital environment. *Clin Lab Med* 2003;**23**(4):885–901.
31. Tenover FC, Arbeit RD, Goering RV. How to select and interpret molecular strain typing methods for epidemiological studies of bacterial infections: A review for health care epidemiologist. *Infect Control Hosp Epidemiol* 1997;**18**(6):426–439.
32. Pfaller MA. Molecular epidemiology in the care of patients. *Arch Pathol Lab Med* 1999; **123**(11):1007–1010.
33. Peterson LR, Noskin GA. New technology for detecting multidrug resistant pathogens in the clinical microbiology laboratory. *Emerg Infect Dis* 2001;**7**:1–12.
34. Tenover FC, Arbeit RD, Goering RV, et al. Interpreting chromosomal DNA restriction patterns produced by pulse-field gel electrophoresis: Criteria for bacterial strain typing. *J Clin Microbiol* 1995;**33**(9):2233–2239.
35. Maslow J, Mulligan ME. Epidemiological typing systems. *Infect Control Hosp Epidemiol* 1996; **17**(9):595–604.
36. Ausubel FM, Brent R, Kingston RE, Moore DD, Seidman JG, Smith JA, Struhl K. (ed.), *Current Protocols in Molecular Biology.* John Wiley & Sons, New York, 1994.
37. Carle GF, Frank M, Olson MV. Electrophoretic separation of large DNA molecules by periodic inversion of electric field. *Science*, 1986;**232**(4746):65–68.
38. Chang N, Chui L. A standardized protocol for the rapid preparation of bacterial DNA for pulse-field gel electrophoresis. *Diagn Microbiol Infect Dis* 1998;**31**:275–279.
39. Sambrook JE, Fritsch F, Maniatis T. *Molecular Cloning; A Laboratory Manual,* 2nd ed. Cold Spring Harbor laboratory Press, Cold Spring Harbor, NY, 1989.
40. Schwartz DC, Saffran W, Welsh J, Haas R, Goldenberg M, Cantor CR. New techniques for purifying large DNA's and studying their properties and packaging. *Cold Spring Harbor Symp Quant Biol* 1983;**47**:189–195.
41. Schwartz DC, Cantor CR. Separation of yeast chromose-sized DNAs by pulse field gradient gel electrophoresi. *Cells* 1984;**37**:67–65.
42. Archer GL, Karchmer AW, Vishniavsky N, Johnston JL. Plasmid-pattern analysis for the differentiation of infecting from non-infecting *Staphylococcus epidermidis*. *J Infect Dis* 1984;**149**:913–920.
43. Eisgruber H, Wiedmann M, Stolle A. Use of plasmid profiling as a typing method for epidemiologically related *Clostridium Perfringes* isolates from food poisoning cases and outbreaks. *Lett Appl Microbiol* 1995;**20**:290–294.
44. Liu PYF, Shi ZY, Lan YJ, Hu BS, Shyr JM, Tsai WS, Lin YH, Tseng CY. Use of restriction endonuclease analysis of polasmids and pulse-field gel electrophoresis to investigate outbreaks of methicillin resistant *Staphylococcus aureus* infection. *Clin Infect Dis* 1996;**22**:86.

45. Schaberg DR, Tompkins LS, Falkow S. Use of agarose gel electrophoresis of plasmid deoxyribonucleic acid to fingerprint Gram-negative bacilli. *J Clin Microbiol* 1981;**13**:1105–1108.
46. Taylor DN, Wachsmuth IK, Shangkuan YH, Schmidt EV. Salmonellosis associated with marijuana: A multistate outbreak traced by plasmid fingerprinting. *N Engl J Med* 1982;**306**: 1249–1253.
47. Tenover FC. Plasmid fingerprinting: A tool for bacterial strain identification and surveillance of nosocomial and community acquired infections. *Clin Lab Med* 1985;**5**:413–436.
48. Donabedian SM, Thal LA, Hershberger E, Perri MB, Chow JW, Bartlett P, Jones R, Johnson J, Zervos MJ. Molecular characterization of gentamicin-resitant enterococci in the United States: Evidence of spread from animals to humans through food. *J Clin Microbiol* 2003;**41**:1109–1113.
49. Feil EJ, Cooper JE, Grundmann H, Robinson DA, Enright MC, Brendt T, Peacock SJ, Smith JM, Murphy M, Spratt BG, Moore CE, Day NP. How clonal is *Staphylococcus aureus*? *J Bacteriol* 2003;**185**:3307–3316.
50. Van Belkum A, Tassios PT, et al. Guidelines for the validation and application of typing methods for the use in bacterial epidemiology. *Clin Microb Infect* 2007;**13**(Suppl 3):1–46.
51. Van Belkum A. DNA fingerprinting of medically important micro-organism by the use of PCR. *Clin Microbiol Rev* 1994;**7**(2):174–184.
52. Mullis KB. The unusual origin of the polymerase chain reaction. *Sci Am* 1990;**262**:56–65.
53. Frenay HM, Bunschoten AE, Schouls LM, Van Leeuwen WJ, Vandenbroucke-Grauls CM, Verhoef J, Mooi FR. Molecular typing of methicillin-resistant *Staphylococcus aureus* on the basis of protein A gene polymorphism. *Eur J Clin Microbiol Infect Dis* 1996;**15**:60–64.
54. Friedman CR, Stoeckle MY, Johnson WD Jr, Riley LW. Double-repetitive-element PCR method for subtyping *Mycobacterium tuberculosis* clinical isolates. *J Clin Microbiol* 1995;**33**:1383–1384.
55. Grimm V, Ezaki S, Susa M, Knabbe C, Schmid RD, Bachmann TT. Use of DNA microarrays for rapid genotyping of TEM beta-lactamases that confer resistance. *J Clin Microbiol* 2004;**42**: 3766–3774.
56. Grundmann H, Schneider C, Hartung D, Daschner FD, Pitt TL. Discriminatory power of three DNA-based typing techniques for *Pseudomonas aeruginosa*. *J Clin Microbiol* 1995;**33**:528–534.
57. Hussain MA, Kauser F, Khan AA, Tiwari S, Habibullah CM, Ahmed N. Implications of molecular genotyping of *Helicobacter pylori* isolates from different human populations by genomic fingerprinting of enterobacterial repetitive intergenic consensus regions for strain identification and geographic evolution. *J Clin Microbiol* 2004;**42**:2372–2378.
58. Kurepina NE, Sreevatsan S, Plikaytis BB, Bifani PJ, Connell ND, Donnelly RJ, van Sooligen D, Musser JM, Kreiswirth BN. Characterization of the phylogenetic distribution and chromosomal insertion sites of five IS6110 elements in *Mycobacterium tuberculosis*: Non-random integration in the dnaA-dnaN region. *Tuber. Lung Dis* 1998;**79**:31–42.
59. Martin IE, Tyler SD, Tyler KD, Khakhria R, Johnson WM. Evaluation of ribotyping as epidemiologic tool for typing *Escherichia coli* serogroup O157 isolates. *J Clin Microbiol* 1996;**34**:720.
60. Nakari UM, Laaksonen K, Korkeila M, Siitonen A. Comparative typing of *Campylobacter jejuni* by heat-stable serotyping and PCR-based restriction fragment length polymorphism analysis. *J Clin Microbiol* 2005;**43**:1166–1170.
61. Nazarowec-White M, Farber JM. Phenotypic and genotypic typing of food and clinical isolates of *Enterobacter sakazakii*. *J Med Microbiol* 1999;**48**:559–567.
62. Stull T, LiPuma JJ, Edlind TD. A broad spectrum probe for molecular epidemiology of bacteria: Ribosomal RNA. *J Infect Dis* 1988;**157**:280–286.
63. Focucault C, LaScola B, Lindross H, Anderson SGE, Raoult D. Multispacer typing technique for sequence-based typing of *Bartonella quintana*. *J Clin Microbiol* 2005;**43**:41–48.

64. Francois P, Renzi G, Pittet D, Bento M, Lewis D, Harbarth S, Vaudaux P, Schrenzel J. A novel multiplex real-time PCR assay for rapid typing of major *Staphylococcus* cassette chromosome mec elements. *J Clin Microbiol* 2004;**42**:3309–3312.

65. Samore MH, Kristjansson M, Venkataraman L, DeGirolami PC, Arbeit RD. Comparison of arbitrarily primed polymerase chain reaction, restriction enzyme analysis and pulsed-field gel electrophoresis for typing *Clostridium difficile*. *J Microbiol Methods* 1996;**25**:215.

66. Louie M, Jayaratne P, Luchsinger I, Devenish J, Yao J, Schlech W, Simor A. Comparison of ribotyping, arbitrarily primed PCR, and pulsed-field gel electrophoresis for molecular typing of *Listeria monocytogenes*. *J Clin Microbiol.* 1996;**34**:15.

67. Killgore GE, Kato H. Use of arbitrary primed PCR to type *Clostridium difficile* and comparison of results with those by immunoblot typing. *J Clin Microbiol* 1994;**32**:1591–1593.

68. Bailey JS, Fedorka-Cray PJ, Stern NJ, Craven SE, Cox NA, Cosby DE. Serotyping and ribotyping of *Salmonella* using restriction enzyme. *J Food Prot* 2002;**65**:1005–1007.

69. Diep BA, Perdreau-Remington F, Sensabaugh GF. Clonal characterization of *Staphylococus aureus* by multilocus restriction fragment typing, a rapid screening approach for molecular epidemiology. *J Clin Microbiol* 2003;**41**:4559–4564.

70. Dunman PM, Mounts W, McAlesse F, Immermann F, Macapagal D, Marsilio E, McDougal L, Tenover FC, Bradford PA, Peterson PJ, Projan SJ, Murphy E. Uses of *Staphylococcus aureus* genechips in genotyping and genetic composition analysis. *J Clin Microbiol* 2004;**42**:4275–4283.

71. Enright MC, Day NPJ, Davies CE, Peacock SJ, Spratt BG. Multilocus sequence typing for characterization of methicillin-resistant and methicillin-susceptible clones of *Staphylococcus aureus*. *J Clin Microbiol* 2000;**38**:1008–1015.

72. Grundmann H, Hori S, Enright MC, Webster C, Tami A, Feil EJ, Pitt T. Determining the genetic structure of the natural population of *Staphylococcus aureus*: A comparison of multilocus sequence typing with pulsed-field gel electrophoresis, randomly amplified polymorphic DNA analysis, and phage typing. *J Clin Microbiol* 2002;**40**:4544–4546.

73. Peacock SJ, de Silva GD, Justice A, Cowland A, Moore CE, Winearls CG, Day NP. Comparison of multilocus sequence typing and pulsed-field gel electrophoresis as tools for typing *Staphylococcus aureus* isolates in microepidemiological setting. *J Clin Microbiol* 2002;**40**:3764–3770.

74. Stampone L, Del Grosso M, Boccia D, Pantosti A. Clonal spread of a vancomycin-resistant *Enterococcus faecium* strain among bloodstream-infecting isolates in Italy. *J Clin Microbiol* 2005;**43**:1575–1580.

75. Tomayko JF, Murray BF. Analysis of *Enterococcus faecalis* isolates from intercontinental sources by multilocus enzyme electrophoresis and pulsed-field gel electrophoresis. *J Clin Microbiol* 1995;**33**:2903.

CHAPTER SIX

Pathogen Elimination: Antibiotic and Disinfectant Use and the Development of Resistance

STEVEN L. FOLEY, BEILEI GE, CARL M. SCHROEDER, AND AARON M. LYNNE

Introduction

Because of the central role of antimicrobial agents and disinfectants in the prevention and control of nosocomial infections, it is important to understand how these agents work. Meanwhile, resistance has developed as a result of use and/or misuse, leading to difficulties in disease management in the healthcare setting. Therefore, a thorough understanding of the resistance mechanisms is necessary. In this chapter, antimicrobial agents are grouped into five categories based on their primary mechanisms of action, which are (i) inhibiting cell wall synthesis (the β-lactams, glycopeptides, and bacitracin); (ii) inhibiting protein synthesis (aminoglycosides, tetracyclines, and macrolides); (iii) inhibiting nucleic acid synthesis (quinolones and rifampicin); (iv) disrupting cell membrane functions (polymyxins); and (v) inhibiting metabolic pathways (sulfonamides and trimethoprim) . The final section of the

Molecular Techniques for the Study of Hospital-Acquired Infection, First Edition. Edited by Steven L. Foley, Anne Y. Chen, Shabbir Simjee, and Marcus J. Zervos.

chapter covers disinfectants. This chapter aims to provide an overview of (i) the basic characteristics of antimicrobial agents and disinfectants that are important for eliminating nosocomial pathogens and (ii) the mechanisms that pathogens adapt and acquire to evade such elimination.

Cell Wall Synthesis Inhibiting Drugs

With few exceptions, a unique and essential element of bacterial structure is the peptidoglycan-containing cell wall, the biosynthesis of which is sophisticated and involves three main stages: (i) synthesis of monomer units composed of disaccharyl pentapeptide in the cytoplasm; (ii) transport of these monomer units coupled with a lipid carrier across the cytoplasmic membrane; and (iii) insertion of nascent peptidoglycans to the preexisting cell wall and cross-linking between individual unit polymers by transpeptidation and transglycosylation, accompanied by the release of the lipid carrier and its recycling to the internal face of the membrane (1, 2). Because the enzymes involved in peptidoglycan synthesis are essential to bacterial cell survival and growth, they have been important clinical targets since the first antibiotic, penicillin, was used in World War II.

BETA-LACTAMS

Beta-lactams comprise a group of natural or semisynthetic small organic molecules with an unusual, highly reactive four-membered lactam ring. This group includes penicillins, cephalosporins, carbapenems, monobactams, and β-lactamase inhibitors. Beta-lactams act on the final stage of peptidoglycan synthesis by forming covalent complexes with enzymes, termed penicillin-binding proteins (PBPs), responsible for cross-linkage of the glycan chains of peptidoglycan (3). The high-molecular-weight PBPs (essential PBPs) tend to be bifunctional transglycosylases/transpeptidases, whereas low-molecular-weight PBPs are usually carboxypeptidases or hydrolases (4). Due to preferential blockage of a subset of PBPs (2), different β-lactams can induce characteristic changes in bacterial cell morphology, such as elongation, chain-like formation, and enlarged or rounded appearance.

Penicillins Penicillins are naturally produced by fungi as secondary metabolites (4). They contain the chemical nucleus 6-aminopenicillanic acid, consisting of a β-lactam ring fused to a five-member sulfur-containing ring (5). Modification of penicillin side chains has been used to generate a range of semisynthetic penicillins with broader spectra of antibacterial activities and improved β-lactamase resistance (Table 6.1) (6). The bactericidal effect of penicillins results from their binding to bacterial PBPs and subsequent interference with the cross-linking reaction of the peptidoglycan synthesis. Currently, there are six groups of penicillins distinguishable by their spectra of activity, route of administration, and susceptibility to β-lactamases (7). Some of the more commonly administered penicillin derivatives include methicillin and oxacillin, which are useful in treating susceptible Gram-positive organisms and ampicillin and amoxicillin, which have a wider activity against Gram-negative organisms (7).

Cephalosporins Cephalosporins are the most widely prescribed and largest-selling class of the β-lactams (4). *Acremonium chrysogenum* produces the cephalosporin

TABLE 6.1 Different categories or generations of common penicillins and cephalosporins

Category	Examples
Penicillins	
Natural	Benzylpenicillin (penicillin G)
	Phenoxymethyl penicillin (penicillin V)
Penicillinase-resistant	Methicillin
Isoxazolyl penicillins	Oxacillin
Broad spectrum	
Aminopenicillins	Ampicillin
	Amoxicillin
Carboxypenicillins	Carbenicillin
	Ticarcillin
Ureidopenicillins	Mezlocillin
	Piperacillin
Penicillin/β-lactamse inhibitor combinations	Ampicillin-sulbactam
	Amoxicillin-clavulanate
Cephalosporins	
Narrow spectrum (first generation)	Cephalothin
	Cefazolin
Expanded spectrum (second generation)	
Cephamycins	Cefoxitin
	Cefuroxime
Extended spectrum (third generation)	Cefoperazone
	Cefotaxime
	Ceftazidime
	Ceftriaxone
New extended spectrum (fourth generation)	Cefepime
	Cefpirome

Source: Adapted from Yao and Moellering (5).

7-aminocephalosporanic acid nucleus, which consists of a β-lactam ring fused to a sulfur-containing six-membered ring (4). Side-chain modifications of cephalosporins have led to multiple drug generations with differential penetrations through cell envelope porins and varied antibacterial and pharmacokinetic properties (Table 6.1) (6). Similar to the penicillins, cephalosporins act by binding to bacterial PBPs and interfering with bacterial peptidoglycan synthesis. Cephalosporins are often grouped into generations (first through fourth), based primarily on their spectrum of activity. The first-generation cephalosporins are primarily active against Gram-positive organisms, with the later generations having increasing activity against Gram-negative organisms. In general, the fourth-generation cephalosporins have the widest spectrum of activity.

Carbapenems The naturally occurring carbapenems are produced by *Streptomyces* spp., with their semisynthetic derivatives imipenem, meropenem, and ertapenem available for clinical use (5). Carbapenems preferentially bind to bacterial PBP1 and PBP2, causing cell elongation and lysis (5). They are stable toward most plasmid- or chromosome-mediated β-lactamases, which aids in their utility for treating a number of penicillin- and cephalosporin-resistant pathogens. Each of the carbapenems has a wide spectrum of activities; however, imipenem is slightly more effective for Gram-positive organisms, while meropenem and ertapenem are more effective for the Gram-negative aerobes (8).

Monobactams Aztreonam is the only monobactam in human clinical use (4). It appears to target the bacterial PBP3 at low concentrations and has low susceptibility to β-lactamases produced by Gram-negative target pathogens (4). Aztreonam has a limited spectrum of activity and is used primarily for the treatment of Gram-negative aerobes.

Beta-Lactamase Inhibitors These compounds include clavulanic acid and sulbactam; they act primarily as, "suicide substrates" by forming an irreversible acyl enzyme complex with the β-lactamase, thereby causing loss of enzyme activity (5). Clavulanic acid is a naturally occurring weak antimicrobial agent initially found in cultures of *Streptomyces clavuligerus* (9). It inhibits β-lactamases from staphylococci and many Gram-negative bacteria. Clinically, clavulanic acid is available for use in combination with oral amoxicillin or ticarcillin. Sulbactam is a semisynthetic derivative with weak antibacterial activity. It also functions as an effective inhibitor of certain plasmid- and chromosome-mediated β-lactamases.

Beta-Lactam Resistance Resistance to β-lactams is generally mediated through one or more of the following mechanisms: (1) drug inactivation by β-lactamase(s) produced by bacterial cells; (2) inability of the drug to reach drug targets, either by reduced permeability of outer membrane or by activated efflux pumps; (3) modification of drug targets, the PBPs . Employment of particular type(s) of mechanism for the resistance to a given β-lactam agent may vary greatly in different bacterial species.

Beta-lactams in clinical isolates, β-lactamases, are a heterogeneous group of enzymes capable of hydrolyzing various β-lactam substrates. Several classification schemes have been proposed over the last two decades according to their hydrolytic spectrum, susceptibility to inhibitors, genetic encoding mechanisms, and amino acid sequences, with two of these schemes—the Ambler (10) and Bush–Jacoby–Medeiros (11)—gaining major influence. These schemes classify the β-lactamases based on their amino acid sequences (Ambler) or substrate and inhibitor profiles (Bush–Jacoby–Medeiros). A number of penicillinases, including members of the TEM and SHV β-lactamases, are able to confer resistance to a range of the penicillins and cephalosporins and thus are termed extended spectrum β-lactamases (ESBLs). Other ESBL types include the CTX-M, OXA, PER, and SFO β-lactamases (12–14). ESBLs have become a problem in a number of Gram-negative pathogens, including *Klebsiella pneumoniae* and *Escherichia coli.* Resistance to third-generation cephalosporins may also be mediated by non-ESBL β-lactamases, such as AmpC-type enzymes (15). Other enzymes such as the metallo-ß-lactamases also target the carbapenems. These enzymes are found in selected species of including *Enterobacter cloacae*, *Serratia marcescens*, *Pseudomonas aeruginosa*, *Stenotrophomonas maltophilia*, and *Acinetobacter baumannii* (16).

Resistance to β-lactams is also mediated through broadly specific drug efflux systems, low outer-membrane permeability, or a combination of both. Observation in *P. aeruginosa* suggested that multiple β-lactam drug resistance occurred through reduced permeability of outer membrane in the absence of activated efflux pumps (17). The role that outer-membrane permeation plays varies in individual bacterial species. For example, wild-type *P. aeruginosa* allows outer membrane permeation of beta-lactam agents at rates of 1–8% of those measured for *E. coli* (18). Activated efflux pump(s), such as the AcrAB–TolC pump, interplay with lower membrane permeation and enhance the effect of preventing drug to reach targets (19). Additionally, modification of PBPs can lead to reduced binding affinity for β-lactams, leading to increased levels of resistance. This resistance mechanism is best exemplified in *Staphylococcus aureus* and *Streptococcus pneumoniae* (20). Though both are Gram-positive cocci, resistance to penicillins in *S. aureus* and *S. penumoniae* is achieved through different mechanisms. Methicillin-resistant *S. aureus* (MRSA) was once largely confined to hospitals and long-term care facilities but is now a significant problem in the community setting (21). MRSA strains harbor *mecA*, which is carried by a unique mobile genetic element, staphylococcal cassette chromosome *mec* (SCC*mec*), which is integrated into the *S. aureus* chromosome (22). The *mecA* gene encodes a methicillin-insensitive transpeptidase, which presumably takes over the physiological function of resident PBPs inhibited by methicillin. Unlike *S. aureus*, *S. pneumoniae* has not been found to produce penicillinase. It appears that most penicillin-resistant isolates of *S. pneumoniae* rely primarily on modifications of resident PBPs, which leads to a significant reduction in the binding affinity of penicillin for these PBPs (23).

GLYCOPEPTIDES

Glycopeptides are large, rigid, heterocyclic molecules consisting of a heptapeptide backbone with various attached sugars (3). Glycopeptides inhibit the late stage of peptidoglycan synthesis by complexing with the D-alanyl-D-alanine (D-Ala-D-Ala) cell wall precursor blocking the required transpeptidation reactions (24). Vancomycin and teicoplanin are the two glycopeptides available for use in clinical medicine. Vancomycin, produced by *Streptomyces orientales*, was introduced into clinical practice 50 years ago. Teicoplanin, produced by *Actinoplanes teichomyceticus*, was launched in Europe in the mid-1980s. Because vancomycin and teicoplanin do not penetrate the pores of Gram-negative outer membranes, they are restricted to treating infections caused by Gram-positive pathogens (4). Because glycopeptides and β-lactams work on two different aspects of peptidoglycan cross-linking, one on cell wall structures and the other on anabolic enzymes, synergistic antibacterial effects are observed when used in combination (4). Vancomycin is a recommended agent for use in the treatment of MRSA (25).

In the Gram-positive bacteria, vancomycin resistance is typically associated with the acquisition of either the *vanA* or *vanB* gene clusters. The gene clusters encode an altered peptidoglycan precursor that contains D-Ala-D-lactate ends instead of the normal ending of D-Ala-D-Ala dipeptide (26). The glycopeptide antibiotics have a 1000-fold lower affinity for the altered precursors compared to the normal peptidoglycan (27). The result is prevention of the glycopeptides from effectively shutting down peptidoglycan synthesis.

BACITRACIN

Bacitracin, widely used in topical applications, consists of a mixture of closely related high-molecular-weight polypeptides produced by *Bacillus licheniformis*, the main component of which (bacitracin A) is a cyclic polypeptide with a peptide side chain (28). Bacitracin inhibits peptidoglycan synthesis by preventing the recycling of the lipid carrier molecule, isoprenyl phosphate (IP), which is needed to effectively carry out peptidoglycan synthesis. Bacitracin also disrupts the bacterial cytoplasmic membrane (5).

Bacitracin resistance has been associated with the products of rhamnose-glucose polysaccharide (RGP) and *mbr* gene clusters. The Mbr proteins appear to have similarity to portions of an ATP-binding cassette (ABC) transporter. This similarity would indicate that the function of the Mbr proteins could be transport of bacitracin inactivation molecules or efflux of the drug itself. The genes that encode RPG synthesis also facilitate the transport of RPG to the cell surface for export. These expressed transport proteins are the IP molecules that are inactivated by bacitracin. The excess IP molecules expressed for polysaccharide export can also be used to transport precursors for peptidoglycan synthesis, thus limiting the effect of bacitracin (29).

Protein Synthesis Inhibiting Drugs

Ribosomes involved in prokaryotic protein synthesis are different from those involved in eukaryotic protein synthesis; thus prokaryote protein-synthesis-inhibiting drugs are an attractive option for combating bacterial infections. Before discussing the classes of protein-synthesis-inhibiting drugs, it is beneficial to briefly review the synthesis process. Bacterial ribosomes, or 70S ribosomes, are composed of two major subunits, the 30S and 50S subunits, each of which is comprised of ribosomal RNA (rRNA) and multiple ribosomal proteins (r-proteins). The 30S subunit is composed of a 16S rRNA molecule and 21 r-proteins, while the 50S subunit is composed of a 5S rRNA and 23S rRNA molecule and 34 r-proteins. The 50S subunit is the target of chloramphenicol, lincosamides, macrolides, and streptogramins; the 30S subunit is the target of the aminoglycosides and tetracyclines (30, 31).

Figure 6.1 briefly illustrates the prokaryotic protein synthesis, which consists of (i) synthesis initiation, (ii) polypeptide elongation, and (iii) synthesis termination. The functional 70S ribosome has three major sites used for binding tRNA molecules in protein synthesis: the acceptor or aminoacyl site (A site), the donor or peptidyl site (P site), and the exit site (E site). Following protein synthesis initiation, amino-acid-carrying tRNAs (aminoacyl tRNA; aa-tRNA) enter the ribosome at the A site. A peptidyl transferase enzyme then moves the elongating polypeptide attached to the tRNA in the P site to the N-terminus of the amino acid on the tRNA in the A site and translocation occurs. Next, the polypeptide-containing tRNA (peptidyl-tRNA) in the A site is translocated to the P site as the empty tRNA from the P site is moved into the E site and is then discharged and recycled. The free A site is now able to receive the next aa-tRNA. The cycle is repeated until each of the codons in the mRNA gene sequence is read and a termination codon is encountered, thereby halting protein synthesis (30, 31). The multifaceted protein assembly apparatus and assembly processes provide multiple targets for different antimicrobial agents to act (30).

AMINOGLYCOSIDES

Aminoglycosides bind to the 30S ribosomal subunit and inhibit protein synthesis by bringing about misreading of mRNA. Aminogylcosides are produced by members of the genus *Streptomyces* and include streptomycin, neomycin, apramycin, spectinomycin,

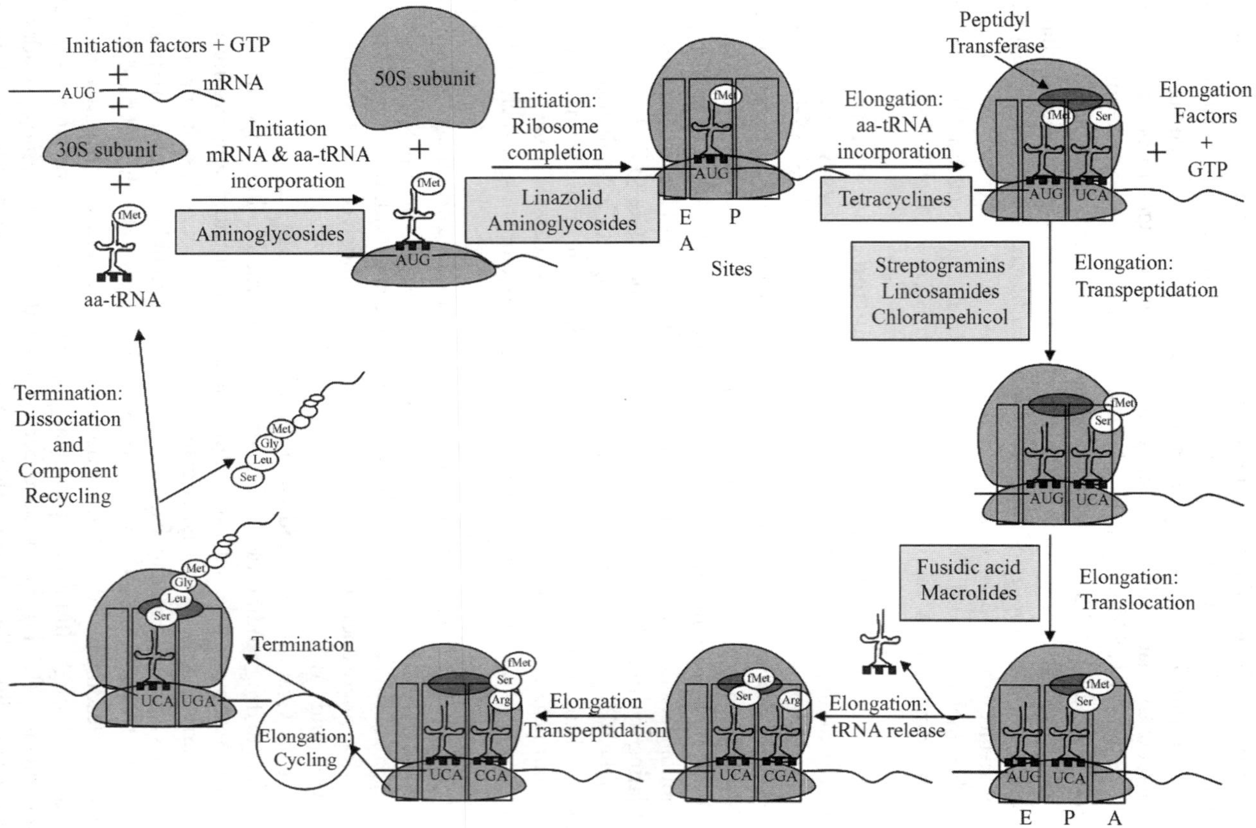

FIGURE 6.1 Schematic diagram for the prokaryotic protein synthesis.

kanamycin, amikacin, gentamicin, and tobramycin (32). The different structures of the individual aminoglycosides likely lead to their variability in spectra of activity. Aminoglycosides tend to be bactericidal. Streptomycin has a broad spectrum of activity against Gram-positive, Gram-negative, and mycobacterial organisms. Gentamicin has a narrower spectrum of activity with primary efficacy against Gram-negatives. An unfavorable characteristic of many aminoglycosides is that they may cause damage to the eighth cranial (vestibulocochlear) nerve and thus lead to hearing loss and kidney impairment or damage (33).

The bactericidal characteristics of aminoglycosides are thought to be attributable to their ability to bind to16S rRNA of the ribosome, which in turn leads to misreading of the mRNA. The binding of the aminoglycosides appears to be sequence-dependent, because variations in 16S rRNA lead to aminoglycoside resistance. A conformational change in the A-site of the ribosome appears to occur following binding of the aminoglycoside to the rRNA. This reduces the amount of energy required for the binding of both correct and incorrect tRNA molecules to the corresponding mRNA codons and thus, because of the lower energy binding of incorrect tRNA molecules, there is a much higher error rate leading to the production of nonfunctional proteins (34).

Resistance to aminoglycoside antibiotics can occur through a number of different mechanisms, including inactivation of the drugs by modifying enzymes, drug efflux, alteration of the ribosome (preventing drug binding), and lowered aminoglycoside entry into the cells. The production of modifying enzymes by many strains of bacteria is able to inactivate the aminoglycosides. The modifying enzymes generally fall into three classes: the aminoglycoside phosphotransferases (APH), the aminoglycoside acetyltransferases (AAC), and the aminoglycoside nucleotidyltransferases (ANT). The APH enzymes function by phosphorylating hydroxyl groups on the aminoglycoside molecules (35).

Many of the APH enzymes confer resistance to multiple agents, including streptomycin, neomycin, and kanamysin. APH enzymes have been found in many human pathogens, including Gram-negative organisms such as *Salmonella* species, *Klebsiella pneumoniae*, *Vibrio cholerae*, and *Campylobacter* species, as well as Gram-positive organisms such as *Staphylococcus aureus* and *Enterococcus* species. The AAC enzymes are associated with resistance to agents such as kanamycin, gentamicin, tobramycin, neomycin, and others and are found within a number of Gram-negative organisms as well as some Gram-positive pathogens. There are five major types of ANT enzymes that are associated with resistance to multiple aminoglycosides. There does not appear to be as great an aminoglycoside cross resistance as with the AAC and APH enzymes; however, the ANTs have been found distributed throughout many Gram-negative and Gram-positive organisms (32).

In addition to drug modification, modification of the drug-binding target has also been associated with resistance to certain aminoglycosides. Certain pathogenic organisms have been found to carry 16S rRNA methylase genes. The methylase enzymes can methylate 16S rRNA, which has been associated with a reduction in susceptibility to the drug streptomycin. Mutations in the 16S rRNA or associated proteins could also affect binding of the drug to the ribosomal target, leading to reduced susceptibility (36). A third mechanism of aminoglycoside resistance is through efflux of the particular drug agent. Efflux pumps in the resistance-nodulation division (RND) family have been shown to remove aminoglycosides (and macrolides, tetracyclines, lincomycin, chloramphenicol, and others) from the cytoplasm of microorganisms. An example of one of the RND multidrug resistance (MDR) pumps is the MexXY in *P. aeruginosa*. In addition to the RND pumps, it appears that an efflux pump (EmrE) in the small multidrug resistance family can also play a role in reduced susceptibility to aminoglycosides (35).

MACROLIDES

The macrolides are produced by members of the genus *Streptomyces*. Erythromycin, the first macrolide, was discovered in 1952. Many macrolides are semisynthetic molecules derived from eythromycin A, including clarithromycin, azithromycin, and telithromycin. Macrolides are important for treatment of infections caused by respiratory pathogens, such as those from *Streptococcus pyogenes, S. pneumoniae, Mycoplasma pneumoniae, Legionella pneumoniae, Chlamydia pneumoniae, Moraxella catarrhalis,* and *Haemophilis influenzae.* They are also used for treating infections caused by Gram-positives, including staphylococci (37). Macrolides function through an interaction with a region near the peptidyl transferase portion of the 23S rRNA, which effectively inhibits the addition of further amino acids leading to premature termination of translation and early discharge of peptidyl-tRNA intermediates (4, 34). The binding of macrolides also prevents the assembly of functional 50S ribosomal subunits (38).

Resistance to the macrolides has been associated with the modification of the ribosomal target, modification of the drugs, and with the presence of MDR efflux pumps. The chromosomal-mediated modification of the ribosome within the 23S rRNA gene prevents the macrolides from binding to the ribosomal target (39). Ribosomal target modification has been seen as a cause of macrolide resistance in a wide variety of bacteria, including Gram-negative and Gram-positive pathogens (40).

Target modification can also occur through methylation of the macrolide-binding region of the ribosome. The methylation enzymes are encoded by the erythomycin ribosome methylase (*erm*) genes and confer resistance to macrolides as well as streptogramin B and lincosamides. Erm methylates one of the same target nucleic acids that codes for the drug-binding site that is associated with the chromosomal-mediated modification resistance discussed above. Methylation of the binding site prevents the drug from efficiently binding to the ribosome and eliciting their antimicrobial activity (40).

Multidrug efflux pumps in some cells may also reduce the susceptibility of microorganisms to macrolide drugs (41). The major pumps that actively remove the macrolides are members of the RND pumps in Gram-negative organisms and the major facilitator (MFS) superfamilies for Gram-positive bacteria. An additional means of macrolide resistance is through modification of the macrolide drugs themselves. Modifying enzymes, including phosphotransferases and esterases, have been discovered that alter some of the different types of macrolides. Most of the organisms that appear to produce these modifying enzymes are Gram-negative enteric organisms; thus drug modification tends to be a lesser cause of clinically relevant macrolide resistance, given that Gram-negative organisms are typically not the target of macrolide therapy (40).

TETRACYCLINES

The tetracyclines were initially isolated from members of the genus *Streptomyces* and now contain a number of semi-synthetic derivatives. The first tetracyclines, oxytetracycline and chlortetracycline, were discovered in the late 1940s. The tetracyclines exhibit a wide spectrum of activity, effective against Gram-positive and Gram-negative bacteria and intracellular pathogens such as rickettsial and chlamydial species. Tetracyclines act by binding to the 30S rRNA subunit near the A site. This prevents the interaction of the aa-tRNA molecule with the ribosome and the addition of amino acid monomers to the elongating polypeptide. There also appear to be secondary binding sites where tetracyclines interact with the bacterial ribosome yet do not interfere with aminoacyl-tRNA binding directly. Binding of these secondary sites likely interferes with a conformational change of the ribosome required for mRNA translation (42).

Resistance to tetracyclines appears to be due to the acquisition of one of the *tet* or *otr* genes, which encode either ribosomal protection proteins that facilitate the removal of the drug from the ribosomal subunit or efflux pumps (43). Resistance can also be associated with the enzymatic degradation of the antimicrobial agents. Many of the *tet* genes can be carried on resistance plasmids and may have the ability to be transferred from one bacterial strain to another, thus spreading resistance (44). Efflux pumps that remove tetracyclines from the bacterial cells are members of the MFS transporter superfamily. The *tet* genes code for the membrane portion of the efflux pumps and have been found in both Gram-positive and Gram-negative organisms. In addition to the membrane protein, the tetracyline efflux mechanism in Gram-negative organisms has a second gene (*tetR*) associated that encodes a repressor molecule. In the absence of tetracycline, the repressor prevents transcription of the efflux pump; however, when tetracyclines are present, the efflux pump expression is induced (45).

Other *tet* genes encode ribosomal protection proteins, which protect the ribosomal target from the antibacterial actions of the tetracyclines. Resistance associated with ribosomal protection proteins appears to confer greater cross-resistance than that of the efflux pumps. The protection proteins share homology with some of the elongation factors that are required for translation to form the functional polypeptide chain. The presence of protection proteins, along with GTP, likely causes the release of tetracycline from the ribosome, allowing the transfer-RNA to deliver amino acid molecules to the acceptor site of the ribosome allowing protein synthesis to progress (45). An additional resistance mechanism that has been associated with tetracycline resistance is enzymatic inactivation of the drug; however, its distribution appears to be limited in many microbial populations (45).

CHLORAMPHENICOL

Chloramphenicol is also derived from members of the genus *Streptomyces*. It is a broad-spectrum drug that has activity against a number of Gram-positives and Gram-negatives, as well as against the mycoplasmas and intracellular bacteria. Clinical use of the drug has been curtailed due to its toxicity; some patients receiving the drug have developed severe hematological complications, including fatal aplastic anemia. While attempts have been made to structurally modify the drug to reduce toxicity, the same modifications have reduced drug efficacy. Chloramphenicol is able to bind to 23S rRNA and block the peptidyl transferase activity needed to transfer the polypeptide from the tRNA molecule in the P site to the aa-tRNA in the A-site during protein synthesis. Chloramphenicol also appears to act by inhibiting the movement of substrates through the ribosome, which leads to disruption of translation termination (46).

Resistance to chloramphenicol has been attributed to both drug efflux and chemical modification of the agent. Many of the resistance determinants associated with chloramphenicol resistance have been found to be located on transferable elements such as integrons and plasmids (47). Chloramphenicol resistance has been associated with different efflux pumps encoded by the *cml* and *flo* genes. In addition to efflux pumps, chloramphenicol resistance has been associated with chemical modification of the drug structure. Likely the most widespread and important modification is the acetylation of the drug by chloramphenicol acetyltransferases, which are coded by the *cat* genes. These enzymes have been detected in a large number of both Gram-negative and Gram-positive organisms, including *E. coli*, *H. influenzae*, *P. aeruginosa*, and *S. aureus* (48).

LINCOSAMIDES

Lincosamides, including lincomycin and clindamycin, are bacteriostatic with activity against many Gram-positives and anaerobes, but have poor activity against Gram-negative aerobes (49). The target for lincosamide binding is on the 23S rRNA molecule and is the same as or located very near the position where the macrolides bind. The lincosamides bind to the 23S rRNA peptidyl transferase site, thus interfering with the positioning of the aa-tRNA molecules and hindering activity of peptidyl transferase enzyme to form new peptide bonds (49). As with macrolides, the products of the Erm methylation block the drug-binding site for the lincosamides on 23rRNA, which leads to reduced antimicrobial activity. Additionally, resistance to lincosamides has been associated with drug modification by lincosamide nucleotidyltransferases that are encoded by *lnuA* and *lnuB*. The acquisition of these nucleotidyltransferase genes has been associated with the development of resistance to lincomycin and with slightly decreased susceptibility in clindamycin. The lincosamide nucleotidyltransferases are typically associated with Gram-positive organisms such as *S. aureus* and *E. faecium* (40). A third mechanism of resistance in the lincosamides is through the acquisition of MDR efflux pumps. Efflux pumps encoded by *lsa* and *lmrP* genes have been associated with resistance to lincosamides, macrolides, and group B streptogramins (50).

STREPTOGRAMINS

The streptogramins are a large group of drugs with complex structures. Based on structure, they are classified into two groups (groups A and B). Combination therapy with a representative of each group produces a strongly synergistic effect. The major representative streptogramins used in human medicine are the combination of quinupristin and dalfopristin (Synercid®) (1). The streptogramins are effective against many Gram-positives, but have limited efficacy against most Gram-negative organisms (51). Like the macrolides and lincosamides, streptogramins bind to 23S rRNA near the peptidyl transferase site and interfere with the protein synthesis (4). The synergistic quinupristin/dalfopristin combination improves antimicrobial action through the binding of dalfopristin to the 50S ribosomal subunit, which causes a conformational change in the ribosome. The conformational change allows quinupristin to bind with greater efficiency to an adjacent site on the ribosome (4). The bound quinupristin/dalfopristin combination inhibits protein synthesis in multiple ways, including inhibition of peptidyl transferase and through the prevention of the release of newly synthesis polypeptide chains (52).

Resistance to the streptogramin antibiotics is most commonly associated with the modification of the ribosomal drug target and with the presence of efflux pumps. As mentioned in previous sections, there is potential for cross-resistance between the macrolides, lincosamides, and the streptogramin antibiotics due to Erm methylase. Multidrug efflux pumps also play a role in streptogramin resistance in some cells (41). The major family of efflux pumps that actively remove type B streptogramins is the ABC transporters (40). ABC transporters also can play a role in the resistance to type A streptogramins. The VgaA and VgaB proteins are components of a pump that is specifically able to export type A streptogramins, which contrasts the Lsa efflux pump that is associated with multidrug resistance (53).

LINEZOLID

The synthetic drug linezolid is a member of the oxazolidinone class of antimicrobial agents. These drugs are structurally unique antimicrobial agents that appear to block the initiation of protein synthesis by binding to the 23S rRNA near the peptidyl transferase site (54). Linezolid is thought to block the initiation of protein synthesis by occupying the P site and disrupting the initial peptide bond formation (4), which prevents the 30S (with fMet tRNA) and 50S subunits from joining to form the functional 70S ribosome (30). Linezolid is used in the treatment of certain infections caused by Gram-positive organisms, including *S. aureus*, *Streptococcus* spp., and vancomycin resistant *E. faecium* (55).

Nucleic Acid Synthesis-Inhibiting Drugs

Other classes of antibiotics function by disrupting different steps in the biosynthesis of DNA and RNA in bacterial pathogens. As with protein synthesis-inhibiting drugs, these groups of antibiotics preferentially target enzymes that are unique in bacterial cells. These targets include the enzymes that relieve supercoiling stress that is generated during the replication of the circular bacterial chromosome and by targeting bacterial RNA polymerase, preventing initiation of transcription.

QUINOLONES/FLUOROQUINOLONES

One of the original quinolones, nalidixic acid, has been commonly used in the laboratory to inhibit bacterial DNA replication, though its clinical use is limited. However, fluorinated quinolones (fluoroquinolones) have proven highly effective for treating bacterial infections, due mainly to their exceptional antibacterial profiles and good pharmacological properties (56). Quinolones work by binding to the type II topoisomerases and trapping DNA during the replication and transcription process and are thus bactericidal. There are two kinds of type II topoisomerases, DNA gyrase and DNA topoisomerase IV, which are involved in DNA unwinding during replication. While DNA gyrase is found in virtually all bacteria, topoisomerase IV is identified only in certain bacteria, including *E. coli*, *Salmonella* spp., *Neisseria gonorrhoeae*, *Staphylococcus aureus*, and *Streptococcus pneumoniae*. Both gyrase and topoisomerase IV are tetrameric structures composed of Gyr(A_2B_2) and Par(C_2E_2) proteins, respectively. A frequent target for quinolone antibiotics is the A subunit of DNA gyrase (57). Because eukaryotic cells do not contain DNA gyrase, the quinolones are specific for prokaryotic cells (56). Early-generation quinolones display relatively poor activity against streptococci and anaerobes; however, recent observations indicate that newer fluoroquinolones, such as ciprofloxacin, moxifloxacin, and gatifloxacin, have enhanced activity against anaerobes (58). Because of their ability to effectively penetrate and accumulate in macrophages and polymorphonucleocytes, the quinolones are useful for targeting infection caused by bacteria capable of surviving in phagocytes (59).

Resistance to quinolones may occur via (i) mutations in DNA toposiomerase genes, (ii) decreased permeability of the bacterial cell wall, or (iii) energy-dependent efflux pumps. DNA mutations conferring quinolone resistance were initially observed for the DNA-gyrase-encoding *gyrA* and *gyrB* genes (60–62). Mutations in these genes reduce the affinity of fluoroquinolone binding to the DNA gyrase. Quinolone resistance mutations have subsequently been discovered in the toposiomerase IV *parC* and *parE* genes (42, 57, 63, 64).

High-level fluoroquinolone resistance has been mapped to mutations in *gyrA* and *parC* primarily. Within these genes is a segment of DNA termed the quinolone resistance-determining region (QRDR). Quinolone resistance mutations in the QRDR of *E. coli* have been shown to occur most often at positions 83(Ser) and 87(Asp) of *gyrA* and at 79(Ser) and 83(Asp) of *parC* (38, 45). Additionally, in some bacterial isolates, the ability of quinolones to enter the bacterial cell is impaired, leading to low-level fluoroquinolone resistance (6, 9, 38). Energy-dependent efflux pumps may also confer fluoroquinolone resistance in Gram-negative and Gram-positive bacteria (65, 66). The AcrA pump appears to be overexpressed in many high-level fluoroquinolone-resistant clinical *E. coli* isolates, but not in fluoroquinolone-susceptible isolates (67). Plasmid-mediated quinolone resistance is mediated by the *qnr* genes (68). The presence of Qnr may reduce the amount of DNA gyrase targets susceptible to quinolone inhibition (69). However, because strains with *qnr* typically display low-level fluoroquinolone resistance, they are difficult to detect using phenotypic assays.

RIFAMPACIN

Rifampacin (rifampin) is a potent and broad-spectrum antibiotic that, along with isoniazid, make up part of the standard six-month-long treatment regimen for infection with *Mycobacterium tuberculosis* (tuberculosis). The rifamycins, of which rifampicin is a semi-synthetic derivative, are structurally complex antibiotics produced by *Streptomyces mediteraranei* (70). They are less effective against Gram-positives than Gram-negatives, presumably due to decreased penetration across the cell membrane (71). Rifampacin works by binding to the DNA-dependent bacterial RNA polymerase and selectively inhibiting bacterial transcription initiation (72). Resistance to rifampicin results from an alteration in the bacterial RNA polymerase. Because rifampicin resistance occurs at a high rate, approximately 10^8–10^9 per bacterium per division, the drug is almost always used in combination, typically with isoniazid to minimize the development of resistance (71, 73). Resistance to rifampicin is most often mediated by mutations in the *rpoB* gene (52, 71, 73, 74). Mutations in *rpoB* lead to decreased affinity of the protein to rifampicin, which, in turn, leads to decreased susceptibility to the drug (71, 75).

NITROIMIDAZOLES

The nitroimidazoles are rooted in the mid-1950s discovery of azomycin and demonstration of its anti-trichomonad effect (76). Subsequently, various nitroimidazoles have been chemically synthesized, including metronidazole, which has been found to have exceptionally high activity against a wide variety of anaerobic protozoa and anaerobic bacteria, including *Trichomonas vaginalis*, *Entamoeba histolytica*, *Bacteroides* spp., *Clostridium* spp., *Helicobacter* spp., and all of the anaerobic cocci (77). Though the precise molecular mechanisms are unclear, nitroimidazoles appear to work by impairment in the helical structure of DNA and subsequent inhibition of DNA synthesis (42, 45). Metronidazole resistance typically results from deficiencies in drug activation, likely due to modification of proteins involved in drug activation (42). Anaerobic resistance to metronidazole has been observed for strains of *T. vaginalis* and *T. foetus*; it appears to result from decreased activity of proteins associated with the hydrogenosome, an unusual organelle and the site of glycolysis in the trichomonads (78).

Cell Membrane Disrupting Drugs

There are many agents that are effective against cell membranes; most, however, do not discriminate between eukaryotic and prokaryotic membranes. This property limits the number of cell membrane disrupting agents that are available for clinical use.

POLYMYXINS

Polymyxins B and E are the primary polymyxins administered systemically in humans. The polymyxins are bactericidal and have broad-spectrum activity. Though they are effective against Gram-positives and Gram-negatives, the drugs appear to have somewhat better activity against the latter. The polymyxins function by disrupting the cell's cytoplasmic membrane, acting on phosphate groups that are exposed on cytoplasmic membrane phospholipids (30). These drugs also appear to have further similar activity against the Gram-negative cell wall. The damage to the cytoplasmic membrane and cell wall causes leakage of cytoplasmic contents leading to cell death (33).

Metabolic Pathway-Inhibiting Drugs

Additional antibiotics function by blocking specific metabolic pathways that are essential for bacterial growth and survival, but not for their human hosts. Pathways such as the one for folate biosynthesis are an effective target for antimicrobial therapy in pathogens that must produce their own folic acid intermediates to survive. The bacterial pathogens are selectively targeted, because humans get their folic acid from preformed sources and do not have the targeted biosynthesis pathway.

SULFONAMIDES

The sulfonamides are structural analogs of *p*-aminobenzoic acid (PABA) that are involved in the synthesis of tetrahydrofolate, which is required for amino acid, pyrimidine, and purine biosynthesis. Sulfonamides block the formation of dihydropteroic acid from pteridine and PABA by competitively inhibiting bacterial dihydropteroate synthase. Bacteria that must synthesize their own folic acid are susceptible to sulfonamides; those that can use preformed folic acid are not. Sulfonamides are typically effective against *Streptococcus pyogenes*, *S. pneumoniae*, *Haemophilus influenzae*, *H. ducreyi*, *Chlamydia trachomatis*, and *Nocardia* and *Avtinomyces* spp. Though sulfonamides have been used for treatment of infection with *Neisseria meningitidis*, most isolates today are resistant (79).

Resistance to the sulfonamides may result from mutations in the biosynthetic pathway of tetrahydrofolate. At least two genes, *sul1* and *sul2*, found in integrons, transposons, and plasmids, have been characterized as expressing dihydropteroate synthases that bypass the blocked step in the metabolic pathway leading to high level sulfonamide resistance (54). Sulfonamide resistance may also occur through alternative means as well. Some sulfonamide-resistant staphylococci have been shown to produce 70 times more PABA than their susceptible counterparts, thus out-competing the effect of the sulfonamides (79).

TRIMETHOPRIM

Trimethoprim acts by competitively inhibiting bacterial dihydrofolate reductase, the enzyme that catalyzes the formation of tetrahydrofolate from dihydrofolate. Trimethoprim blocks a step in the tetrahydrofolate biosynthetic pathway that is downstream of the one blocked by sulfonamides. Trimethoprim used in combination with sulfonamides (trimethoprim-sulfamethoxazole, also called co-trimoxazole) produces a synergistic antibacterial effect (80). Trimethoprim exhibits a spectrum of activity similar to that of sulfamethoxazole and is effective against most Gram-negative and Gram-positive bacteria; however, resistance to trimethoprim frequently develops when the drug is used by itself. Trimethoprim-sulfamethoxazole may be effective against those organisms that are resistant to each drug alone, an important example of which is the MRSA.

Trimethoprim resistance emerged shortly after the introduction of trimethoprim-sulfamethoxazole for clinical use in the early 1970s (57). Among the Gram-negative organisms, resistance to trimethoprim is typically associated with carriage of a plasmid encoding an altered dihydrofolate reductase (81). Upwards of 20 different genes that express drug-resistant dihydrofolate reductases (*dfr* genes) have been characterized thus far. These *dfr* genes are commonly located on integrons, transposons, and plasmids; consequently, they may be transferred throughout bacterial populations (24). Trimethoprim resistance also arises as a result of mutations in chromosomal genes that lead to the overproduction of a dihydrofolate reductase, thus minimizing the impact of trimethoprim on tetrahydrofolate production.

Chemical Disinfectants

In addition to the antimicrobials mentioned above and used for treatment of infections, disinfectants are widely used to control pathogens in the healthcare environment. In this section, a number of important classes of disinfectants are reviewed along with a section on the mechanisms of disinfectant resistance.

ALCOHOLS

Alcohols are bacteriocidal chemical compounds characterized by their hydroxyl group, which is bound to carbon atom of alkyl group. The optimum bacteriocidal concentrations for alcohols are between 60% and 90% (82). Ethyl alcohol is the most common and most effective alcohol used as a disinfectant (83). At a concentration of 70%, ethyl alcohol is effective at killing most vegetative bacteria as well as many fungi and viruses. The mode of action for the antimicrobial properties of alcohol is likely the denaturation of proteins (84). When ethyl alcohol is mixed with water, proteins denature more quickly than in absolute ethyl alcohol (82). Alcohols have been used to disinfect a number of hospital instruments but are generally not recommended for sterilization of medical equipment due to their lack of ability to kill spores (84). There is also concern with using alcohols because they may damage certain equipment. Prolonged use of alcohols can damage the shellac mountings of lensed instruments and swell and harden rubber and plastic tubing (84).

ALDEHYDES

Aldehydes are organic compounds containing a terminal carbonyl group. Common aldehydes used as disinfectants are formaldehyde and glutaraldehyde (84). Formaldehyde is sold under the name formalin, which is an aqueous-based solution of 37% formaldehyde. Formaldehyde is considered a potential carcinogen, and limits have been set by Occupational Safety and Health Administration (OSHA) on employee exposure time. Its exact mode of action is unknown but is thought to act as an alkylating agent by reaction with carboxyl, sufhydryl, and hydroxyl groups (85). Glutaraldehyde is a dialdehyde and is an important disinfectant. It has a broad spectrum of activity against microorganisms. In aqueous solutions, the glutaraldehydes are acidic and generally not sporicidal (84); however, by adjusting the pH to alkaline levels, the solution becomes sporicidal. Numerous reviews have been published detailing the modes of action of the glutaraldehyde on different microorganisms (1, 86). Glutaraldehyde is commonly used as a disinfectant for various types of medical equipment. Unlike alcohols, glutaraldehyde does not damage the lenses on certain instruments. Like formaldehyde, prolonged exposure to glutaraldehyde can be toxic.

OXIDIZING AGENTS

A number of oxidizing agents are used as disinfectants. In general, oxidizing agents oxidize the cell membrane of microorganisms, thereby causing lysis and death. Common ozidixing agents used in healthcare include sodium hypochlorite, iodine and iodophors, hydrogen peroxide, and peracetic acid. Sodium hypochlorite (bleach) is widely used to disinfect innate surfaces and can be used to disinfect blood spills. The exact mode of action for sodium hypochlorite is unknown but thought to destroy cellular protein activity due to its high oxidizing potential. Additionally, tinctures of iodine have long been used in healthcare settings as antiseptics. Iodophors (combination of iodine and a solubilizing agent) have been used both as antiseptics and disinfectants. Aqueous solutions of iodine are generally unstable, whereas iodophors are considered more stable due to the solubilzing agent acting as a carrier of "free" iodine (85). Similar to chlorine compounds, iodine displays rapid antimicrobial properties. The mode of action is thought to be through disruption of the structure and synthesis of proteins and nucleic acids.

Hydrogen peroxide is a widely used disinfectant and antiseptic. Hydrogen peroxide produces hydroxyl free radicals that disrupt thiol groups of proteins and enzymes (85). It is effective against a wide range of microorganisms and is available in a wide range of concentrations (3–90%). A 3% solution is effective when used on inanimate surfaces (84). Higher concentrations and longer contact times are needed for hydrogen peroxide to be sporicidal (85). Catalase-producing microorganisms may be protected from hydrogen peroxide in low concentrations by degrading it to water and oxygen. This defense can be offset by concentrations (3% or greater) used for disinfection (87). Conversely, peracetic acid is more potent than hydrogen peroxide, even at lower concentrations. A 0.3% solution of peracetic acid is sporicidal, bactericidal, virucidal, and fungicidal. It is mainly used to sterilize a variety of medical, surgical, and dental devices such as flexible scopes and hemodialyzers. Although not completely understood, the mode of action for peracetic acid is thought to be similar to that of hydrogen peroxide (84).

PHENOLICS

Phenolics have long been used in the hospital setting. Phenol is one of the oldest known disinfectants and has been used in healthcare settings since its initial use by Lister. Phenol's mode of action at high concentrations is to disrupt the cell membrane and precipitate the cellular proteins (84). Phenol derivatives, such as bis-phenols (triclosan, hexachlorophene) and halophenols (chloroxylenol), also disrupt the cellular membrane components (85). Many phenolic disinfectants can be used on environmental surfaces, but concerns about toxicity in neonates has limited their use (84, 85).

QUATERNARY AMMONIUM COMPOUNDS

Quanternary ammonium compounds (QACs) are cationic surfactants and have been used for a variety of applications. QACs are generally bactericidal, fungicidal, and virucidal against select viruses (84). The cell membrane is the target site for QACs, and bactericidal activity is attributed to membrane disorganization, denaturation of cell proteins and nucleic acids, and leakage of low-molecular-weight intracellular material (85). QACs are commonly used for sanitation of noncritical surfaces with certain QACs approved for use with medical equipment that comes in contact with skin.

MECHANISMS OF RESISTANCE TO DISINFECTANTS

Microorganisms often differ in their response to disinfectants based upon factors such as cellular structure and physiology. In general, infectious agents such as prions, coccidia, spores, and mycobacterium tend to be the most resistant to disinfectants, while large nonenveloped viruses, bacteria, and lipid-enveloped viruses tend to be the most susceptible (88). Among the bacteria, the Gram-negative organisms tend to be more resistant than vegetative Gram-positive bacteria, due in large part to the barrier formed by the outer membrane. Bacterial spores are resistant to many types of disinfectants due to the spore coat, causing a barrier to entry of chemical agent. Likewise, the waxy cell wall of mycobacteria also provides a barrier limiting the effectiveness of disinfectants such as QACs and glutaraldehyde.

Acquired resistance to QACs is often due to an efflux pump encoded by the *qac*AB and *qac*CD families of genes (88). The *qac*AB family of genes encodes a proton-dependent efflux system with high affinity for QAC and other cations (89). This efflux system shows great homology to tetracycline efflux systems found in tetracycline-resistant bacteria (90). Efflux systems have also been described for many other disinfectants, including silver compounds, ethidium bromide, orthophenylphenol, chlorhexidine salts, acridimes, and diamidines (85, 91, 92).

Acquired resistance to mercurial compounds is due to inactivation of organic or inorganic mercury to nontoxic elemental mercury encoded by genes of the *mer* operon (4). Resistance can be classified as narrow spectrum (inorganic mercury) or broad spectrum (organomercurials) (4). Genes of the *mer* operon are often plasmid-encoded and sometimes present in mobile genetic elements. Other disinfectants can also be inactivated by the products of plasmid-encoded-genes, including the aldehydes and chlorhexadine salts (85).

Concluding Remarks

In the healthcare setting, the development and dissemination of antimicrobial- and disinfectant-resistant microorganisms creates challenges in the management and elimination of nosocomial infections. A better understanding of the mechanisms of action and the mechanisms of resistance development of different groups of antimicrobials and disinfectants will allow for more rational approaches to control nosocomial pathogens.

REFERENCES

1. Gorman SP, Scott EM, Russell AD. Antimicrobial activity, uses and mechanism of action of glutaraldehyde. *J Appl Bacteriol* 1980;**48**:161–190.
2. Greenwood D. *Antimicrobial Chemotherapy.* Oxford University Press, Oxford, 2000.
3. McDermott PF, Walker RD, White DG. Antimicrobials: Modes of action and mechanisms of resistance. *Int J Toxicol* 2003;**22**:135–143.
4. Walsh C. *Antibiotics Actions, Origins, Resistance.* ASM Press, Washington, DC, 2003.
5. Yao J, Moellering RC. Antibacterial agents. In Murray PR, Baron EJ, Pfaller MA, Tenover FC, Yolken RH (eds.), *Manual of Clinical Microbiology,* 8th ed. ASM Press, Washington, DC, 2003.
6. Scholar EM, Pratt WB. *The Antimicrobial Drugs.* Oxford University Press, New York, 2000.
7. Bush K. B-lactam antibiotics: Penicillins. In Greenwood D, Whitley RJ, Finch RG, Greenwood D, Norrby SR, Whitley RJ (eds.), *Antibiotic and Chemotherapy Anti-infective agents and their use in therapy,* Vol. 8. Chuchill Livingstone, London, 2003, pp. 224–259.
8. Chambers HF. Other B-lactam antibiotics. In Mandell GL, Bennett JE, Dolin R (eds.), *Principles and Practice of Infectious Diseases,* 6th ed., Vol. 2. Elsevier Churchill Livingstone, Philadelphia, 2005, pp. 311–318.
9. Reading C, Cole M. Clavulanic acid: A beta-lactamase-inhiting beta-lactam from *Streptomyces clavuligerus. Antimicrob Agents Chemother* 1977;**11**:852–857.
10. Ambler RP. The structure of beta-lactamases. *Philos Trans R Soc Lond B Biol Sci* 1980;**289**:321–331.
11. Bush K, Jacoby GA, Medeiros AA. A functional classification scheme for beta-lactamases and its correlation with molecular structure. *Antimicrob Agents Chemother* 1995;**39**:1211–1233.
12. Du Bois SK, Marriott MS, Amyes SG. TEM- and SHV-derived extended-spectrum beta-lactamases: Relationship between selection, structure and function. *J Antimicrob Chemother* 1995;**35**:7–22.
13. Nordmann P. Trends in beta-lactam resistance among Enterobacteriaceae. *Clin Infect Dis* 1998; *27*(Suppl 1): S100–S106.
14. Tenover FC, Raney PM, Williams PP, Rasheed JK, Biddle JW, Oliver A, Fridkin SK, Jevitt L, McGowan JE Jr., Evaluation of the NCCLS extended-spectrum beta-lactamase confirmation methods for *Escherichia coli* with isolates collected during Project ICARE. *J Clin Microbiol* 2003;**41**:3142–3146.
15. Philippon A, Arlet G, Jacoby GA. Plasmid-determined AmpC-type beta-lactamases. *Antimicrob Agents Chemother* 2002;**46**:1–11.
16. Bush K. Metallo-beta-lactamases: A class apart. *Clin Infect Dis* 1998; *27*(Suppl 1): S48–S53.
17. Kadry AA. Lack of efflux mechanism in a clinical isolate of Pseudomonas aeruginosa highly resistant to beta-lactams and imipenem. Folia Microbiol (Praha) 2003;**48**:529–533.

18. Woodruff WA, Hancock RE. Construction and characterization of *Pseudomonas aeruginosa* protein F-deficient mutants after *in vitro* and *in vivo* insertion mutagenesis of the cloned gene. *J Bacteriol* 1988;**170**:2592–2598.
19. Murakami S, Nakashima R, Yamashita E, Yamaguchi A. Crystal structure of bacterial multidrug efflux transporter AcrB. *Nature* 2002;**419**:587–593.
20. Spratt BG, Cromie KD. Penicillin-binding proteins of Gram-negative bacteria. *Rev Infect Dis* 1988;**10**:699–711.
21. Palavecino E. Community-acquired methicillin-resistant *Staphylococcus aureus* infections. *Clin Lab Med* 2004;**24**:403–418.
22. Hiramatsu K, Katayama Y, Yuzawa H, Ito T. Molecular genetics of methicillin-resistant *Staphylococcus aureus. Int J Med Microbiol* 2002;**292**:67–74.
23. Hakenbeck R, Coyette J. Resistant penicillin-binding proteins. *Cell Mol Life Sci* 1998;**54**:332–340.
24. Van Bambeke F, Van Laethem Y, Courvalin P, Tulkens PM. Glycopeptide antibiotics: from conventional molecules to new derivatives. *Drugs* 2004;**64**:913–936.
25. Gilbert DN, Moellering RC, Eliopoulos GM, Sande MA. *The Sanford Guide to Antimicrobial Therapy*, 34th ed. Antimicrobial Therapy, Inc, Hyde Park, VT, 2004.
26. Arthur M, Quintiliani R Jr., Regulation of VanA- and VanB-type glycopeptide resistance in enterococci. *Antimicrob Agents Chemother* 2001;**45**:375–381.
27. Wright GD. Mechanisms of resistance to antibiotics. *Curr Opin Chem Biol* 2003;**7**:563–569.
28. Stone KJ, Strominger JL. Mechanism of action of bacitracin: Complexation with metal ion and C 55-isoprenyl pyrophosphate. *Proc Natl Acad Sci USA* 1971;**68**:3223–3227.
29. Tsuda H, Yamashita Y, Shibata Y, Nakano Y, Koga T. Genes involved in bacitracin resistance in *Streptococcus mutans. Antimicrob Agents Chemother* 2002;**46**:3756–3764.
30. Greenwood D, Whitley RJ. Modes of action. In Finch RG, Greenwood D, Norrby SR, Whitley RJ (eds.), *Antibiotic and Chemotherapy Anti-infective Agents and Their Use in Therapy*, Vol. 8. Chuchill Livingstone, London, 2003, pp. 11–24.
31. Prescott LM, Harley JP, Klein DA. *Microbiology*. McGraw-Hill Higher Education, Dubuque, IA, 2005.
32. Vakulenko SB, Mobashery S. Versatility of aminoglycosides and prospects for their future. *Clin Microbiol Rev* 2003;**16**:430–450.
33. Katzung BG. *Basic & Clinical Pharmacology*. Appleton & Lange, Norwalk, CT, 1992.
34. Zhanel GG, Walters M, Noreddin A, Vercaigne LM, Wierzbowski A, Embil JM, Gin AS, Douthwaite S, Hoban DJ. The ketolides: A critical review. *Drugs* 2002;**62**:1771–1804.
35. Poole K. Aminoglycoside resistance in *Pseudomonas aeruginosa. Antimicrob Agents Chemother* 2005;**49**:479–487.
36. Sigmund CD, Ettayebi M, Morgan EA. Antibiotic resistance mutations in 16S and 23S ribosomal RNA genes of *Escherichia coli. Nucleic Acids Res* 1984;**12**:4653–4663.
37. Farrington E. Macrolide antibiotics. *Pediatr Nurs* 1998;**24**:433–446.
38. Garza-Ramos G, Xiong L, Zhong P, Mankin A. Binding site of macrolide antibiotics on the ribosome: New resistance mutation identifies a specific interaction of ketolides with rRNA. *J Bacteriol* 2001;**183**:6898–6907.
39. Kapusnik-Uner JE, Sande MA, Chambers HF. Tetracyclines, chloramphenicol, erythromycin, and miscellaneous antibacterial agents. In Hardman JG, Limbird LE, Molinoff PB, Ruddon RW, Gilman AG (eds.), *Goodman & Gilman's The Pharmacological Basis of Therapeutics*, 9th ed. McGraw-Hill, Health Professions Division, New York, 1996, pp. 1123–1153.
40. Leclercq R. Mechanisms of resistance to macrolides and lincosamides: Nature of the resistance elements and their clinical implications. *Clin Infect Dis* 2002;**34**:482–492.

41. Charvalos E, Tselentis Y, Hamzehpour MM, Kohler T, Pechere JC. Evidence for an efflux pump in multidrug-resistant *Campylobacter jejuni. Antimicrob Agents Chemother* 1995;**39**:2019–2022.

42. Brodersen DE, Clemons WM Jr, Carter AP, Morgan-Warren RJ, Wimberly BT, Ramakrishnan V. The structural basis for the action of the antibiotics tetracycline, pactamycin, and hygromycin B on the 30S ribosomal subunit. *Cell* 2000;**103**:1143–1154.

43. Connell SR, Trieber CA, Dinos GP, Einfeldt E, Taylor DE, Nierhaus KH. Mechanism of Tet(O)-mediated tetracycline resistance. *Embo J* 2003;**22**:945–953.

44. Bacon DJ, Alm RA, Burr DH, Hu L, Kopecko DJ, Ewing CP, Trust TJ, Guerry P. Involvement of a plasmid in virulence of *Campylobacter jejuni* 81–176. *Infect Immun* 2000;**68**:4384–4390.

45. Chopra I, Roberts M. Tetracycline antibiotics: Mode of action, applications, molecular biology, and epidemiology of bacterial resistance. *Microbiol Mol Biol Rev* 2001;**65**:232–260; second page, table of contents.

46. Xaplanteri MA, Andreou A, Dinos GP, Kalpaxis DL. Effect of polyamines on the inhibition of peptidyltransferase by antibiotics: Revisiting the mechanism of chloramphenicol action. *Nucleic Acids Res* 2003;**31**:5074–5083.

47. Struelens MJ, Finch RG, Greenwood D, Norrby SR, Whitley RJ. The problem of resistance. *Antibiotic and Chemotherapy Anti-Infective Agents and Their Use in Therapy*, Vol. 8. Chuchill Livingstone, London, 2003, pp. 25–47.

48. Murray IA, Shaw WV. *O*-Acetyltransferases for chloramphenicol and other natural products. *Antimicrob Agents Chemother* 1997;**41**:1–6.

49. Spizek J, Rezanka T. Lincomycin, clindamycin and their applications. *Appl Microbiol Biotechnol* 2004;**64**:455–464.

50. Putman M, van Veen HW, Degener JE, Konings WN. The lactococcal secondary multidrug transporter LmrP confers resistance to lincosamides, macrolides, streptogramins and tetracyclines. *Microbiology* 2001;**147**:2873–2880.

51. Delgado, G Jr, Neuhauser MM, Bearden DT, Danziger LH. Quinupristin-dalfopristin: An overview. *Pharmacotherapy* 2000;**20**:1469–1485.

52. Allington DR, Rivey MP. Quinupristin/dalfopristin: A therapeutic review. *Clin Ther* 2001;**23**:24–44.

53. Butaye P, Cloeckaert A, Schwarz S. Mobile genes coding for efflux-mediated antimicrobial resistance in Gram-positive and Gram-negative bacteria. *Int J Antimicrob Agents* 2003;**22**:205–210.

54. Wesson KM, Lerner DS, Silverberg NB, Weinberg JM. Linezolid, quinupristin/dalfopristin, and daptomycin in dermatology. *Clin Dermatol* 2003;**21**:64–70.

55. Donowitz GE. Oxazolidinones. In Mandell GL, Bennett JE, Dolin R (eds.), *Principles and Practice of Infectious Diseases*, 6th ed., Vol. 2. Elsevier Churchill Livingstone, 2005, Philadelphia, pp. 436–440.

56. Campbell EA, Korzheva N, Mustaev A, Murakami K, Nair S, Goldfarb A, Darst SA. Structural mechanism for rifampicin inhibition of bacterial RNA polymerase. *Cell* 2001;**104**:901–912.

57. Saif YM. *Diseases of Poultry.* Iowa State Press, Ames, Ia, 2003.

58. Dalhoff A, Schmitz FJ. *In vitro* antibacterial activity and pharmacodynamics of new quinolones. *Eur J Clin Microbiol Infect Dis* 2003;**22**:203–221.

59. Lambert MP, Neuhaus FC. Mechanism of D-cycloserine action: alanine racemase from *Escherichia coli* W. *J Bacteriol* 1972;**110**:978–987.

60. Fisher LM, Lawrence JM, Josty IC, Hopewell R, Margerrison EE, Cullen ME. Ciprofloxacin and the fluoroquinolones. New concepts on the mechanism of action and resistance. *Am J Med* 1989;**87**:2S–8S.

61. Heisig P. High-level fluoroquinolone resistance in a *Salmonella typhimurium* isolate due to alterations in both gyrA and gyrB genes. *J Antimicrob Chemother* 1993;**32**:367–377.

62. Heisig P, Tschorny R. Characterization of fluoroquinolone-resistant mutants of *Escherichia coli* selected *in vitro. Antimicrob Agents Chemother* 1994;**38**:1284–1291.

63. Barnard FM, Maxwell A. Interaction between DNA gyrase and quinolones: Effects of alanine mutations at GyrA subunit residues Ser(83) and Asp(87). *Antimicrob Agents Chemother* 2001;**45**:1994–2000.

64. McClure WR, Cech CL. On the mechanism of rifampicin inhibition of RNA synthesis. *J Biol Chem* 1978;**253**:8949–8956.

65. Ma D, Cook DN, Alberti M, Pon NG, Nikaido H, Hearst JE. Genes *acrA* and *acrB* encode a stress-induced efflux system of *Escherichia coli. Mol Microbiol* 1995;**16**:45–55.

66. Ma D, Cook DN, Alberti M, Pon NG, Nikaido H, Hearst JE. Molecular cloning and characterization of *acrA* and *acrE* genes of *Escherichia coli. J Bacteriol* 1993;**175**:6299–6313.

67. Mazzariol A, Tokue Y, Kanegawa TM, Cornaglia G, Nikaido H. High-level fluoroquinolone-resistant clinical isolates of *Escherichia coli* overproduce multidrug efflux protein AcrA. *Antimicrob Agents Chemother* 2000;**44**:3441–3443.

68. Tran JH, Jacoby GA. Mechanism of plasmid-mediated quinolone resistance. *Proc Natl Acad Sci USA* 2002;**99**:5638–5642.

69. Tran JH, Jacoby GA, Hooper DC. Interaction of the plasmid-encoded quinolone resistance protein Qnr with *Escherichia coli* DNA gyrase. *Antimicrob Agents Chemother* 2005;**49**:118–125.

70. Mandell GL, Sande MA. Drugs used in the chemotherapy of tuberculosis and leprosy. In Hardman JG, Limbird LE, Molinoff PB, Ruddon RW, Gilman AG (eds.), *Goodman & Gilman's The Pharmacological Basis of Therapeutics*, 6th ed. McGraw-Hill, Health Professions Division, New York, 1980, pp. 1200–1221.

71. Floss HG, Yu TW. Rifamycin-mode of action, resistance, and biosynthesis. *Chem Rev* 2005;**105**:621–632.

72. Hartmann G, Honikel KO, Knusel F, Nuesch J. The specific inhibition of the DNA-directed RNA synthesis by rifamycin. *Biochim Biophys Acta* 1967;**145**:843–844.

73. Lambert R, Provenzale D, Ectors N, Vainio H, Dixon MF, Atkin W, Werner M, Franceschi S, Watanabe H, Tytgat GN, Axon AT, Neuhaus H. Early diagnosis and prevention of sporadic colorectal cancer. *Endoscopy* 2001;**33**:1042–1064.

74. Heil A, Zillig W. Reconstitution of bacterial DNA-dependent RNA-polymerase from isolated subunits as a tool for the elucidation of the role of the subunits in transcription. *FEBS Lett* 1970;**11**:165–168.

75. Wehrli W. Rifampin: Mechanisms of action and resistance. *Rev Infect Dis* 1983;**5**(Suppl 3): S407–S411.

76. Horie H. Anti-Trichomonas effect of azomycin. *J Antibiot (Tokyo)* 1956;**9**:168.

77. Tracy JW, Webster LJ. Trypanosomiasis, leishmaniasis, amebiasis, giardiasis, trichomoniasis, and other protozoal infections. In Hardman JG, Limbird LE, Molinoff PB, Ruddon RW, Gilman AG (eds.), *Goodman & Gilman's the Pharmacological Basis of Therapeutics*, 9th ed. McGraw-Hill, Health Professions Division, New York, 1996, pp. 987–1008.

78. Quon DV, d'Oliveira CE, Johnson PJ. Reduced transcription of the ferredoxin gene in metronidazole-resistant Trichomonas vaginalis. *Proc Natl Acad Sci USA* 1992;**89**:4402–4406.

79. Mandell GL, Petri W. Sulfonamides, trimethoprim-sulfamethoxazole, quinolones, and agents for urinary tract infections. In Hardman JG, Limbird LE, Molinoff PB, Ruddon RW, Gilman AG (eds.), *Goodman & Gilman's The Pharmacological Basis of Therapeutics*, 9th ed. McGraw-Hill, Health Professions Division, New York, 1996, pp. 1057–1072.

80. Christopher T, Walsh BLB, Nathan CF, O'Brien TF, Riley M, White RJ, Wright GD. *Treating Infectious Diseases in a Microbial World.* National Academy of Sciences, Washington, DC, 2006.

81. Oethinger M, Kern WV, Jellen-Ritter AS, McMurry LM, Levy SB. Ineffectiveness of topoisomerase mutations in mediating clinically significant fluoroquinolone resistance in *Escherichia coli* in the absence of the AcrAB efflux pump. *Antimicrob Agents Chemother* 2000;**44**:10–13.

82. Morton HE. *Alcohols*. Lea & Febiger, Philadelphia, 1983.

83. Morton HE. *The Relationship of Concentration and Germicidal Efficiency of Ethyl Alcohol*. Annals of the New York Academy of Science 53, 1950, pp. 191–196.

84. Rutala W, Weber DJ. Selection and use of disinfectants in healthcare. In Mayhall CG (ed.), *Hospital Epidemiology and Infection Control*, 3rd ed. Lippincott Williams and Wilkins, Philadelphia, 2004, pp. 1473–1522.

85. McDonnell G, Russell AD. Antiseptics and disinfectants: Activity, action, and resistance. *Clin Microbiol Rev* 1999;**12**:147–179.

86. Scott EM, Gorman SP. Glutaraldeyde. In Block SS (ed.), *Disinfection, Sterilization, and Peservation*. Lippincott Williams & Wilkins, Philadelphia, 2001, pp. 361–381.

87. Block SS. Peroxygen compounds. In Block SS (ed.), *Disinfection, Sterilization, and Preservation*. Lippincott Williams & Wilkins, Philadelphia, 2001, pp. 185–204.

88. Russell AD. Bacterial resistance to disinfectants: Present knowledge and future problems. *J Hosp Infect* 1999;**43**(Suppl): S57–S68.

89. Amavisit P, Markham PF, Lightfoot D, Whithear KG, Browning GF. Molecular epidemiology of Salmonella Heidelberg in an equine hospital. *Vet Microbiol* 2001;**80**:85–98.

90. Del Vecchio VG, Petroziello JM, Gress MJ, McCleskey FK, Melcher GP, Crouch HK, Lupski JR. Molecular genotyping of methicillin-resistant *Staphylococcus aureus* via fluorophore-enhanced repetitive-sequence PCR. *J Clin Microbiol* 1995;**33**:2141–2144.

91. Gupta A, Matsui K, Lo JF, Silver S. Molecular basis for resistance to silver cations in *Salmonella*. *Nat Med* 1999;**5**:183–188.

92. Thorrold CA, Letsoalo ME, Duse AG, Marais E. Efflux pump activity in fluoroquinolone and tetracycline resistant *Salmonella* and *E. coli* implicated in reduced susceptibility to household antimicrobial cleaning agents. *Int J Food Microbiol* 2007;**113**:315–320.

PART TWO

Techniques to Characterize Nosocomial Pathogens

CHAPTER SEVEN

Rapid PCR Screening Methods

NGOLELA ESTHER BABADY, FRANKLIN R. COCKERILL, AND ROBIN PATEL

Introduction to Real-Time PCR

The invention of the polymerase chain reaction (PCR) by Mullis and colleagues at Cetus Corporation revolutionized the field of molecular microbiology. The concept that DNA could be exponentially amplified *in vitro* followed an earlier report describing steps required for DNA amplification, including DNA denaturation, excess primers, and repeat cycling (1). The first PCR report, published in 1985 (2) (with the specifics of the reaction published two years later (3)), described the amplification of specific target sequences of the β-globin gene for diagnosis of sickle cell anemia. This marked a major improvement in DNA detection, which previously relied strictly on the amount of natural DNA that could be extracted from specimens. PCR has served as an important tool in basic applied research and has been broadly applied to the diagnosis of human disease states and infections.

The first PCR assay amplified 1 μg of DNA using 20 amplification cycles. Amplified product was detected by gel electrophoresis and by Southern blot analysis using a radioactive ^{32}P probe (2). The entire process required over 24 hours to complete. Several improvements have simplified and shortened the process. First, methods to detect amplified DNA (i.e., other than Southern blot analysis) reduced the time for detection from over 24 hours to 8 hours (i.e., the time necessary to run an agarose gel) (Table 7.1). Another major improvement was the substitution of the temperature susceptible Klenow fragment of *Escherichia coli* DNA polymerase I with the thermostable *Thermus aquaticus (Taq)* DNA polymerase (4, 5), which can withstand prolonged incubation at temperatures of 95°C. This

Molecular Techniques for the Study of Hospital-Acquired Infection, First Edition. Edited by Steven L. Foley, Anne Y. Chen, Shabbir Simjee, and Marcus J. Zervos.

TABLE 7.1 Examples of detection methods used for conventional PCR

Methods	DNA probe label	Detection	Sensitivity	Reference
Autoradiography	^{32}Phosphorus	Nylon membrane incubated with ^{32}P probe and exposed to X-ray film	1–5 pg	92
Chemiluminescence	Peroxidase Digoxigenin	Nylon membrane incubated with DNA probe, followed by incubation with luminol or dioxetane, and exposure to X-ray film or measurement with a luminometer	100 fg	93, 94
Fluorescence	Ethidium bromide	Agarose gel visualized under UV light after gel electrophoresis	1–5 ng	95, 96
	Carbofluorescein, rhodamine, and coumarine TOTO and YOYO	Fluorescent dye incorporated in primers used for amplification; detection occurs after gel electrophoresis under UV light or laser excitation followed by fluorescence detection	4 pg	97, 98
Enzyme immunoassay	Biotinylated RNA probe	β-Galactosidase-labeled monoclonal antibody to DNA–RNA hybrid used for detection and quantization with a fluorogenic substrate	5 pg	99
Colorimetry	Biotin Digoxigenin	Nylon membrane incubated with DNA probes, followed by incubation with anti-conjugate antibodies and addition of substrate (BCIP or NBT); color formation detected with a densitometer	1–10 pg	100–102

UV, ultraviolet; BCIP, 5-bromo-4-chloro-3-indolyphosphate *p*-toluidine salt; NBT, nitro-blue tetrazolium chloride; TOTO, thiazole orange homodimer; YOYO, oxazole yellow homodimer.

novel polymerase eliminated the need for constant addition of DNA polymerase during the amplification procedure. The development of the thermal cycler instrument permitted automation of the amplification process and improved reproducibility of results (6). Further improvements in automation occurred in the early 1990s with the introduction of rapid-cycle PCR. This method permitted completion of 30 amplification cycles in 10–30 minutes, depending on the size of the product (6–9). More rapid heat exchange of the reaction mix, accomplished by increasing the surface-to-volume ratio of the sample using capillary tubes and the capability of thermal cyclers to rapidly alter temperature in the reaction chambers, facilitated shorter amplification cycling times. Subsequently, denaturation and annealing time was reduced to less than 1 second. The introduction of rapid thermal cyclers was followed by the addition of ethidium bromide to the amplification mix for simultaneous amplification and detection of the PCR product (10, 11). This method was referred to as "rapid-cycle, real-time" PCR and later simply referred to as "real-time" PCR. Detection probes, labeled with fluorescent reporter molecules, were subsequently introduced for real-time monitoring of DNA amplification, which continues to be used to this day.

Real-time PCR represents a substantial improvement over conventional PCR. Since amplification and detection of DNA occur simultaneously, real-time PCR permits continuous monitoring of DNA amplification and eliminates the need for post-amplification analysis. This results in a faster and generally more sensitive and more specific assay than with conventional PCR. Additionally, because real-time PCR testing platforms use closed systems, the chances for carryover of amplified product (contamination) is considerably less than conventional PCR. These properties have facilitated the use of PCR in diagnostic clinical microbiology laboratories. One of the first studies on the potential use of PCR for diagnostic clinical microbiology reported the detection of HIV proviral DNA in established infected cell lines and in cells cultured from infected individuals (12). Today, a literature search of real-time PCR assays for clinical diagnostic purposes yields thousands of papers, emphasizing the extensive use of real-time PCR in the field of diagnostic clinical microbiology. This chapter will focus on technologies available for real-time PCR, including instrumentation and detection chemistries, primer design and assay development, quality control and quality assurance issues, and cost. Finally, clinical applications of real-time PCR, focused on the detection nosocomial pathogens, will be presented.

Real-Time PCR Instrumentation

The first commercially available real-time PCR instrument, the GeneAmp SDS 5700, was developed by Applied Biosystems (Foster City, CA) in 1997. Today, several companies manufacture real-time PCR instruments and a variety of features are available for the user (Table 7.2). Some of the important differing characteristics of a real-time PCR instrument include fluorescence excitation sources and ranges, optical detection modes and ranges, thermocycler system, and ramp rate (rate at which the temperature is achieved), as well as cost and reaction number capacity.

FLUORESCENCE EXCITATION

The light source necessary to provide the excitation energy for the fluorophore can be a halogen lamp, a light-emitting diode (LED), or a laser. The excitation energy provided

TABLE 7.2 Examples of real-time PCR instruments

Manufacturer	Model	Light source	Optical detector	Excitation range (number of filters)	Detection range (number of filters)
Abbott	m2000rt	THL	CCD	5	5
Applied Biosystems (ABI)	Prism SDS 7000	THL	CCD	350–790	4
	Prism SDS 7300	THL	CCD	1	4
	Prism SDS 7500	THL	CCD	5	5
	Prism SDS 7900	Laser	CCD	488	500–600
Bioer	Line-Gene	LED	PMT	470	530–710 (3)
	Line-Gene 2	LED	PMT	470	4
Bio-Rad	MiniOpticon	LED	Two photodiodes	470–500 (1)	523–700 (2)
	MyiQ	THL	CCD	475–495 (1)	515–545 (1)
	Opticon 2	LED	2-PMTs	470–505 (1)	523–700 (2)
	Chromo4	LED	Four photodiodes	450–650 (4)	515–730 (4)
	iQ5	THL	CCD	475–645 (5)	515–700 (5)
	iCycler iQ	THL	CCD	480–650 (5)	515–720 (5)
Cepheid	SmartCycler I	LED	SPD	450–650 (4)	510–750 (4)
	SmartCycler II	LED	SPD	450–650 (4)	510–750 (4)
Corbett Research	Rotor-Gene 2000	LED	PMT	470–625 (4)	510–610 (6)
	Rotor-Gene 3000	LED	PMT	470–625 (4)	510–610 (4)
	Rotor-Gene 6000	LED	PMT	365–680 (7)	460–712 (6)
Eppendorf	MasterCycler ep realplex 2	LED	1-PMT	470	520 & 550 (2)
	MasterCycler ep realplex 4	LED	2-PMT	470	520–605 (4)
Roche	LightCycler 2.0	LED	Six photodiodes	470	530–710 (6)
	LightCycler 480	Xenon lamp	CCD	450–615 (5)	500–670 (6)
Stratagene	Mx3000P	THL	PMT	350–750 (4)	350–700 (4)
	Mx30005P	THL	PMT	350–750 (5)	350–700 (5)
	Mx4000	THL	PMT	350–750	350–830
Techne	Quantica	THL	PMT	470–650 (4)	500–710 (4)

THL, tungsten halogen lamp; LED, light-emitting diode; CCD, charged couple device; PMT, photomultipler tube; SPD, silicon photodiode.

by the halogen lamp is a broad-range spectrum that can be filtered to accommodate a wide range of fluorophores. However, since the energy is not focused, the intensity of the light passing through a filter is decreased, which may result in decreased intensity. LED and laser sources emit narrower-spectra, exciting fluorophores at specific wavelengths. To increase their excitation capabilities, some instruments use multiple LED sources (Table 7.2).

OPTICAL DETECTION

Detection of the light emitted from excited fluorophores is accomplished by photodetectors that convert emitted light into an electric signal (either current or voltage). Photodetectors can be charge-couple device (CCD) cameras (semiconductor detectors), photomultiplier tubes (which multiply the signal produced by emitted light and contain a photocathode that emits electrons when illuminated), photodiodes (which are similar to semiconductors), silicon detectors, or fluorimeters. A set of optical filters can be used to increase the number of detectable wavelengths and therefore the diversity of detectable fluorophores.

THERMAL CYCLER

The ability of a thermal cycler to maintain a uniform temperature in all reaction wells and to quickly change from one temperature to another (ramping) greatly impacts the reproducibility and speed of the associated assays. Heating and cooling can be accomplished using either a heating block or surrounding air. Heating block cylcers are based on Peltier technology in which current passed through the junction between two (n- and p-type thermoelectric) semiconductors results in transfer of heat from one side of the junction to the other (13). Cooling can be accomplished by use of either a refrigerant or a water bath. Ramping in the heating block method is limited by the thermal mass and low thermal conductivity of the heat block (13). Air themocyclers use (a) either a light bulb or a heating coil as a source of heat, which is directed by movement of air, and (b) a fan to expel the hot air and introduce cooler air into a reaction chamber. Narrow-gauged tubes (e.g., capillary tubes) in the reaction chamber are exposed to rapid changes in temperatures, resulting in a considerably shorter ramping rate (14–16).

PCR Detection Chemistries

The first reporter molecules used for real-time detection of PCR product involved addition of ethidium bromide into the reaction mix. The amplification was continuously monitored by taking video images of each amplification cycle with a CCD camera and analyzing those images at the end of each run (10). Ethidium bromide is carcinogenic and was eventually replaced with safer and more sensitive alternatives, including other nonspecific, as well as sequence-specific, reporter molecules (probes).

NONSPECIFIC FLUORESCENT DYES

Nonspecific fluorescent dyes (including ethidium bromide) bind to double-stranded DNA regardless of the sequence. The dyes specifically bind to the minor groove of double-stranded DNA and do not discriminate between amplified DNA and artifacts such as primer dimers; these dyes are therefore not optimal for multiplexing by color (17). Despite their lack of specificity, these dyes are useful when the goal is to simply detect DNA amplification since they will only fluoresce when bound to double-stranded DNA. Furthermore, they are inexpensive and easy to use and do not require probe design. Although SYBR Green I is the most commonly used nonspecific dye, a recent study by Gudnason and colleagues comparing the performance of various double-stranded DNA binding dyes suggests that

TABLE 7.3 Examples of fluorescent dyes used for real-time PCR

Manufacturer	Dyes	Excitation (nm)	Emission (nm)	References	Website
Molecular Probes	SYBR Green I	280, 502	530	17	www.probes.com
Molecular Probes	Pico Green	502	523	103	www.probes.com
Molecular Probes	YO-PRO-1	491	509	104	www.probes.com
Molecular Probes	SYTO-9	483	498	18,105	www.probes.com
Idaho Technology	LC Green I	440–470	470–520	106–108	www.idahotech.com
TataaBiocenter	BEBO	470	510	109	www.tataa.com

SYTO-82 and SYTO-13 are better choices for real-time PCR, since unlike SYBR Green I, these dyes do not significantly inhibit PCR, bind preferentially to GC-rich regions, or affect the melting temperature of the amplified product (18). Commercially available fluorescent dyes are provided in Table 7.3.

SPECIFIC PROBES

Specific fluorescent probes are based on fluorescence (or Förster) resonance energy transfer (FRET), a process that relies on the proximity of a donor (high-energy) fluorophore to an acceptor or quenching fluorophore (low energy). The low-energy fluorophore is called an acceptor, if it receives energy emitted from the donor fluorophore and fluoresces at a lower wavelength, or a quencher, if it prevents the donor from emitting light until the two are separated. An overlap between donor emission spectrum and quencher/acceptor absorption spectrum is necessary for FRET to occur. Upon light excitation, the donor fluorophore will emit light that will be absorbed by the acceptor/quenching fluorophore if they are in close proximity to one another. In the case of acceptor probes, the result is acceptor probe emission of fluorescence at a longer wavelength. In the case of quencher probes, the donor and quencher are located in close proximity with the result that donor fluorescence is quenched. Upon separation, as occurs once such probes bind specific DNA, the donor probe fluorescence can be detected and measured.

A variety of probes operate on the FRET principle, including molecular beacons, Taqman (5′ nuclease) probes, hybridization probes, sunrise primers, scorpion primers, and light-up probes (19–25). The first three are the most commonly used and will be reviewed here.

Molecular beacons are oligonucleotide probes, which are folded upon themselves in a hairpin structure that positions the donor fluorophore on the 5′ end close to the quencher fluorophore on the 3′ end. The two regions at the ends of the probes are designed to be complementary to each other and, in the absence of complementary DNA, will stay bound to one another. When DNA complementary to the loop is present, the molecular beacon probes anneal to their complementary sequences forcing the hairpin structure to open. The result is separation of the donor dye at the 5′ end from quencher dye at the 3′ end. A fluorescent signal from the donor dye can therefore be measured because it is no longer quenched by the quencher dye (Figure 7.1A).

Taqman oligonucleotide probes also have a donor fluorophore on their 5′ end and a quencher fluorophore on their 3′ end. The probe anneals to complementary amplified

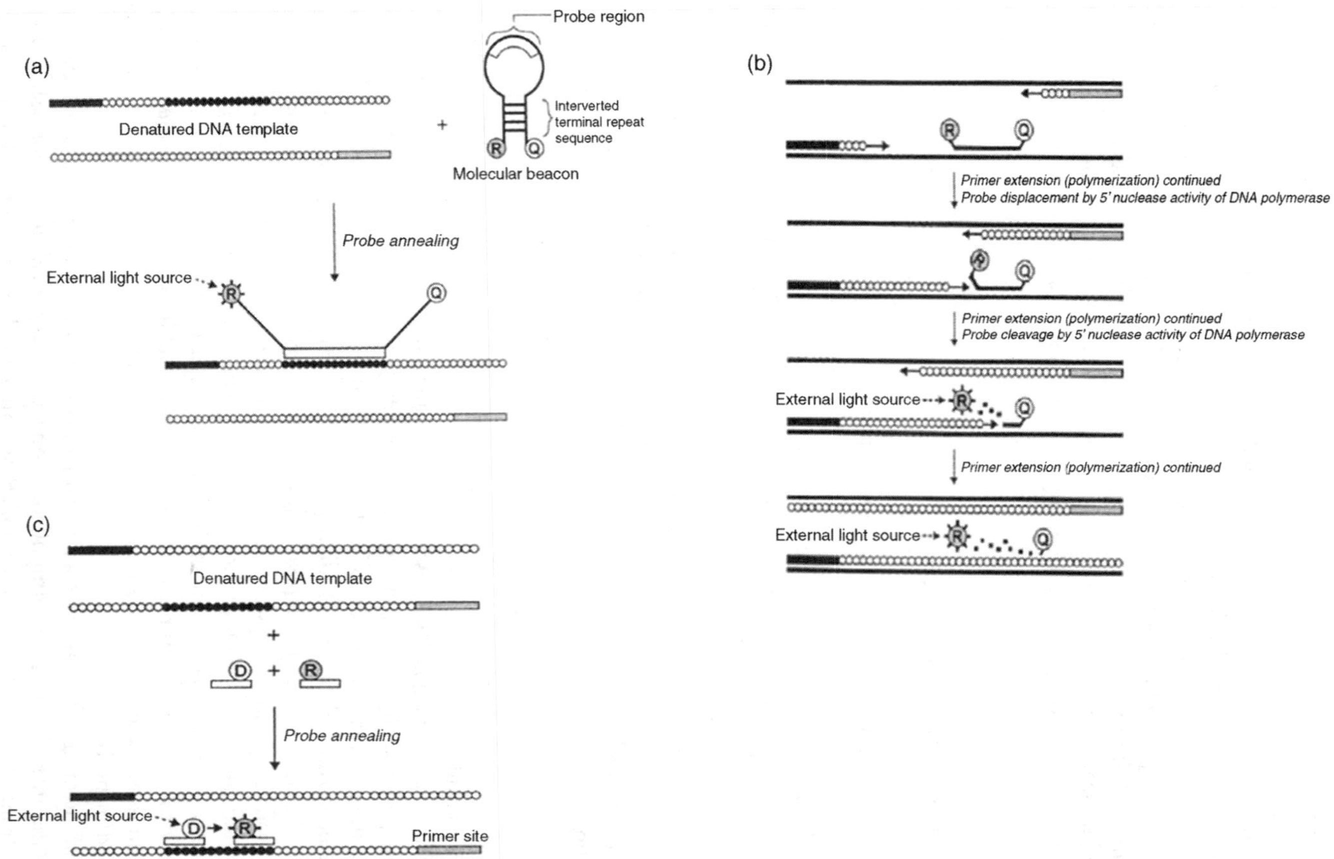

FIGURE 7.1 Examples of real-time PCR detection chemistries. R, reporter/donor fluorophore; Q, quencher/acceptor fluorophore. (A) Molecular beacon, (B) 5′-nuclease (Taqman) probe, (C) FRET hybridization probe. Reprinted from reference 38, with permission.

DNA and is cleaved during primer extension by the 5′ nuclease activity of *Taq* polymerase, releasing and separating the donor from the quencher fluorophore and allowing fluorescence. One of the advantages of Taqman probes is that fluorescence can be detected anytime during the PCR process since the fluorescent donor accumulates after each cycle (Figure 7.1B).

FRET hybridization probe technology involves the use of two probes: One probe has a fluorescent donor dye at the 3′ end of the oligonucleotide, and the other one has an acceptor dye at the 5′ end. The two dyes are designed to bind to adjacent sequences on the amplified DNA product. Upon binding to target DNA, the donor and acceptor fluorophores will be in close proximity to each other; upon light excitation, the donor will emit fluorescence that will be absorbed by the acceptor, which will become excited and, in turn, emit light at a longer, third wavelength, which is then detected by the instrument (Figure 7.1C).

Primer and Probe Design

Several guidelines exist for optimal design of primers and probes (15, 26–28). These guidelines include recommendations on (a) the size of the amplified DNA and (b) the length, GC content, and melting temperature (Tm) of the primers and probes. In general, the amplified DNA is best kept between 150 and 500 base pairs (bp). Primers and probes should be between 17 and 25 bp, although longer sequences can sometimes contribute to higher specificity. Optimally, the 3′ end of both primers should end with AA or TT to prevent stable primer dimer formation and avoid complementary 3′ ends, which can be extended by DNA polymerase and result in decreased PCR efficiency. To ensure that the melting temperature (Tm) of the primers is not too high, their GC content should be less than 60%. Probes are usually designed to have a Tm approximately 5°C higher than the Tm of the primers. The Tm of both primers should be within a degree of each other to ensure that they have similar annealing temperatures (usually 60 ± 5°C). Attention should be paid to avoid secondary structures, such as hairpin loops and primer and probe dimers.

Although useful, the guidelines listed above are only a starting point; primers and probes should be experimentally optimized. Primers and probes can be designed either manually or using computer software (e.g., OLIGO (www.oligo.net), LightCycler software (Hybridization) (Roche Applied Science, Indianapolis, IN), Primer express (Applied Biosystems, Foster City, CA), Genescript (Taqman) (https://www.genscript.com/ssl-bin/app/primer), Primer Biosoft (TaqMan®, TaqMan®MGB, molecular beacons, and FRET) (http://www.premierbiosoft.com), and PRIMO (http://www.changbioscience.com/primo/primo.html). Many of these programs have features that allow the user to set parameters and will yield primer and probe sets based on the user's parameters. In addition, these software programs have functions that screen for potential secondary structures and dimer formation between primers and/or probes.

One of the most important factors in primer design is primer specificity, which ensures that only the intended target is amplified. Using the basic local alignment search tool (BLAST) from the National Center for Biotechnology Information (NCBI), primer specificity can be checked *in silico* against sequences available in the NCBI database. Alternatively or additionally, one can BLAST the gene of interest to identify a unique region that can then be used for primer and probe design. Once primers have been designed, a specificity panel should be tested *in vitro* using DNA from relevant sources to exclude cross-reactivity with other organisms.

Assay Optimization

Optimization involves the titration of each component of the PCR reaction to determine the conditions that will yield the best results. The optimal concentration of primers, probes, magnesium ions, DNA polymerase, deoxyribonucleotide triphosphates (dNTPs), and the optimal number of amplification cycles need to be determined. Commercial master mix kits available from various manufacturers (i.e., Roche Applied Science (FastStart DNA HybProbe), Cepheid (SmartMix™, Sunnyvale, CA) are designed to facilitate assay optimization by including some of the necessary reagents reagent such as dNTPs, *Taq* DNA polymerase, and fluorescent dyes (i.e., SYBR Green 1) in predetermined concentrations. This allows users to focus on optimization of primers, probes, and $MgCl_2$ concentration. Primer and probe design software programs such as the Lightcycler Probe design 2.0 (Roche Applied Science, Indianapolis, IN) have default experimental concentrations for primers, probes, and Mg^{2+} concentrations, depending on the reaction settings selected providing a starting point from which optimization can be carried out.

For primers and probes, concentrations are typically varied from 0.1 to 0.5 μM. When designing primers and probes, one typically begins with the concentration chosen by the software, which in most cases is 0.2 μM, and then optimizes from there. The concentration of magnesium is crucial since Mg^{2+} affects DNA polymerase enzyme activity and binds to deoxynucleotide triphosphates (dNTPs) (26, 29). Titration of $MgCl_2$ concentration (i.e., from 0.5 to 5 mM) early in assay development is recommended (29, 30). An optimal concentration of the thermostable *Taq* DNA polymerase will ensure that the assay proceeds to completion without loss of efficiency and sensitivity (i.e., if the concentration is too low) or loss of specificity (i.e., if the concentration is too high) (26, 29). Hot start PCR, a modification of conventional PCR, can prevent formation on nonspecific product by only starting the amplification process at temperatures above which primer mismatch will not occur. This technique, which uses thermostable *Taq* DNA polymerase or anti-*Taq* DNA polymerase antibodies in the master mix, helps increase the sensitivity of the assay and prevents formation of unwanted primer dimers (30).

As for conventional PCR, appropriate thermal cycling parameters are necessary for successful amplification. Cycling conditions depend, to a certain extent, on the platform and chemistry being used. Most real-time PCR instruments have set default programs that can be modified by the user. In general, the number of cycles should be between 25 and 35 to prevent formation of nonspecific products; the length of the cycle depends on the expected length of the amplified DNA (26, 29).

Another variable to consider is the concentration of DNA template. A template concentration that is too high might inhibit the reaction, whereas a template concentration that is too low might not result in any detectable product (and thus a false-negative result). Since the copy numbers of target in patient specimens cannot be predicted and vary from one patient to another, the assay should be designed to detect the lowest amount of target possible. Analytical assay sensitivity is determined by serially diluting a positive control until no product is detected. Ideally, the crossing point (Cp) or crossing threshold (CT), which is the point at which amplified DNA is detected, should be between 10 and 30 cycles (30).

Another factor that influences assay performance is the presence of inhibitors in the specimens being tested. The effect of these inhibitors can be attenuated by dilution of the specimen. Specimens such as blood and stool are notorious for affecting the outcome of a reaction and should be diluted, if possible, to dilute inhibitors. Purification and preparation of specimens for PCR can be performed manually using commercially available kits (e.g., QIAamp DNA mini (Qiagen, Valencia, CA), Puregene DNA Purification and Generation Capture Column (Gentra System, Minneapolis, MN), NucliSens isolation (bioMerieux, Durham, NC), Wizard Genomic DNA Purification (Promega, Madison, WI), High Pure PCR Template Preparation (Roche Applied Sciences, Indianapolis, IN), NucleoSpin Tissue (Macherey-Nagel, Bethlehem, PA), GFX Genomic blood DNA Purification (GE Healthcare Bio-Sciences, Piscataway, NJ), UltraClean DNA (MoBio, Carlsbad, CA), MasterPure DNA purification (EpicentreTechnologies, Madison, WI), IsoQuick nucleic acid extraction (MicroProbe, Carlsbad, CA)). Several of these kits have been evaluated and compared (31, 32). Their efficiency in recovering DNA from specific specimens may vary and should be considered when choosing a kit. For high-volume laboratories, the use of automated DNA purification systems can be beneficial not only in terms of time saved and ergonomic issues, but also in terms of reproducibility and decreased human errors, which occur with repetitive, high-volume tasks. Several choices are available, which vary in specimen capacity and run time (Table 7.4).

TABLE 7.4 Examples of automated nucleic acids extraction and purification systems

Manufacturer	Instrument	Maximum capacity	Maximum run time (min)	Web site
Applied Biosystems	ABI Prism 6100	96	30	www.appliedbiosystems.com
	ABI Prism 6700	96	75	
biomerieux	NucliSens Extractor	10	45	www.biomerieux-usa.com
Corbett Life Sciences	X-tractore Gene	96		www.corbettlifescience.com
Promega	Maxwell 16	16	45	www.promega.com
Qiagen	BioRobot EZ1	6	20	www.qiagen.com
	BioRobot M48	48	306	
	BioRobot M96	96		
	BioRobot MDx	96	150	
Roche Applied Science	MagNA Pure Compact	8	30	www.roche-applied-science.com
	MagNA Pure LC	32	90	
Taigen Bioscience Corporation	Lab Turbo 36	36	60	www.labturbo.com
	Lab Turbo 96	96	60	
	Lab Turbo 496	4 (96)	90	

Quality Control and Quality Assurance

Once an assay has been developed, it should be validated to ensure that the results are accurate and reproducible. Several validation experiments need to be performed before the implementation of a new test. The College of American Pathologists (CAP) Molecular Pathology checklist (33) and the Clinical Laboratory Improvement Amendments (CLIA) 1988 revised document (34) have guidelines that specifically address assay validation, including determination of analytical and clinical sensitivities, test accuracy, precision, and analytical specificity (33, 34). These documents also include guidelines relating to (a) the use of a positive and negative control with every run for both qualitative and quantitative assays and (b) the use of standards for quantitative assays (33). In most instances, the negative control for a real-time PCR assay consists of the master mix plus water (i.e., instead of DNA template). However, once the assay has been developed, it is preferable that the negative control be DNA extracted from an organism other than the target organism for which the assay was developed. The positive control may consist of a plasmid that contains the amplification target. The concentration of the positive control should be kept close to the lower end of detection of the assay to ensure that specimens containing a low copy number of the infecting organisms will be positive (24). As mentioned above, the limit of detection of an assay can be determined by making a serial dilution of the positive control template until no amplification product is detected. This assessment, referred to as "analytical sensitivity," will help in predicting the clinical sensitivity of the assay when it is tested on raw specimens instead of purified DNA template known to carry the target of interest.

In addition to positive and negative controls, both internal and external controls may be included with each assay. An internal control ensures that true-positive results are not missed, by indirectly assessing the presence of inhibitors in the reaction. The internal control can be either a completely different target or the same target with primers and probes that will yield either a product with a different Tm or a product detected at a different wavelength. This can be accomplished by modifying the internal DNA sequence of the target by either inserting into or deleting a portion of the internal DNA sequence and using different sets of probes for detection of native and altered target. This type of internal control is called a homologous internal control. When the internal control is a completely different target, such as a housekeeping gene (e.g., actin), it is referred to as a heterologous control (24, 35). The internal control can either be added to the PCR master mix (homologous) or, in the case of a housekeeping gene, be endogenous to the specimen and therefore part of the total DNA extract. Care should be taken during the development stage to ensure that the concentration of the internal control does not affect the sensitivity of the assay. External controls, on the other hand, are not included in the same reaction mix as the target DNA. Instead, they are detected in a separate vessel and control for thermocycling efficiency and not, necessarily, for false-negativity (35).

Measures should also be set in place to prevent and detect possible false-positive results. False positivity can result from specimen to specimen contamination or from specimen contamination by amplified DNA. In order to prevent specimen cross-contamination, CAP guidelines suggest that testing samples be loaded in the following order: patient, followed by the positive control(s), and then the negative control(s) (33). Amplified product contamination can be prevented by physically separating the specimen extraction, reagent preparation, and specimen amplification work areas. Addition of uracil-*N*-glycosylase (UNG) and deoxyuridine triphosphate (dUTP) in the master mix can also be used to prevent carryover of amplified product (i.e., contamination by amplified DNA) (36). UNG removes uracil from the amplified DNA rendering it susceptible to hydrolysis at high temperature and thus creating an inefficient template for further amplification. Finally, good laboratory techniques, such as frequent glove changes and bleaching of work areas before and after testing, should always be used to help prevent contamination.

Quality assurance in the laboratory ensures that the result obtained from a patient specimen is accurate. In addition to CAP and CLIA, the World Health Organization (WHO) has established guidelines (37) that summarize parameters to consider in order to ensure quality of laboratory results. Although not specifically aimed at molecular techniques, such guidelines can be applied to real-time PCR. These guidelines address preanalytical, analytical, and post-analytical parameters including specimen collection and transportation, standard operating procedures, personnel qualification, quality control records, reporting of patient results, external and internal quality assessment testing, equipment performance, and quality of reagents used for testing. It is recommended that only specimen sources for which an assay has been validated be tested; all other specimen types should be rejected. Standard operating procedures should contain all information necessary to perform and interpret the test and should provide information on acceptable results. These documents should be reviewed annually. Quality control records should be retained and reviewed; corrective action should be taken and should be documented when problems arise. The quality of the reagents used for real-time PCR is obviously important. Primers and probes, as well as any other reagents used in the assay, should always be purified and stored at the proper temperature. Commercial kits should be used prior to their expiration dates and according to manufacturers' instructions; any deviation from manufacturers' instructions should be documented. Finally, frequent monitoring of test results is recommended in order to establish trends and therefore be aware when there is a change in a trend, which needs to be investigated to ensure that it is not due to a quality failure (38).

Real-Time PCR in the Clinical Microbiology Laboratory

Clinical microbiology laboratories have traditionally relied on methods such as conventional culture, direct microscopy, and serology, including antigen and antibody detection, for diagnosis of infectious diseases. In most instances, these methods are still considered the gold standard and any novel real-time PCR test developed needs to be compared to these methods for determination of analytical sensitivity and specificity. However, the introduction of conventional PCR, followed by real-time PCR, has significantly changed the way that microorganisms are detected in clinical microbiology laboratories.

At first, real-time PCR assay development was focused on organisms that were fastidious or uncultivable (39, 40). For example, our laboratory developed a real-time PCR assay for the detection of both *Bordetella pertussis* and *Bordetella parapertussis* in nasopharyngeal swabs (41). Detection of *B. pertussis* had been traditionally done by culture, which took 3–7 days and lacked sensitivity, or by direct fluorescent antibody testing, which, similar to culture, lacked sensitivity (41). This real-time PCR assay was developed to detect either the insertion sequence IS*481* of *B. pertussis* or the insertion sequence IS*1001* of *B. parapertussis*. When compared to culture and direct fluorescent antibody testing, the assay was more sensitive (less than one organism per reaction), and decreased the analytical time from 3–7 days to 45 minutes (post-nucleic acid extraction); further, the assay was able to differentiate between *B. pertussis* and *B. parapertussis*, both of which can cause whooping cough. This example illustrates not only the impact of real-time PCR on turnaround time [which is defined as the total time between (a) accessioning of the specimen in the laboratory and (b) issuance of the final report (40)], but also its impact on test sensitivity and the ability to distinguish between two very similar pathogens. Currently at the Mayo Clinic, real-time PCR has completely replaced culture for the detection of *B. pertussis* and *B. parapertussis*.

Another example of real-time PCR replacing conventional methods is its use in the detection of *Mycoplasma pneumoniae*, a common agent of community-acquired pneumonia in children. *M. pneumoniae* culture requires special media and can take as long as three weeks, having little clinical value (42). Serological diagnosis of *M. pneumoniae*, by complement fixation or enzyme-linked immunosorbent assay, relies on detection of IgG and IgM. However, this method lacks sensitivity, especially in the acute phase of the infection, when antibodies are not yet present, necessitating the use of paired sera (acute and convalescent), and rendering serology useful only for retrospective diagnosis (42, 43). Several real-time PCR assays for detection of *M. pneumoniae* have been developed (44–46), and all have shown higher sensitivity than serological methods.

Today, real-time PCR assays are not just used to detect slow-growing or uncultivable organisms. They have been applied to the detection of any organism whose faster or more accurate detection can have an impact on patient care, including but not limited to groups A and B streptococci, *Bacillus anthracis*, *Escherichia coli*, *Staphylococcus aureus*, and enterovirus (40, 47). In addition to rapid turnaround time and increased sensitivity, real-time PCR has been used to detect antimicrobial resistance genes [e.g., in vancomycin resistant enterococcus (VRE), methicillin-resistant *Staphylococcus aureus* (MRSA)], to quantify viral load [e.g., human immunodeficiency virus (HIV), hepatitis B virus (HBV)], and to differentiate species of a single genus in a single assay through multiplexing (i.e., *B. pertussis* and *B. parapertussis*). Furthermore, in many cases, real-time PCR is a safer alternative to culture, is easier to use, and is not subject to the intralaboratory variability of culture (40). These advantages allow faster and better patient care. Some of the disadvantages of real-time PCR include the inability to distinguish between dead or live organisms and between infection and/or colonization.

Several real-time PCR tests are now commercially available in addition to the multitude of "home-brewed" tests that have been developed in individual clinical microbiology laboratories. It is imperative that careful analysis and validation be undertaken by individual laboratories before implementation of a real-time PCR assay. Some of the variables to consider include (a) establishing if a need exists for the test and (b) assessing laboratory capabilities such as personnel skills, work space availability, and integration of the new test into current work flow (24, 48, 49). As for any new test, employees that will be performing the test need to be adequately trained not only on the necessary molecular technical skills (such as proper pipetting), but also on the background theory and principles of the test as well as annual review of the standard operating procedures. Initial training should include observation of the entire procedure as performed by a competent technologist, performance of the test while being observed by a competent technologist, and competency assessment before independent testing. As previously mentioned, physical separation of the various steps is optimal to minimize contamination. Preferably, a "clean room" should be dedicated for reagent storage and master mix preparation, away from specimen extraction, instrument setup and loading, and target amplification spaces (24). Another variable to keep in mind is the effect of introducing any new test on the laboratory workflow and the design of the flow so that results are obtained in a timely fashion. An example that illustrates this point is our implementation of a real-time PCR test for the detection of influenza virus types A and

B (50). We showed that real-time PCR had greater sensitivity and faster turnaround time (a few hours) than both shell vial assay (1–2 days) and cell culture (several days) in detecting influenza viruses (24, 50). Since influenza viruses are highly contagious, rapid diagnosis is essential for both infection control and proper treatment. A process was put in place that involves a PCR testing four times a day. Throat swabs are received in the clinical microbiology laboratory along with a prescription filled out for oseltamivir. Patients select a pharmacy to which their prescription can be faxed in case of a positive test result. This workflow process has an average turnaround time of 5.5 hours, which allows physicians to target therapy and patients to start treatment in a timely manner (50).

Costs of Real-Time PCR in the Clinical Microbiology Laboratory

The issue of cost of real-time PCR cannot be disregarded. Elements factored in the total cost of a test include the price of equipment (nucleic acid extraction systems and thermocycler instruments), the price of the reagents and supplies, the cost of royalties to be paid for use of patented technologies, and personnel time (24, 48, 51).

The approximate listed prices for nucleic acid extraction systems can vary from \$12,000 to \$170,000 (49), while thermocycler prices vary from \$76,000 to \$130,000 (52). The prices of reagents (e.g., enzymes, dNTPs, primers, probes) and supplies (e.g., pipettes, pipette tips, capillaries, plates, or rotors) also vary, depending on the manufacturers and the platforms used. A right to-use search should be performed prior to implementation to determine if the target that will be used for the assay has been patented and to decide if the royalties will be affordable. Royalties might also have to be paid for the use of PCR technology itself (24).

Workload recording, the process of collecting information on the effort and resources involved in performing a test, should be done for both the real-time PCR test and the test that will be replaced. Comparison of the overall costs between the two tests can partly support (or not support) the implementation of PCR in the laboratory (40, 51). This analysis has to take into account the fact that instruments can be used for more than one test and that, with batching, technologists can run multiple specimens at the same time. Something that is difficult to assess in workload recording is the bedside savings that result from increased sensitivity and turnaround time, which, in turn, may result in shorter hospital stays or in more appropriate use of isolation and antimicrobial agents (53–55).

APPLICATION OF THE REAL-TIME TECHNOLOGY TO THE DIAGNOSIS OF NOSOCOMIAL PATHOGENS

Nosocomial infections, also termed healthcare-associated infections, are characterized by high morbidity and mortality. In the United States, 1.7 million nosocomial infections occurred in 2002 and were associated with 99,000 deaths (56). These infections include urinary tract infection, bloodstream infection, pneumonia, and surgical site infection, and their cost is estimated at \$6.7 billion per year (56, 57). Therefore, it is important to establish measures to prevent and treat nosocomial infections, including prompt identification of responsible pathogens and their antimicrobial susceptibilities, in order to initiate effective therapy and prevent their spread.

TABLE 7.5 Examples of real-time PCR assays for nosocomial pathogens

Pathogens	Amplification targets	Specimen type	Platform	References
Staphylococcus aureus	*Sa442*	Nasal swabs	LightCycler	91
	Proprietary	Blood culture	SmartCycler	75
	nuc	Blood culture	SmartCycler	110
	23S ribosomal RNA gene	Hand "juice"	ABI Prism	111
	tuf	Blood culture	LightCycler	112
Methicillin-resistant *Staphylococcus aureus* (MRSA)	*mecA*	Blood culture	SmartCycler	110
	SCCmec and *orfX*	Blood culture and nasal swabs	SmartCycler	75, 113–115
	SCCmec and *orfX*	Nasal swabs	LightCycler	116
Vancomycin-resistant *Enterococcus* species (VRE)	*vanA*, *vanB*, *vanC1*, and *vanC2/C3*	Rectal swabs	LightCycler	117
	vanA, *vanB*, and *vanB2/3*	Perianal swabs	LightCycler	118
	vanA and/or *vanB*	Fecal swabs	Smartcycler	119
	vanA and *vanB*	Rectal swabs	LightCycler	120, 121
Streptococcus pneumoniae	*plyA*	CSF, blood, serum, and plasma	ABI Prism	122, 123
	lytA, *ply*, and *psaA*	Serum, middle ear fluid, and CSF	Mx3000P/ ABI Prism	124
	lytA	CSF, sputum, and blood	ABI Prism	125
Pseudomonas aeruginosa	*oprL*	Blood culture	LightCycler	126
	gyrB	Sputum	LightCycler	127
	gyrB, *oprI*, *algD*, and exotoxin A	Sputum, oropharyngeal swabs, and BAL	iCYCLER	128
Escherichia coli	*uspA*	Urine	ABI Prism	129
	uidA	Amniotic fluid (spiked)	LightCycler	130
Escherichia coli (ETEC)	LT1 and ST1	Stool (spiked)	LightCycler	131
Escherichia coli (EHEC)	stx_1, stx_2 and stx_{2e}	Stool	LightCycler	132, 133
	stx_1 and stx_2, E-*hly*, *eae*	Stool (spiked)	LightCycler	134
	stx_1 and stx_2	Stool	SmartCycler	135
	$rfb_{E.coli\ O157}$ and stx_2	Stool (spiked)	ABI Prism	136
Mycobacterium tuberculosis	IS*6110*	Respiratory	Smartcycler	137, 138
	16S ribosomal RNA gene	Respiratory and nonrespiratory	Lightcycler	139
	ITS	Respiratory	Lightcycler	140
	16S ribosomal RNA gene	Sputum and tissue biopsies	ABI Prism	141

(continued)

TABLE 7.5 (*Continued*)

Pathogens	Amplification targets	Specimen type	Platform	References
Clostridium difficile	*tcdB*	Stool	LightCycler	142
	tcdB	Stool	iCycler IQ	143, 144
	tcdA and *tcdB*	Stool	SmartCycler	145
Klebsiella pneumoniae	16S ribosomal RNA gene	Blood culture	LightCycler	146
Acinetobacter species	16S ribosomal RNA gene	Blood culture	LightCycler	147
Legionella species	16S ribosomal RNA gene and *mip*	Sputum, endotracheal aspirates, lung biopsy, and bronchoscopic specimens	ABI Prism	148
	5S ribosomal RNA gene, 16S ribosomal RNA gene and *mip*	Serum	ABI Prism	149
	16S ribosomal RNA gene	Throat swabs, BAL, nasopharyngeal aspirates (NPA), sputum, and bronchus aspirates	NucliSens EasyQ	150
	5S ribosomal RNA gene, 16S ribosomal RNA gene and *mip*	BAL or lung biopsy specimens	Lightcycler	151
	23S-5S ribosomal RNA gene spacer	Sputum	ABI Prism	152
	16S ribosomal RNA gene	BAL and throat swabs	iCycler IQ	153
	mip	BAL and sputum	LightCycler	154
	16S ribosomal RNA gene	BAL	LightCycler	155
	16S ribosomal RNA gene	BAL and sputum	LightCycler	156
Aspergillus species	ITS2	BAL, bronchial and tracheal secretions, blood, and tissues	LightCycler	157
	28S ribosomal RNA gene	Lung tissues, blood, and bronchotracheal secretions	ABI Prism	158
	18S SSU ribosomal RNA gene	Blood	LightCycler	159
	Cytochrome b gene	BAL and blood	LightCycler	160
	mtDNA	BAL and tissues	LightCycler	161

TABLE 7.5 (*Continued*)

Pathogens	Amplification targets	Specimen type	Platform	References
Candida species	ITS2	BAL, bronchial and tracheal secretions, blood, and tissues	LightCycler	157
	28S ribosomal RNA gene	Lung tissues, blood, and bronchotracheal secretions	ABI Prism	158
	18S SSU ribosomal RNA gene	Blood	LightCycler	159
	ITS2	Blood culture	LightCycler	162
	RPR1	Blood	Rotor-Gene	163

Respiratory specimens included: sputum, bronchial, and tracheal aspirates, bronchial and tracheal secretions, and bronchoalveolar lavage fluid. Nonrespiratory specimens included: biopsy, blood, gastric fluid, stool, urine, cerebrospinal fluid, and wound secretion.

Some of the most common pathogens associated with healthcare-associated infections include *Staphylococcus aureus*, *Enterococcus* species (especially vancomycin-resistant enterococci, VRE), *Escherichia coli*, *Pseudomonas aeruginosa*, *Acinetobacter baumanii*, *Clostridium difficile*, *Legionella* species, *Mycobacterium tuberculosis*, *Klebsiella pneumoniae*, *Aspergillus* species, *Zygomycete* species, *Candida* species, and various viruses, including influenza virus types A and B (58–63). An assay developed by Roche diagnostics (www.roche.com), LightCycler® SeptiFast, has the potential to detect and differentiate up to 25 organisms causing nosocomial infections directly from blood, including several of those listed above. References to other assays developed to detect the above-mentioned pathogens are listed in Table 7.5. This list is not inclusive and only represents a sample of numerous published assays. Real-time PCR assays for methicillin-resistant *S. aureus* (MRSA) and *M. tuberculosis* are described in more detail below.

METHICILLIN-RESISTANT *Staphylococcus aureus*

S. aureus is one of the most common pathogens responsible for both community-acquired infections, such as skin and soft tissue infections (64), and nosocomial infections, especially in patients with recent surgery or indwelling devices, such as ventilators or catheters (65). Although *S. aureus* can transiently colonize the skin and nares, especially of young children (66), in some individuals carriage can be persistent (67, 68). A break in the skin, as occurs during surgical procedures, can result in introduction of *S. aureus* from skin flora into wounds (69, 70).

The emergence of MRSA (71, 72) has increased the need for (a) faster identification, to allow better infection control, (b) decolonization of carriers prior to surgery as necessary, and (c) informed and appropriate antimicrobial agent selection (70). At the Mayo Clinic, long-term care facility residents are kept in strict isolation upon hospital admission until their nasal screen for MRSA (performed on admission) is negative. Culture-based methods for detection of MRSA take between 24 and 96 hours (73). By using real-time PCR, the turnaround time for detection can be reduced to less than one hour (74). At the time this chapter was written, two FDA-approved real-time PCR were available for detecting MRSA: the Xpert™ MRSA test (Cepheid, Sunnyvale, CA), which runs on the GeneXpert® system (Cepheid, Sunnyvale, CA), and the GeneOhm StaphSR (Becton Dickinson, Franklin, Lakes, NJ), which runs on the Smartcycler system (Cepheid, Sunnyvale, CA), and is able to detect and differentiate between *S. aureus* and MRSA. The Xpert™ MRSA test detects MRSA from swabs, while the GeneOhm StaphSR is FDA approved for detection of *S. aureus* and MRSA from positive blood cultures (75). Becton Dickinson also has a commercially available MRSA test (GeneOhm™ MRSA) that can detect MRSA from nasal swabs and was used by Paule et al. (76) for screening of admissions at Evanston Northwestern Healthcare. However, this test was not FDA approved when this chapter was written. References to examples of "home-brewed" tests are listed in Table 7.5.

Mycobacterium tuberculosis

The incidence of tuberculosis in 2006 was 9.2 million new cases with an estimated 0.5 million cases of drug-resistant TB and 1.7 million deaths worldwide (77). Transmission of *M. tuberculosis* occurs person-to-person through inhalation of aerosolized droplet nuclei containing *M. tuberculosis* bacilli spread by an individual with active pulmonary tuberculosis. As such, in hospital settings, patients with possible tuberculosis are placed under airborne isolation until they no longer pose a risk (78–80). Healthcare workers, as well as visitors entering isolation rooms, are required to wear a protective respirator (e.g., N95 tight-fitted respirator, powered air-purifying respirator) (79). Such measures were recommended following an increase in hospital-acquired tuberculosis and the rise in incidence of multidrug-resistant tuberculosis (81–83). Conventional methods for the detection of *M. tuberculosis* include Ziehl–Neelsen, Kinyoun, and auramine– rhodamine stains of smear for the detection of acid-fast bacilli and culture, which are nonspecific and lengthy, respectively. Additional methods used for identification of mycobacteria include hybridization probes (Gen-Probe, Inc., San Diego, CA) (84) and the amplified *Mycobacterium tuberculosis* direct (MTD) test (Gen-Probe, Inc., San Diego, CA). The latter can identify *M. tuberculosis* directly from respiratory clinical specimens (15, 85, 86). The hybridization probes are used only on organisms growing on culture, and it can take several weeks to obtain enough growth for the test. The MTD test is sensitive and specific but is a cumbersome process with several steps; it is an expensive test and it has the potential to produce false-positive results with other mycobacteria including *M. celatum*, *M. leprae*, *M. kansasii*, and *M. avium* (87–90). The need for sensitive, specific, and faster methods of detection has resulted in the development of several real-time PCR tests to complement existing testing methods (Table 7.5). However, at the time this chapter was written, no real-time PCR assay had been approved by the FDA for clinical diagnostic purposes.

The application of rapid real-time PCR technology to the identification of nosocomial pathogens will certainly have a positive impact on infection control in hospitals by improving the time to diagnosis and therefore result in better patient care and reduction in the overall cost of care for hospitalized patients (91).

Summary

Rapid real-time PCR has greatly improved the detection of pathogens in clinical microbiology laboratories by increasing accuracy, efficiency, and turnaround time of testing. Manufacturers are releasing a wide variety of instruments that will cater to both small and large diagnostic laboratories. As more laboratories adopt real-time PCR and other molecular techniques and as more assays become commercially available, careful attention to quality and standardization of will be needed. Ultimately, it is likely that more traditional assays will be replaced with real-time PCR assays, which will benefit patient care.

REFERENCES

1. Kleppe K, et al. Studies on polynucleotides. XCVI. Repair replications of short synthetic DNA's as catalyzed by DNA polymerases. *J Mol Biol* 1971;**56**(2):341–361.
2. Saiki RK, et al. Enzymatic amplification of beta-globin genomic sequences and restriction site analysis for diagnosis of sickle cell anemia. *Science* 1985;**230**(4732):1350–1354.
3. Mullis KB, Faloona FA. Specific synthesis of DNA *in vitro* via a polymerase-catalyzed chain reaction. *Methods Enzymol* 1987;**155**:335–350.
4. Kogan SC, Doherty M, Gitschier J. An improved method for prenatal diagnosis of genetic diseases by analysis of amplified DNA sequences. Application to hemophilia A. *N Engl J Med* 1987;**317**(16):985–990.
5. Saiki RK, et al. Primer-directed enzymatic amplification of DNA with a thermostable DNA polymerase. *Science* 1988;**239**(4839):487–491.
6. Wittwer CT, Fillmore GC, Hillyard DR. Automated polymerase chain reaction in capillary tubes with hot air. *Nucleic Acids Res* 1989;**17**(11):4353–4357.
7. Wittwer CT, Fillmore GC, Garling DJ. Minimizing the time required for DNA amplification by efficient heat transfer to small samples. *Anal Biochem* 1990;**186**(2):328–331.
8. Wittwer CT, Garling DJ. Rapid cycle DNA amplification: Time and temperature optimization. *Biotechniques* 1991;**10**(1):76–83.
9. Wittwer CT, et al. Rapid cycle allele-specific amplification: Studies with the cystic fibrosis delta F508 locus. *Clin Chem* 1993;**39**(5):804–809.
10. Higuchi R, et al. Kinetic PCR analysis: Real-time monitoring of DNA amplification reactions. *Biotechnology (NY)* 1993;**11**(9):1026–1030.
11. Higuchi R, et al. Simultaneous amplification and detection of specific DNA sequences. *Biotechnology (NY)* 1992;**10**(4):413–417.
12. Kwok S, et al. Identification of human immunodeficiency virus sequences by using *in vitro* enzymatic amplification and oligomer cleavage detection. *J Virol* 1987;**61**(5):1690–1694.
13. Qiu X, Yuan J. Temperature control for PCR thermocyclers based on peltier-effect thermoelectric. *Conf Proc IEEE Eng Med Biol Soc* 2005;**7**:7509–7512.
14. Logan JMJ, Edwards KJ. An overview of real-time PCR platforms. In Edwards K, Logan J, Saunders N (eds.), Real-Time PCR: *An Essential Guide*. Horizon Biosciences, Norfolk, UK, 2004, pp. 13–29.
15. McPherson MJ, Moller SG. Chapter 3: Reagents and instrumentation. Chapter 4: Optimization of PCR. In Owens E. (ed.), *PCR*, 2nd ed. Taylor & Francis, New York, 2006, pp. 55–62, 65–74.
16. Chapin K, Lauderdale TL. Evaluation of a rapid air thermal cycler for detection of *Mycobacterium tuberculosis*. *J Clin Microbiol* 1997;**35**(8):2157–2159.
17. Wittwer CT, et al. Continuous fluorescence monitoring of rapid cycle DNA amplification. *Biotechniques* 1997;**22**(1):130–131, 134–138.

18. Gudnason H, et al. Comparison of multiple DNA dyes for real-time PCR: Effects of dye concentration and sequence composition on DNA amplification and melting temperature. *Nucleic Acids Res* 2007;**35**(19):e127.
19. Whitcombe D, et al. Detection of PCR products using self-probing amplicons and fluorescence. *Nat Biotechnol* 1999;**17**(8):804–807.
20. Nazarenko IA, Bhatnagar SK, Hohman RJ. A closed tube format for amplification and detection of DNA based on energy transfer. *Nucleic Acids Res* 1997;**25**(12):2516–2521.
21. Isacsson J, et al. Rapid and specific detection of PCR products using light-up probes. *Mol Cell Probes* 2000;**14**(5):321–328.
22. Heid CA, et al. Real time quantitative PCR. *Genome Res* 1996;**6**(10):986–994.
23. Kostrikis LG, et al. Spectral genotyping of human alleles. *Science* 1998;**279**(5354): 1228–1229.
24. Espy MJ, et al. Real-time PCR in clinical microbiology: Applications for routine laboratory testing. *Clin Microbiol Rev* 2006;**19**(1):165–256.
25. Valasek MA, Repa JJ. The power of real-time PCR. *Adv Physiol Educ* 2005;**29**(3):151–159.
26. Edwards KJ. Performing real-time PCR. In Edwards KJ, Logan J, Saunders N (eds.), *Real-Time PCR: An Essential Guide*. Horizon Bioscience, Norfolk, UK, 2004, pp. 71–83.
27. SantaLucia, J. Chapter 1: Physical principles and visual-OMP software for optimal PCR design. In Yuryev, A. (ed.), *PCR Primer Design*. In Walker JM (series ed.), *Methods in Molecular Biology*, Vol. 402. Humana Press, Totowa, NJ, 2007, pp. 3–33.
28. Wu JS, et al. Primer design using genetic algorithm. *Bioinformatics* 2004;**20**(11):1710–1717.
29. Rolfs A, Schuller I, Finckh U, Weber-Rolfs I. *PCR: Clinical Diagnostics and Research*. Springer-Verlag, Berlin, 1992.
30. Technical note LC 9/2000. Roche Molecular Biochemicals, Indianapolis, IN, 2000.
31. Queipo-Ortuno MI, et al. Comparison of seven commercial DNA extraction kits for the recovery of *Brucella* DNA from spiked human serum samples using real-time PCR. *Eur J Clin Microbiol Infect Dis* 2008;**27**(2):109–114.
32. Fahle GA, Fischer SH. Comparison of six commercial DNA extraction kits for recovery of cytomegalovirus DNA from spiked human specimens. *J Clin Microbiol* 2000;**38**(10): 3860–3863.
33. College of American Pathologists. *Molecular Pathology Checklist*. College of American Pathologists, Northfield, IL, 2006.
34. CLSI/NCCLS. *User Protocol for Evaluation of Qualitative Test Performance*; *Approved Guidelines*, 2nd ed. Document EP12-A2, Vol. 28, #3. NCCLS, Wayne, PA, 2002.
35. Lee MA, Leslie DL, Squirrell DJ. Internal and external controls for reagent validation. In Edwards, KJ, Logan, J, Saunders N (eds.), *Real-Time PCR: An Essential Guide*. Horizon Bioscience, Norfolk, UK, 2004, pp. 85–101.
36. *Uracile DNA Glycosylase*. Invitrogen Life Technologies, 2008.
37. Kumari S, Bhatia, R. *Quality Assurance in Bacteriology and Immunology*, 2nd ed. World Health Organization, New Dehli, India, 2003.
38. Sloan LM. Real-time PCR in clinical microbiology: Verification, validation, and contamination control. *Clin Microbiol Newsletter* 2007;**29**(12):87–95.
39. Wolk D, Mitchell S, Patel R. Principles of molecular microbiology testing methods. *Infect Dis Clin North Am* 2001;**15**(4):1157–1204.
40. Cockerill FR, Uhl JR. Applications and challenges of real-time PCR for the clinical microbiology laboratory. In Reisch U, Wittwer C, Cockerill FR (eds.), *Rapid Cycle Real-Time PCR Methods and Applications*, Springer Verlag, Heidelberg, Germany, 2002, pp. 3–27.

41. Sloan LM, et al. Multiplex LightCycler PCR assay for detection and differentiation of *Bordetella pertussis* and *Bordetella parapertussis* in nasopharyngeal specimens. *J Clin Microbiol* 2002;**40** (1):96–100.
42. Ferwerda A, Moll HA, de Groot R. Respiratory tract infections by *Mycoplasma pneumoniae* in children: A review of diagnostic and therapeutic measures. *Eur J Pediatr* 2001;**160**(8):483–491.
43. Sillis M. Modern methods for the diagnosis of *Mycoplasma pneumoniae* pneumonia. *Rev Med Microbiol* 1993;**4**:24–28.
44. Templeton KE, et al. Comparison and evaluation of real-time PCR, real-time nucleic acid sequence-based amplification, conventional PCR, and serology for diagnosis of *Mycoplasma pneumoniae*. *J Clin Microbiol* 2003;**41**(9):4366–4371.
45. Pitcher D, et al. Real-time detection of *Mycoplasma pneumoniae* in respiratory samples with an internal processing control. *J Med Microbiol*, 2006;**55**(Pt 2):149–155.
46. Ursi D, et al. Detection of *Mycoplasma pneumoniae* in respiratory samples by real-time PCR using an inhibition control. *J Microbiol Methods* 2003;**55**(1):149–153.
47. Sails AD. Applications of real-time PCR in clinical microbiology. In Edwards KJ, Logan J, Saunders, N (eds.), *Real-Time PCR: An Essential Guide*. Horizon Bioscience, Norfolk, UK, 2004, pp. 247–326.
48. Forbes BA. Introducing a molecular test into the clinical microbiology laboratory: Development, evaluation, and validation. *Arch Pathol Lab Med* 2003;**127**(9):1106–1111.
49. Mothershed EA, Whitney AM. Nucleic acid-based methods for the detection of bacterial pathogens: Present and future considerations for the clinical laboratory. *Clin Chim Acta* 2006;**363**(1–2):206–220.
50. Zitterkopf NL, et al. Relevance of influenza a virus detection by PCR, shell vial assay, and tube cell culture to rapid reporting procedures. *J Clin Microbiol* 2006;**44**(9):3366–3367.
51. Smith TF, Uhl JR, Espy MJ, Sloan LM, Vetter EA, Jones MF, Rosenblatt JE, Cockerill F.R. III, Development, implementation, and trend analysis of real-time PCR tests for the clinical microbiology laboratory. *Clin Microbiol Newsletter* 2004;**26**(19):145–153.
52. Bell AS, Ranford-Cartwright LC. Real-time quantitative PCR in parasitology. *Trends Parasitol* 2002;**18**(8):337–342.
53. Doern GV, et al. Clinical impact of rapid *in vitro* susceptibility testing and bacterial identification. *J Clin Microbiol* 1994;**32**(7):1757–1762.
54. Barenfanger J, et al. Clinical and financial benefits of rapid detection of respiratory viruses: An outcomes study. *J Clin Microbiol* 2000;**38**(8):2824–2828.
55. Barenfanger J, Drake C, Kacich G. Clinical and financial benefits of rapid bacterial identification and antimicrobial susceptibility testing. *J Clin Microbiol* 1999;**37**(5):1415–1418.
56. Klevens RM, et al. Estimating health care-associated infections and deaths in U.S. hospitals, 2002. *Public Health Rep* 2007;**122**(2):160–166.
57. Graves N. Economics and preventing hospital-acquired infection. *Emerg Infect Dis* 2004;**10** (4):561–566.
58. Jones RN. Resistance patterns among nosocomial pathogens: Trends over the past few years. *Chest* 2001;**119**(2 Suppl): 397S–404S.
59. Yerly S, et al. Nosocomial outbreak of multiple bloodborne viral infections. *J Infect Dis* 2001;**184**(3):369–372.
60. Walsh TJ, Pizzo PA. Nosocomial fungal infections: A classification for hospital-acquired fungal infections and mycoses arising from endogenous flora or reactivation. *Annu Rev Microbiol* 1988;**42**:517–545.
61. Perlroth J, Choi B, Spellberg B. Nosocomial fungal infections: Epidemiology, diagnosis, and treatment. *Med Mycol* 2007;**45**(4):321–346.

62. Goldmann DA. Nosocomial viral infections: Recent developments and new strategies. *Eur J Clin Microbiol Infect Dis* 1989;**8**(1):75–81.
63. Anderson LJ. Major trends in nosocomial viral infections. *Am J Med* 1991;**91**(3B): 107S–111S.
64. McCaig LF, et al. *Staphylococcus aureus*-associated skin and soft tissue infections in ambulatory care. *Emerg Infect Dis* 2006;**12**(11):1715–1723.
65. National Nosocomial Infections Surveillance (NNIS) System Report, Data Summary from January 1992–June 2001, issued August 2001. *Am J Infect Control* 2001;**29**(6):404–421.
66. Kuehnert MJ, et al. Prevalence of *Staphylococcus aureus* nasal colonization in the United States, 2001–2002. *J Infect Dis* 2006;**193**(2):172–179.
67. Nouwen JL, et al. Predicting the *Staphylococcus aureus* nasal carrier state: Derivation and validation of a "culture rule". *Clin Infect Dis* 2004;**39**(6):806–811.
68. Nouwen J, et al. *Staphylococcus aureus* carriage patterns and the risk of infections associated with continuous peritoneal dialysis. *J Clin Microbiol* 2006;**44**(6):2233–2236.
69. Kluytmans JA, Wertheim HF. Nasal carriage of *Staphylococcus aureus* and prevention of nosocomial infections. *Infection* 2005;**33**(1):3–8.
70. Wertheim HF, et al. The role of nasal carriage in *Staphylococcus aureus* infections. *Lancet Infect Dis* 2005;**5**(12):751–762.
71. Kuehnert MJ, et al. Methicillin-resistant-*Staphylococcus aureus* hospitalizations, United States. *Emerg Infect Dis* 2005;**11**(6):868–872.
72. Klevens RM, et al. Invasive methicillin-resistant *Staphylococcus aureus* infections in the United States. *JAMA* 2007;**298**(15):1763–1771.
73. Safdar N, et al. Comparison of culture screening methods for detection of nasal carriage of methicillin-resistant *Staphylococcus aureus*: A prospective study comparing 32 methods. *J Clin Microbiol* 2003;**41**(7):3163–3166.
74. Huletsky A, et al. Identification of methicillin-resistant *Staphylococcus aureus* carriage in less than 1 hour during a hospital surveillance program. *Clin Infect Dis* 2005;**40**(7):976–981.
75. Stamper PD, et al. Clinical validation of the molecular BD GeneOhm StaphSR assay for direct detection of *Staphylococcus aureus* and methicillin-resistant *Staphylococcus aureus* in positive blood cultures. *J Clin Microbiol* 2007;**45**(7):2191–2196.
76. Paule SM, et al. Performance of the BD GeneOhm methicillin-resistant *Staphylococcus aureus* test before and during high-volume clinical use. *J Clin Microbiol* 2007; **45**(9):2993–2998.
77. WHO. Global tuberculosis control—Surveillance, planning, financing. In *WHO/HTM/TB*. World Health Organization, Geneva, Switzerland, 2008, pp. 15–20.
78. Bennett CL, Hounshell JB, Chmiel JS. Hospital measures for prevention of tuberculosis transmission in U.S. cities with and without previous nosocomial tuberculosis outbreaks. *Ann Intern Med* 2000;**133**(6):486.
79. Guidelines for preventing the transmission of *Mycobacterium tuberculosis* in health-care facilities, 1994—CDC. Notice of final revisions to the "Guidelines for preventing the transmission of *Mycobacterium tuberculosis* in health-care facilities, 1994". *Fed Regist* 1994;**59** (208):54242–54303.
80. Control of tuberculosis transmission in health care settings. A joint statement of the International Union Against Tuberculosis and Lung Disease (IUATLD) and the Tuberculosis Programme of the World Health Organization (WHO). *Tuber Lung Dis* 1994; **75**(2):94–95.
81. McGowan JE, Jr. Resurgent nosocomial tuberculosis: Consequences and actions for hospital epidemiologists. *Infect Control Hosp Epidemiol* 1992;**13**(10):575–578.

82. Nosocomial transmission of multidrug-resistant tuberculosis to health-care workers and HIV-infected patients in an urban hospital—Florida. *MMWR Morb Mortal Wkly Rep* 1990;**39**(40):718–722.
83. Lee EH, et al. Nosocomial transmission of *Mycobacterium tuberculosis* in a children's hospital. *Int J Tuberc Lung Dis* 2005;**9**(6):689–692.
84. Musial CE, et al. Identification of mycobacteria from culture by using the Gen-Probe Rapid Diagnostic System for *Mycobacterium avium* complex and *Mycobacterium tuberculosis* complex. *J Clin Microbiol* 1988;**26**(10):2120–2123.
85. Chedore P, Jamieson FB. Rapid molecular diagnosis of tuberculous meningitis using the Gen-probe Amplified *Mycobacterium tuberculosis* direct test in a large Canadian public health laboratory. *Int J Tuberc Lung Dis* 2002;**6**(10):913–919.
86. O'Sullivan CE, et al. Evaluation of Gen-Probe amplified *Mycobacterium tuberculosis* direct test by using respiratory and nonrespiratory specimens in a tertiary care center laboratory. *J Clin Microbiol* 2002;**40**(5):1723–1727.
87. Chedore P, et al. False-positive amplified *Mycobacterium tuberculosis* direct test results for samples containing *Mycobacterium leprae*. *J Clin Microbiol* 2006;**44**(2):612–613.
88. Christiansen DC, Roberts GD, Patel R. *Mycobacterium celatum*, an emerging pathogen and cause of false positive amplified *Mycobacterium tuberculosis* direct test. *Diagn Microbiol Infect Dis* 2004;**49**(1):19–24.
89. Tjhie JH, et al. Misidentification and diagnostic delay caused by a false-positive amplified *Mycobacterium tuberculosis* direct test in an immunocompetent patient with a *Mycobacterium celatum* infection. *J Clin Microbiol* 2001;**39**(6):2311–2312.
90. Jorgensen JH, et al. False-positive Gen-Probe direct *Mycobacterium tuberculosis* amplification test results for patients with pulmonary *M. kansasii* and M. avium infections. *J Clin Microbiol* 1999;**37**(1):175–178.
91. Shrestha NK, et al. Predictive value and cost-effectiveness analysis of a rapid polymerase chain reaction for preoperative detection of nasal carriage of *Staphylococcus aureus*. *Infect Control Hosp Epidemiol* 2003;**24**(5):327–333.
92. Geuskens M, Ficq A. Detection of DNA by an autoradiographic method after "staining" with radioactive actinomycin D and high-resolution autoradiography. *Acta Histochem Suppl* 1968;**8**:135–136.
93. Rihn B, et al. Evaluation of non-radioactive labelling and detection of deoxyribonucleic acids. Part One: Chemiluminescent methods. *J Biochem Biophys Methods* 1995; **30**(2–3):91–102.
94. Dubitsky A, Brown J, Brandwein H. Chemiluminescent detection of DNA on nylon membranes. *Biotechniques* 1992;**13**(3):392–400.
95. Morgan AR, et al. Review: Ethidium fluorescence assays. Part 1. Physicochemical studies. *Nucleic Acids Res* 1979;**7**(3):547–569.
96. LePecq JB, Paoletti C. A fluorescent complex between ethidium bromide and nucleic acids. Physical–chemical characterization. *J Mol Biol* 1967;**27**(1):87–106.
97. Rye HS, et al. Stable fluorescent complexes of double-stranded DNA with bis-intercalating asymmetric cyanine dyes: Properties and applications. *Nucleic Acids Res* 1992;**20**(11): 2803–2812.
98. Chehab FF, Kan YW. Detection of specific DNA sequences by fluorescence amplification: A color complementation assay. *Proc Natl Acad Sci USA*, 1989;**86** (23):9178–9182.
99. Coutlee F, et al. Immunodetection of DNA with biotinylated RNA probes: A study of reactivity of a monoclonal antibody to DNA–RNA hybrids. *Anal Biochem* 1991;**198**(1):217.

100. Leary JJ, Brigati DJ, Ward DC. Rapid and sensitive colorimetric method for visualizing biotin-labeled DNA probes hybridized to DNA or RNA immobilized on nitrocellulose: Bio-blots. *Proc Natl Acad Sci USA*, 1983;**80**(13):4045–4049.

101. Rihn B, et al. Evaluation of non-radioactive labelling and detection of deoxyribonucleic acids. Part Two: Colorigenic methods and comparison with chemiluminescent methods. *J Biochem Biophys Methods*, 1995;**30**(2–3):103–112.

102. Kemp DJ, et al. Colorimetric detection of specific DNA segments amplified by polymerase chain reactions. *Proc Natl Acad Sci USA* 1989;**86**(7):2423–2427.

103. Blotta I, et al. Quantitative assay of total dsDNA with PicoGreen reagent and real-time fluorescent detection. *Ann Ist Super Sanita* 2005;**41**(1):119–123.

104. Ishiguro T, et al. Homogeneous quantitative assay of hepatitis C virus RNA by polymerase chain reaction in the presence of a fluorescent intercalater. *Anal Biochem* 1995;**229**(2):207–213.

105. Monis PT, Giglio S, Saint CP. Comparison of SYTO9 and SYBR Green I for real-time polymerase chain reaction and investigation of the effect of dye concentration on amplification and DNA melting curve analysis. *Anal Biochem* 2005;**340**(1):24–34.

106. Cheng JC, et al. Rapid detection and identification of clinically important bacteria by high-resolution melting analysis after broad-range ribosomal RNA real-time PCR. *Clin Chem* 2006;**52**(11):1997–2004.

107. Dames S, et al. Unlabeled probes for the detection and typing of herpes simplex virus. *Clin Chem* 2007;**53**(10):1847–1854.

108. Lin JH, et al. Rapid differentiation of influenza A virus subtypes and genetic screening for virus variants by high-resolution melting analysis. *J Clin Microbiol* 2008.

109. Bengtsson M, et al. A new minor groove binding asymmetric cyanine reporter dye for real-time PCR. *Nucleic Acids Res* 2003;**31**(8):e45.

110. Thomas LC, et al. Development of a real-time *Staphylococcus aureus* and MRSA (SAM-) PCR for routine blood culture. *J Microbiol Methods* 2007;**68**(2):296–302.

111. Horn P, Schouenborg PO, Brandslund I. Quantification of Staphylococcus aureus and Staphylococcus epidermidis on the hands of health-care workers using a real-time polymerase chain reaction method. *Scand J Clin Lab Invest* 2007;**67**(2):165–177.

112. Sakai H, et al. Simultaneous detection of Staphylococcus aureus and coagulase-negative staphylococci in positive blood cultures by real-time PCR with two fluorescence resonance energy transfer probe sets. *J Clin Microbiol* 2004;**42**(12):5739–5744.

113. Oberdorfer K, et al. Evaluation of a single-locus real-time polymerase chain reaction as a screening test for specific detection of methicillin-resistant *Staphylococcus aureus* in ICU patients. *Eur J Clin Microbiol Infect Dis* 2006;**25**(10):657–663.

114. Ornskov D, et al. Screening for methicillin-resistant *Staphylococcus aureus* in clinical swabs using a high-throughput real-time PCR-based method. *Clin Microbiol Infect* 2008;**14**(1):22–28.

115. Huletsky A, et al. New real-time PCR assay for rapid detection of methicillin-resistant *Staphylococcus aureus* directly from specimens containing a mixture of staphylococci. *J Clin Microbiol* 2004;**42**(5):1875–1884.

116. Hougardy N, Louahabi A, Goffinet P. Direct and fast detection of methicillin resistant *Staphylococcus aureus* carriage by automated nucleic acid extraction and real time PCR. *Pathol Biol (Paris)*, 2006;**54**(8–9):477–481.

117. Al-Mohri HA, et al. Utility of direct, real-time PCR in the management of a nosocomial outbreak of vancomycin-resistant *Enterococcus faecium* (*vanB* genotype). *Eur J Clin Microbiol Infect Dis* 2007.

118. Sloan LM, et al. Comparison of the Roche LightCycler vanA/vanB detection assay and culture for detection of vancomycin-resistant enterococci from perianal swabs. *J Clin Microbiol* 2004; **42**(6):2636–2643.
119. Stamper PD, et al. Comparison of the BD GeneOhm VanR assay to culture for identification of vancomycin-resistant enterococci in rectal and stool specimens. *J Clin Microbiol* 2007;**45** (10):3360–3365.
120. Palladino S, et al. Rapid detection of *vanA* and *vanB* genes directly from clinical specimens and enrichment broths by real-time multiplex PCR assay. *J Clin Microbiol* 2003;**41**(6):2483–2486.
121. Palladino S, et al. Real-time PCR for the rapid detection of *vanA* and *vanB* genes. *Diagn Microbiol Infect Dis* 2003;**45**(1):81–84.
122. Corless CE, et al. Development and evaluation of a "real-time" RT-PCR for the detection of enterovirus and parechovirus RNA in CSF and throat swab samples. *J Med Virol* 2002;**67** (4):555–562.
123. Van Gastel E, et al. Evaluation of a real-time polymerase chain reaction assay for the diagnosis of pneumococcal and meningococcal meningitis in a tertiary care hospital. *Eur J Clin Microbiol Infect Dis* 2007;**26**(9):651–653.
124. Carvalho Mda G, et al. Evaluation and improvement of real-time PCR assays targeting lytA, ply, and psaA genes for detection of pneumococcal DNA. *J Clin Microbiol* 2007;**45**(8):2460–2466.
125. Sheppard CL, et al. Autolysin-targeted LightCycler assay including internal process control for detection of *Streptococcus pneumoniae* DNA in clinical samples. *J Med Microbiol* 2004;**53** (Pt 3):189–195.
126. Jaffe RI, Lane JD, Bates CW. Real-time identification of *Pseudomonas aeruginosa* direct from clinical samples using a rapid extraction method and polymerase chain reaction (PCR). *J Clin Lab Anal*, 2001;**15**(3):131–137.
127. Motoshima M, et al. Rapid and accurate detection of *Pseudomonas aeruginosa* by real-time polymerase chain reaction with melting curve analysis targeting *gyrB* gene. *Diagn Microbiol Infect Dis* 2007;**58**(1):53–58.
128. Qin X, et al. Use of real-time PCR with multiple targets to identify *Pseudomonas aeruginosa* and other nonfermenting Gram-negative bacilli from patients with cystic fibrosis. *J Clin Microbiol* 2003;**41**(9):4312–4317.
129. Hinata N, et al. Quantitative detection of *Escherichia coli* from urine of patients with bacteriuria by real-time PCR. *Mol Diagn* 2004;**8**(3):179–184.
130. Straka M, et al. Rapid detection of group B streptococcus and *Escherichia coli* in amniotic fluid using real-time fluorescent PCR. *Infect Dis Obstet Gynecol* 2004;**12**(3–4):109–114.
131. Reischl U, et al. Real-time fluorescence PCR assays for detection and characterization of heat-labile I and heat-stable I enterotoxin genes from enterotoxigenic *Escherichia coli*. *J Clin Microbiol* 2004;**42**(9):4092–4100.
132. Bellin T, et al. Rapid detection of enterohemorrhagic *Escherichia coli* by real-time PCR with fluorescent hybridization probes. *J Clin Microbiol* 2001;**39**(1):370–374.
133. Pulz M, et al. Comparison of a shiga toxin enzyme-linked immunosorbent assay and two types of PCR for detection of shiga toxin-producing *Escherichia coli* in human stool specimens. *J Clin Microbiol* 2003;**41**(10):4671–4675.
134. Reischl U, et al. Real-time fluorescence PCR assays for detection and characterization of Shiga toxin, intimin, and enterohemolysin genes from Shiga toxin-producing *Escherichia coli*. *J Clin Microbiol* 2002;**40**(7):2555–2565.
135. Belanger SD, et al. Rapid detection of Shiga toxin-producing bacteria in feces by multiplex PCR with molecular beacons on the smart cycler. *J Clin Microbiol* 2002;**40**(4): 1436–1440.

136. Hsu CF, Tsai TY, Pan TM. Use of the duplex TaqMan PCR system for detection of Shiga-like toxin-producing *Escherichia coli* O157. *J Clin Microbiol* 2005;**43**(6):2668–2673.
137. Cleary TJ, et al. Rapid and specific detection of Mycobacterium tuberculosis by using the Smart Cycler instrument and a specific fluorogenic probe. *J Clin Microbiol* 2003;**41** (10):4783–4786.
138. Pounder JI, Aldous WK, Woods GL. Comparison of real-time polymerase chain reaction using the Smart Cycler and the Gen-Probe amplified *Mycobacterium tuberculosis* direct test for detection of M. tuberculosis complex in clinical specimens. *Diagn Microbiol Infect Dis* 2006;**54** (3):217–222.
139. Burggraf S, et al. Comparison of an internally controlled, large-volume LightCycler assay for detection of *Mycobacterium tuberculosis* in clinical samples with the COBAS AMPLICOR assay. *J Clin Microbiol* 2005;**43**(4):1564–1569.
140. Miller N, et al. Rapid and specific detection of *Mycobacterium tuberculosis* from acid-fast bacillus smear-positive respiratory specimens and BacT/ALERT MP culture bottles by using fluorogenic probes and real-time PCR. *J Clin Microbiol* 2002;**40**(11):4143–4147.
141. Drosten C, Panning M, Kramme S. Detection of *Mycobacterium tuberculosis* by real-time PCR using pan-mycobacterial primers and a pair of fluorescence resonance energy transfer probes specific for the *M. tuberculosis* complex. *Clin Chem* 2003;**49**(10):1659–1661.
142. Peterson LR, et al. Detection of toxigenic *Clostridium difficile* in stool samples by real-time polymerase chain reaction for the diagnosis of C. difficile-associated diarrhea. *Clin Infect Dis* 2007;**45**(9):1152–1160.
143. van den Berg RJ, et al. Rapid diagnosis of toxinogenic *Clostridium difficile* in faecal samples with internally controlled real-time PCR. *Clin Microbiol Infect* 2006;**12**(2):184–186.
144. van den Berg RJ, et al. Evaluation of real-time PCR and conventional diagnostic methods for the detection of *Clostridium difficile*-associated diarrhoea in a prospective multicentre study. *J Med Microbiol* 2007;**56**(Pt 1): 36–42.
145. Belanger SD, et al. Rapid detection of *Clostridium difficile* in feces by real-time PCR. *J Clin Microbiol* 2003;**41**(2):730–734.
146. Kurupati P, et al. Rapid detection of Klebsiella pneumoniae from blood culture bottles by real-time PCR. *J Clin Microbiol* 2004;**42**(3):1337–1340.
147. Wellinghausen N, et al. Algorithm for the identification of bacterial pathogens in positive blood cultures by real-time LightCycler polymerase chain reaction (PCR) with sequence-specific probes. *Diagn Microbiol Infect Dis* 2004;**48**(4):229–241.
148. Diederen BM, et al. Utility of real-time PCR for diagnosis of Legionnaires' disease in routine clinical practice. *J Clin Microbiol* 2008;**46**(2):671–677.
149. Diederen BM, et al. Evaluation of real-time PCR for the early detection of Legionella pneumophila DNA in serum samples. *J Med Microbiol* 2007;**56**(Pt 1): 94–101.
150. Loens K, et al. Development of conventional and real-time NASBA for the detection of *Legionella* species in respiratory specimens. *J Microbiol Methods* 2006;**67**(3):408–415.
151. Hayden RT, et al. Direct detection of Legionella species from bronchoalveolar lavage and open lung biopsy specimens: comparison of LightCycler PCR, *in situ* hybridization, direct fluorescence antigen detection, and culture. *J Clin Microbiol* 2001;**39** (7):2618–2626.
152. Herpers BL, et al. Real-time PCR assay targets the 23S-5S spacer for direct detection and differentiation of *Legionella* spp. and *Legionella pneumophila*. *J Clin Microbiol* 2003;**41** (10):4815–4816.
153. Templeton KE, et al. Development and clinical evaluation of an internally controlled, single-tube multiplex real-time PCR assay for detection of *Legionella pneumophila* and other *Legionella* species. *J Clin Microbiol* 2003;**41**(9):4016–4021.

154. Wilson DA, et al. Detection of *Legionella pneumophila* by real-time PCR for the mip gene. *J Clin Microbiol* 2003;**41**(7):3327–3330.

155. Reischl U, et al. Direct detection and differentiation of *Legionella* spp. and *Legionella pneumophila* in clinical specimens by dual-color real-time PCR and melting curve analysis. *J Clin Microbiol* 2002;**40**(10):3814–3817.

156. Rantakokko-Jalava K, Jalava J. Development of conventional and real-time PCR assays for detection of *Legionella* DNA in respiratory specimens. *J Clin Microbiol* 2001;**39**(8):2904–2910.

157. Schabereiter-Gurtner C, et al. Development of novel real-time PCR assays for detection and differentiation of eleven medically important *Aspergillus* and *Candida* species in clinical specimens. *J Clin Microbiol* 2007;**45**(3):906–914.

158. Baskova L, et al. The Pan-AC assay: A single-reaction real-time PCR test for quantitative detection of a broad range of *Aspergillus* and *Candida* species. *J Med Microbiol* 2007;**56**(Pt 9): 1167–1173.

159. Pryce TM, et al. Real-time automated polymerase chain reaction (PCR) to detect *Candida albicans* and *Aspergillus fumigatus* DNA in whole blood from high-risk patients. *Diagn Microbiol Infect Dis* 2003;**47**(3):487–496.

160. Spiess B, et al. Development of a LightCycler PCR assay for detection and quantification of *Aspergillus fumigatus* DNA in clinical samples from neutropenic patients. *J Clin Microbiol* 2003;**41**(5):1811–1818.

161. Rantakokko-Jalava K, et al. Semiquantitative detection by real-time PCR of *Aspergillus fumigatus* in bronchoalveolar lavage fluids and tissue biopsy specimens from patients with invasive aspergillosis. *J Clin Microbiol* 2003;**41**(9):4304–4311.

162. Selvarangan R, et al. Rapid identification of commonly encountered *Candida* species directly from blood culture bottles. *J Clin Microbiol* 2003;**41**(12):5660–5664.

163. Innings A, et al. Multiplex real-time PCR targeting the RNase P RNA gene for detection and identification of *Candida* species in blood. *J Clin Microbiol* 2007;**45**(3):874–880.

CHAPTER EIGHT

Restriction Analysis Techniques

RICHARD V. GOERING, MARY E. STEMPER,
SANJAY K. SHUKLA, AND STEVEN L. FOLEY

Introduction

Historically, the epidemiological evaluation of healthcare-associated infection has relied on modifications of phenotypic analyses, discussed elsewhere in this book, which have traditionally served as the basis for microbial identification and taxonomic classification. However, the advent of molecular biology brought with it increasing realization that all phenotypic analyses generally suffer from the disadvantage that observable characteristics represent an expression of underlying genotype several molecular levels removed from the true genetic identity of the organism. Thus, based on the principle that the "chromosome" is the most fundamental molecule of identity in the cell, techniques originally developed in the molecular biology laboratory began to find application in clinically relevant areas, including epidemiological analysis (1, 2). This chapter explores a subset of those methods, concentrating on techniques employing restriction enzymes and electrophoretic analysis with specific reference to problem bacterial pathogens. One of the restriction-enzyme analysis methods that plays a vital role in many investigations of nosocomial infections is pulsed-field gel electrophoresis (PFGE) and is covered in extensive detail in chapter 9.

Molecular Techniques for the Study of Hospital-Acquired Infection, First Edition. Edited by Steven L. Foley, Anne Y. Chen, Shabbir Simjee, and Marcus J. Zervos.

Chromosomal Restriction-Enzyme Analysis (REA)

Conceptually, REA is a very straightforward approach to epidemiological typing. Chromosomal DNA is purified by relatively simple (e.g., kit-based) methods from isolates of interest. The DNA is digested with one of several commonly available restriction enzymes (e.g., *Eco*RI, *Hin*dIII, etc.). The resulting chromosomal restriction fragments are then separated by conventional agarose-gel electrophoresis to yield a pattern which, based on the spatial distribution of restriction sites around the chromosome, represents a genomic "fingerprint" of the organism which can be compared with other isolates as an indicator of potential relatedness. The method is attractive in its simplicity and potential widespread

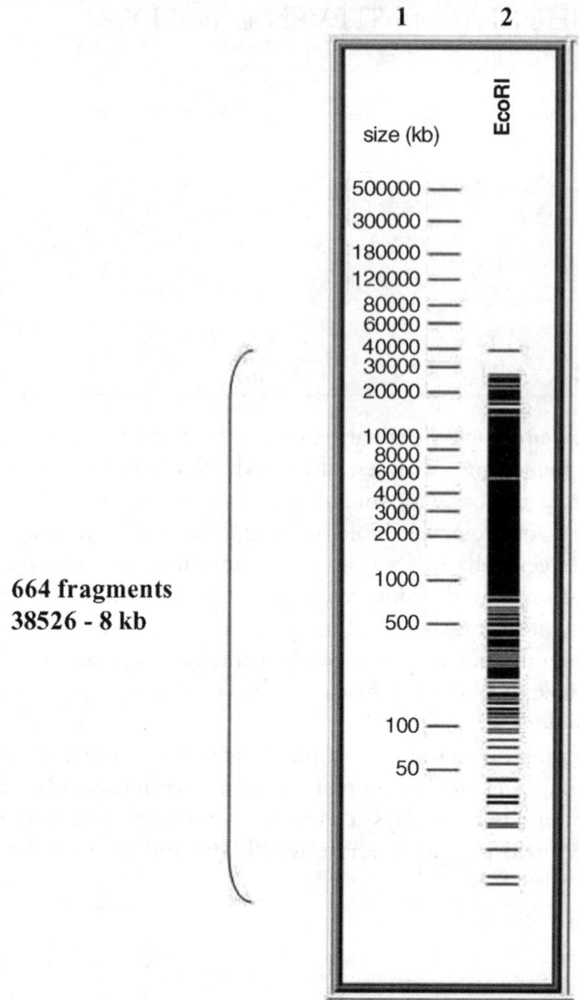

FIGURE 8.1 Diagrammatic representation of REA with *S. aureus* USA300-FPR3757 chromosomal DNA digested with the restriction enzyme *Eco*RI. Data were generated by output from the Comprehensive Microbial Resource section of the J. Craig Venter Institute web site: http://cmr.jcvi.org/tigr-scripts/CMR/CmrHomePage.cgi.

application since the chromosome represents an essential feature of all bacterial pathogens. In experienced hands, REA is a useful approach to assessing isolate interrelationships (e.g., *Clostridium difficile*, *Enterococcus faecium*, etc.) (3–6). However, as shown in Figure 8.1, digesting a 2 to 3 Mb bacterial chromosome (e.g., *Staphylococcus aureus* USA300-FPR3757) with a frequent-cutting restriction enzyme may generate >600 fragments. During electrophoresis, considerable potential exists for bands of similar size to cluster and comigrate — a challenge for accurate pattern-to-pattern comparison (e.g., what constitutes a significant difference) and nomenclature. In addition, REA patterns do not readily lend themselves to database storage and sharing between laboratories.

REA and Plasmid Analysis

One of the most important methodological discoveries of molecular biology has been the ability to rapidly and inexpensively analyze bacterial cells for plasmid content by agarose gel electrophoresis (7). While initially developed to monitor the results of recombinant DNA cloning experiments, the method has also been used to analyze plasmid carriage in clinical bacterial isolates (8–10). For epidemiological analysis the rationale has been that related isolates would likely exhibit the same plasmid content. However, plasmids are "molecular transients" in the cell that may be gained, lost, and otherwise rearranged over time, presenting difficulties regarding data interpretation. In addition, similar plasmid agarose-gel profiles in different bacterial isolates do not automatically equate with identical plasmid carriage, only indicating that the plasmids are of similar size. This issue is partially addressed when the plasmid DNA is subjected to restriction-enzyme digestion prior to electrophoresis which, as with chromosomal analysis, yields sequence-based patterns determined by restriction-site distribution. However, cells containing large plasmids may generate restriction-fragment numbers that still represent a challenge to interpret. Beyond this, plasmid analysis (with or without REA) does not address the most fundamental epidemiological question of isolate chromosomal relatedness. In addition, some clinical isolates may carry only one or no detectable plasmids, thus further limiting the overall utility of this approach for assessing epidemiological relatedness.

REA and Probes

One of the most important techniques to emerge from the molecular biology laboratory has been the use of DNA probes. The understanding that "target" DNA molecules could be denatured to single-stranded form, immobilized on a surface and then queried for a specific sequence by hybridization with a labeled single-stranded DNA probe, was a revolutionary scientific milestone (11). In recent years, commercial probe-based methods have found multiple clinical applications, especially in the area of diagnostics. In a related manner, protocols have been developed combining REA with probes aimed at examining specific subsets of chromosomal fragments for potentially useful information regarding isolate interrelationships. As shown in Figure 8.2, in its most common application, genomic DNA is digested with a frequent-cutting restriction enzyme as for REA. However, after electrophoresis, the resulting fragment pattern is transferred (also referred to as blotting) *in situ* to a nitrocellulose or nylon membrane in a manner that preserves the spatial distribution of the fragments in a denatured (i.e., single-stranded) state (11). The transferred

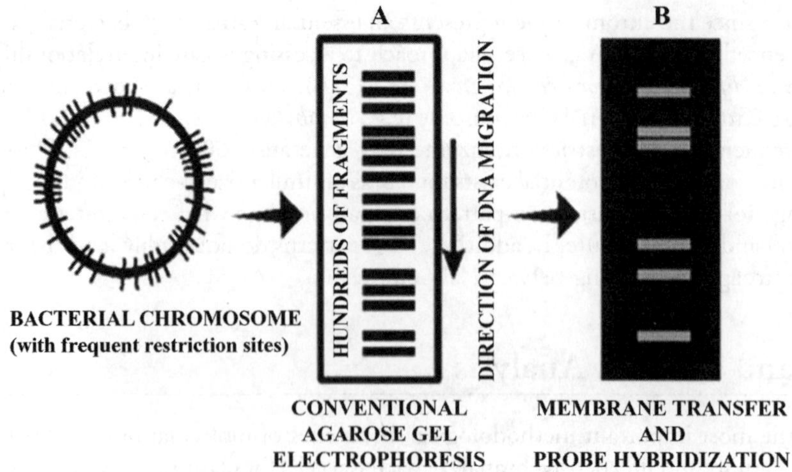

FIGURE 8.2 **Diagrammatic representation of REA with further analysis using a probe and Southern hybridization.**

(membrane-bound) DNA pattern is then queried utilizing an appropriate single-stranded DNA sequence (i.e., probe) complementary to one found at multiple locations on the bacterial chromosome and thus on different restriction fragments. Under proper conditions, the probe (labeled either colorimetrically or radioactively) hybridizes to its chromosomal complements, resulting in banding patterns [restriction fragment-length polymorphisms (RFLPs)] that are visualized based on the probe label. Thus, the discriminatory power of this method is directly related to the copy number and distribution of the targeted sequence around the bacterial chromosome. Issues of nomenclature and pattern-to-pattern comparison, noted above for REA, potentially also apply to REA–probe combinations. Thus, in its classic form this approach is currently not widely used in the epidemiological analysis of healthcare-associated pathogens. However, an interesting exception is the usefulness of REA with probes for the insertion sequence IS*6110* in the epidemiological analysis of *Mycobacterium tuberculosis* (12, 13). Probes have also been employed with REA of plasmids (see above), although this application most commonly relates to investigating plasmid carriage and transfer of specific genes (e.g., for antibiotic resistance) (14–16) rather than to studies of bacterial epidemiological relatedness. An additional commonly used application of REA and Southern hybridization involves analysis of variation in bacterial ribosomal RNA (rRNA) genes as a measure of epidemiological relatedness. Ribotyping is more fully explored in the following section.

Ribotyping

Ribotyping takes advantage of the fact that bacteria typically contain multiple rRNA gene copies (i.e., 1–15) distributed at different locations around the bacterial chromosome. Isolate-to-isolate sequence differences in neutral housekeeping genes flanking rRNA genes may affect restriction-enzyme recognition sites producing different RFLP hybridization patterns with rRNA probes (17). Ribotyping has been utilized to genotype a wide array of pathogens that have been associated with hospital-acquired infections. These include *E. coli, K. pneumoniae, A. baumanii, Enterobacter* spp., *L. pneumophila, Pseudomonas* spp., *Moraxella catarrhalis, Enterococcus* spp., *Streptococcus* spp., and *Staphylococcus* spp. The basic procedural elements of ribotyping begin with the isolation of total cellular DNA from the isolate being analyzed. The DNA is restricted with a frequent cutting enzyme, such as *Eco*RI, *Pst*I, *Hind*III, *Sma*I, and *Pvu*II (18). The DNA fragments are separated by electrophoresis and the restriction fragments are transferred to a nylon membrane and incubated with a probe that is targeted to the conserved regions of rRNA operon (19). Some ribotyping schemes utilize probes that will target regions of the 16S rRNA genes, while others also probe for sequences of the 5S and/or 23S rRNA genes as well (18). Restriction fragments containing the conserved regions of an rRNA gene will be detected and provide a profile that can be used to genotype strains. Differences in band sizes are due to the number of rRNA gene sequences present and the location of restriction sites adjacent to the rRNA gene (20, 21).

For larger clinical diagnostic laboratory settings, it may be feasible to utilize an automated ribotyping system, such as the RiboPrinter Microbial Characterization System (Qualicon, Inc., Wilmington, DE). Automated systems reduce the number of manual steps, which helps to improve reproducibility and reduces labor costs. With the RiboPrinter, the laboratory personal prepares the initial cell suspensions and loads them into the instrument for cell lysis, restriction digestion, electrophoresis, and Southern blotting. The resultant DNA fingerprints are processed and the banding profiles are prepared for importation into an analysis program such as BioNumerics. The overall advantages of using the Riboprinter System must be weighed against disadvantages, including increased cost and potentially reduced discrimination due to DNA fragment comigration resulting from the short agarose gel lengths employed (17). Overall, the discriminatory ability of ribotyping appears to be lower than PFGE and some of the PCR-based methods. This is especially true in bacterial species with fewer rRNA operons in the genome. Typically, the sensitivity of ribotyping using a single restriction enzyme corresponds to the results obtained by serotyping in enteric pathogens (22). Another potential difficulty that may be encountered in difference strains is that if a bacterial genome is modified by methylation, there will be poor restriction of the genomic DNA leading to little or no band separation (23).

REA and PCR

The above discussion has centered on approaches to molecular typing based on REA as the "foundation" protocol. However, restriction enzymes may also be useful for analyzing chromosomal sequence subsets rather than total genomic DNA. In this regard, PCR is commonly used as a first step with specific amplicons further analyzed by REA to generate RFLP patterns with potential epidemiologic application (i.e., PCR–RFLP analysis) (24–27). Another method for the characterization of nosocomial pathogens that relies on a combination of restriction digest analysis and PCR to distinguish among unrelated strains is amplified fragment-length polymorphism (AFLP). AFLP is described in detail in the following section.

Amplified Fragment-Length Polymorphism

Amplified fragment-length polymorphism (AFLP) is a method that combines restriction digest analysis and PCR to distinguish among unrelated strains. ALFP has been used successfully to type a wide range of bacterial pathogens, including the Gram negative pathogens *E. coli*, *Klebsiella pneumoniae*, *Acinetobacter baumannii*, *Legionella pneumophila*, and *Pseudomonas aeruginosa* as well as the Gram positives *Enterococcus* spp., *Streptococcus* spp., and *Staphylococcus* spp.

In AFLP analysis, the bacterial DNA is isolated and frequent cutting restriction enzymes, often *Eco*RI and *Mse*I, are used to restrict the genome into a large number of fragments. Following restriction, there typically are too many fragments to resolve by standard electrophoresis; thus a second set of procedures is used to reduce the number and increase the signal strength of fragments for analysis. This signal amplification occurs by ligating short adapter or linker sequences containing sequence complementary to the restriction enzyme overhangs on the free ends of the restriction fragments (Figure 8.3). D'Agata et al. (28) used the adapters, 5′-CTCGTAGACTGCGTACC-3′ and 5′-AATTGG-TACGCAGTCTAC-3′ for the *Eco*RI restriction ends and used 5′-GACGATGAGTCCT-GAG-3′ and 5′-GACTGCGTACCAATTCA-3′ for the *Mse*I ends (28). The adapters serve as templates for PCR primer binding which is used to originate product amplification. The PCR primers that are complementary to the linker sequence typically contain one or more additional bases at their 3′ end that interact with the restriction fragment sequence adjacent to the linker sequence. In the procedure evaluated by D'Agata et al. (28), an *Eco*RI-adapter targeted primer (5′ GACTGCGTACCAATTCA-3′) was used for each species examined. Separate *Mse*I adapter targeted primers (5′-ACGATGAGTCCTGAGTC-3′) were used for *P. aeruginosa* and *A. baumannii* and (5′-GATGAGTCCTGAGTAAC-3′) *Enterococcus* spp. (28). The inclusion of additional template-independent bases on the primer serves to cut down on the number of products that are amplified. The PCR process is carried out with very high stringency, which prevents amplification from primers with imperfect matches. The result is that for each additional base added to the primer, the number of PCR products is reduced by an average of four (29).

The resultant PCR products are separated to generate an amplification product profile that can be used to genotype the isolates (30, 31). A frequent modification to the basic AFLP procedure is the use of PCR primers containing a fluorescent tag, which is often referred to as fluorescent-AFLP (f-AFLP). Following PCR, the fluorescent-labeled products can be separated using an automated DNA sequencer containing fragment analysis software. During separation, an internal size standard is typically included in each of the PCR product mixes that allows for enhanced ability to compare the profiles and improved phylogenetic analysis (32). A potential drawback of AFLP in a healthcare setting laboratory is access to an automated DNA sequencer for efficient. This characteristic has probably limited the utility of this method in clinical molecular epidemiology. However, as more laboratories begin to utilize 16S rRNA gene sequencing for pathogen identification, the DNA sequencer may become more readily available to them. One of the attractions of AFLP over a method such as PFGE is that the time from bacterial isolation to genotype results is reduced, which may be useful in trying to identify pathogen transmission characteristics and ultimately limit disease outbreaks within the healthcare setting (33, 34).

There have been a number of studies that have evaluated the use of AFLP for bacterial typing. In the healthcare setting, Fontana et al. (35) used f-AFLP in combination with a computer-based epidemiological monitoring system. The software system was used to monitor clinical laboratory data and alert hospital personnel of potential hospital-acquired infections that would require further attention. When likely outbreak(s) occurred, f-AFLP was used successfully to identify members of specific outbreaks. The study found that f-AFLP appeared to work well for typing Gram-negative organisms such as *P. aeruginosa*, ESBL-producing *E. coli*, *K. pneumoniae*, and *Enterobacter cloacae* and Gram-positive

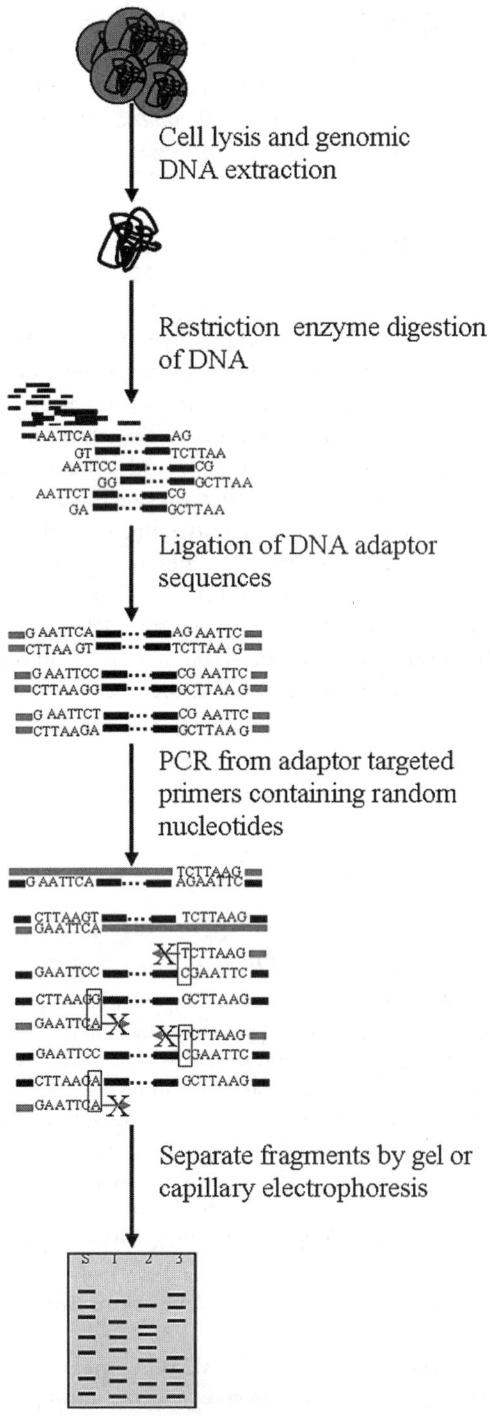

FIGURE 8.3 Major procedural steps to carry out amplified fragment-length polymorphism (AFLP) analysis. The, "X" represents restriction fragments where PCR amplification failed due to a mismatch of the PCR primers contain added base(s) that were not complementary to the template sequence. Adapted from Foley et al. (36).

organisms such as *E. faecium* and *S. epidermidis* and the fungal pathogen *Candida parapsilosis* (35). In another study when f-AFLP was compared to PFGE in clinical epidemiological investigation of *P. aeruginosa*, *E. faecium*, and *A. baumanii* (28) both methods worked well for *P. aeruginosa* and *A. baumanii*. However, PFGE had a higher discriminatory ability than f-AFLP for *E. faecium*.

REA Analysis and the Future

The number of bacterial pathogens with totally sequenced chromosomes is growing at an amazing rate. These data are driving important new sequence-based approaches to the epidemiological analysis of healthcare-associated infections. However, REA-based methods will likely continue to have an important potential role in outbreak investigation. This is due, in part, to the fact that all epidemiological analysis operates within the confines of the available epidemiological window where rarely, if ever, does the index organism or case readily identify itself. Thus, no matter how sophisticated the strain typing technology, the fact remains that one is attempting to determine probable cause, transmission, etc., with an incomplete dataset. In this regard, having a visual overview of isolate relatedness may provide information and insight not as readily available by other methods including sequence-based approaches. Nevertheless, the value of any approach to molecular typing, including REA-based approaches, is not as a stand-alone method but rather as part of an overall investigation that includes all available molecular, clinical, and epidemiological data and has the greatest chance of achieving a reliable and clinically useful answer.

REFERENCES

1. Goering RV. The molecular epidemiology of nosocomial infection: Past, present, and future. *Rev Med Microbiol* 2000;**11**:145–152.
2. Singh A, Goering RV, Simjee S, Foley SL, Zervos MJ. Application of molecular techniques to the study of hospital infection. *Clin Microbiol Rev* 2006;**19**:512–530.
3. Killgore G, Thompson A, Johnson S, Brazier J, Kuijper E, Pepin J, et al. Comparison of seven techniques for typing international epidemic strains of *Clostridium difficile*: Restriction endonuclease analysis, pulsed-field gel electrophoresis, PCR-ribotyping, multilocus sequence typing, multilocus variable-number tandem-repeat analysis, amplified fragment length polymorphism, and surface layer protein A gene sequence typing. *J Clin Microbiol* 2008;**46**:431–437.
4. Mikasova E, Oravcova K, Kaclikova E, Kuchta T, Drahovska H. Typing of food-borne *Listeria monocytogenes* by polymerase chain reaction-restriction enzyme analysis and amplified fragment length polymorphism. *New Microbiol* 2005;**28**:265–270.
5. Price CS, Huynh H, Paule S, Hollis RJ, Noskin GA, Pfaller MA, et al. Comparison of an automated ribotyping system to restriction endonuclease analysis and pulsed-field gel electrophoresis for differentiating vancomycin-resistant *Enterococcus faecium* isolates. *J Clin Microbiol* 2002;**40**:1858–1861.
6. Savor C, Pfaller MA, Kruszynski JA, Hollis RJ, Noskin GA, Peterson LR. Comparison of genomic methods for differentiating strains of *Enterococcus faecium*: assessment using clinical epidemiologic data. *J Clin Microbiol* 1998;**36**:3327–3331.
7. Meyers JA, Sanchez D, Elwell LP, Falkow S. Simple agarose gel electrophoretic method for the identification and characterization of plasmid deoxyribonucleic acid. *J Bacteriol* 1976;**127**:1529–1537.

8. Kropec A, Hubner J, Daschner FD. Comparison of three typing methods in hospital outbreaks of *Acinetobacter calcoaceticus* infection. *J Hosp Infect* 1993;**23**:133–141.
9. Schaberg DR, Tompkins LS, Falkow S. Use of agarose gel electrophoresis of plasmid deoxyribonucleic acid to fingerprint gram-negative bacilli. *J Clin Microbiol* 1981;**13**:1105–1108.
10. Taylor DN, Wachsmuth IK, Shangkuan YH, Schmidt EV, Barrett TJ, Schrader JS, et al. Salmonellosis associated with marijuana: A multistate outbreak traced by plasmid fingerprinting. *N Engl J Med* 1982;**306**:1249–1253.
11. Southern EM. Detection of specific sequences among DNA fragments separated by gel electrophoresis. *J Mol Biol* 1975;**98**:503–517.
12. Farnia P, Masjedi MR, Varahram M, Mirsaeidi M, Ahmadi M, Khazampour M, et al. The recent-transmission of *Mycobacterium tuberculosis* strains among Iranian and Afghan relapse cases: A DNA-fingerprinting using RFLP and spoligotyping. *BMC Infect Dis* 2008;**8**:109.
13. Phyu S, Stavrum R, Lwin T, Svendsen OS, Ti T, Grewal HM. Predominance of *Mycobacterium tuberculosis* EAI and Beijing lineages in Yangon, Myanmar. *J Clin Microbiol* 2009;**47**:335–344.
14. Girlich D, Poirel L, Leelaporn A, Karim A, Tribuddharat C, Fennewald M, et al. Molecular epidemiology of the integron-located VEB-1 extended-spectrum beta-lactamase in nosocomial enterobacterial isolates in Bangkok, Thailand. *J Clin Microbiol* 2001;**39**:175–182.
15. Markovska R, Schneider I, Keuleyan E, Sredkova M, Ivanova D, Markova B, et al. Extended-spectrum beta-lactamase-producing Enterobacteriaceae in Bulgarian hospitals. *Microb Drug Resist* 2008;**14**:119–128.
16. Mulvey MR, Susky E, McCracken M, Morck DW, Read RR. Similar cefoxitin-resistance plasmids circulating in *Escherichia coli* from human and animal sources. *Vet Microbiol* 2009;**134**:279–287.
17. Bouchet V, Huot H, Goldstein R. Molecular genetic basis of ribotyping. *Clin Microbiol Rev* 2008;**21**:262–273.
18. Bingen EH, Denamur E, Elion J. Use of ribotyping in epidemiological surveillance of nosocomial outbreaks. *Clin Microbiol Rev* 1994;**7**:311–327.
19. Chisholm SA, Crichton PB, Knight HI, Old DC. Molecular typing of *Salmonella* serotype Thompson strains isolated from human and animal sources. *Epidemiol. Infect* 1999;**122**:33–39.
20. Gendel SM, Ulaszek J. Ribotype analysis of strain distribution in *Listeria monocytogenes*. *J Food Prot* 2000;**63**:179–185.
21. Snipes KP, Hirsh DC, Kasten RW, Hansen LM, Hird DW, Carpenter TE, et al. Use of an rRNA probe and restriction endonuclease analysis to fingerprint *Pasteurella multocida* isolated from turkeys and wildlife. *J Clin Microbiol* 1989;**27**:1847–1853.
22. Kumao T, Ba-Thein W, Hayashi H. Molecular subtyping methods for detection of *Salmonella enterica* serovar Oranienburg outbreaks. *J Clin Microbiol* 2002;**40**:2057–2061.
23. Olive DM, Bean P. Principles and applications of methods for DNA-based typing of microbial organisms. *J Clin Microbiol* 1999;**37**:1661–1669.
24. Nishimura M, Nukina M, Yuan JM, Shen BQ, Ma JJ, Ohta M, et al. PCR-based restriction fragment length polymorphism (RFLP) analysis and serotyping of *Campylobacter jejuni* isolates from diarrheic patients in China and Japan. *FEMS Microbiol Lett* 1996;**142**:133–138.
25. de la Puente Redondo VA, Navas Mendez J, Garcia del Blanco N, Ladron Boronat N, Gutierrez Martin CB, Rodriguez Ferri EF. Typing of *Haemophilus parasuis* strains by PCR-RFLP analysis of the *tbpA* gene. *Vet Microbiol* 2003;**92**:253–262.
26. Shima K, Kawamura N, Hinenoya A, Sugimoto N, Wu Y, Asakura M, et al. Rapid culture-free identification and molecular typing of Shiga toxin-producing *Escherichia coli* by PCR-RFLP. *Microbiol Immunol* 2008;**52**:310–313.

27. Waleron M, Waleron K, Podhajska AJ, Lojkowska E. Genotyping of bacteria belonging to the former *Erwinia* genus by PCR-RFLP analysis of a *recA* gene fragment. *Microbiology* 2002;**148**:583–595.

28. D'Agata EM, Gerrits MM, Tang YW, Samore M, Kusters JG. Comparison of pulsed-field gel electrophoresis and amplified fragment-length polymorphism for epidemiological investigations of common nosocomial pathogens. *Infect. Control Hosp. Epidemiol.* 2001;**22**:550–554.

29. Savelkoul PH, Aarts HJ, de Haas J, Dijkshoorn L, Duim B, Otsen M, et al. Amplified-fragment length polymorphism analysis: the state of an art. *J. Clin. Microbiol.* 1999;**37**:3083–3091.

30. Mueller UG, Wolfenbarger LL. AFLP genotyping and fingerprinting. *Trends Ecol. Evolut.* 1999;**14**:389–394.

31. Vos P, Hogers R, Bleeker M, Reijans M, van de Lee T, Hornes M, et al. AFLP: a new technique for DNA fingerprinting. *Nucleic Acids Res* 1995;**23**:4407–4414.

32. Tamada Y, Nakaoka Y, Nishimori K, Doi A, Kumaki T, Uemura N, et al. Molecular typing and epidemiological study of *Salmonella enterica* serotype Typhimurium isolates from cattle by fluorescent amplified-fragment length polymorphism fingerprinting and pulsed-field gel electrophoresis. *J Clin Microbiol* 2001;**39**:1057–1066.

33. Lindstedt BA, Heir E, Vardund T, Kapperud G. Fluorescent amplified-fragment length polymorphism genotyping of *Salmonella enterica* subsp. *enterica serovars* and comparison with pulsed-field gel electrophoresis typing. *J. Clin. Microbiol.* 2000;**38**:1623–1627.

34. Scott F, Threlfall J, Stanley J, Arnold C. Fluorescent amplified fragment length polymorphism genotyping of *Salmonella* Enteritidis: a method suitable for rapid outbreak recognition. *Clin. Microbiol. Infect.* 2001;**7**:479–485.

35. Fontana C, Favaro M, Pistoia ES, Minelli S, Bossa MC, Altieri A, et al. The combined use of VIGI@ct (bioMerieux) and fluorescent amplified length fragment polymorphisms in the investigation of potential outbreaks. *J. Hosp. Infect.* 2007;**66**:262–268.

36. Foley SL, Zhao S, Walker RD. Molecular typing methods for the discrimination of *Salmonella* foodborne pathogens. *Foodborne Pathogens and Diseases.* 2007;**4**:253–276.

CHAPTER NINE

Pulsed-Field Gel Electrophoresis

MARY E. STEMPER, STEVEN L. FOLEY, RICHARD V. GOERING, AND SANJAY K. SHUKLA

Introduction

Nosocomial infections are a serious concern in modern hospitals, and infection control practitioners are constantly challenged to minimize the potential of cross-transmission among patients and from healthcare providers. In order to accomplish this, they primarily rely on diagnostic microbiology laboratories to determine the source(s) of an outbreak or infection in patients. In other words, they seek to determine whether a patient, a healthcare provider, or a hospital environment is the source of infection(s) in other patients over a short- or long-term period of time in their institution. Monitoring this transmission dynamic is complicated because the standard and policies of healthcare practices vary among individuals and hospitals. A number of tools are available to microbiology laboratories to determine how two bacterial strains are related to each other in a given space and time. These approaches include comparing biochemical profiles, antimicrobial susceptibility patterns, and more recently the use of pulsed-field gel electrophoresis (PFGE). In PFGE, genomic DNA patterns of two strains are compared to determine how similar or dissimilar their patterns are, thereby characterizing them as related, somewhat related, or unrelated. It is often considered a gold standard for typing of bacterial pathogens because it is relatively straightforward in its approach, use, and interpretation.

PFGE is the most common epidemiological typing method for healthcare-associated bacteria because of its utility for a broad range of pathogens (see Table 9.1

Molecular Techniques for the Study of Hospital-Acquired Infection, First Edition. Edited by Steven L. Foley, Anne Y. Chen, Shabbir Simjee, and Marcus J. Zervos.

TABLE 9.1 Optimal conditions for specific nosocomial agents based on current literature[a]

Organism	Plug preparation and lytic enzymes[a]	Lysis buffer[b]	Restriction enzymes
Methicillin-resistant *Staphylococcus aureus*	Harvest cells from ON growth on BAP, resuspend, add lysostaphin and 1% Gold agarose	EC and ESP	*Sma*I
Coagulase-negative *Staphylococcus*	Harvest cells from ON growth in BHI or LB, resuspend, add lysostaphin, lysozyme, and 1% Gold agarose	EC and ESP	*Sma*I
Vancomycin-resistant *Enterococcus*	Harvest cells from ON growth in BHI or LB, resuspend, add lysozyme, mutanolysin, and 1% Gold agarose	EC and ESP	*Sma*I
Clostridium difficile	Harvest cells from ON growth in BHI in anaerobic conditions, resuspend, add Lysostaphin, lysozyme and 1% Gold agarose containing 1% SDS	EC and ESP	*Sma*I[c]
Escherichia coli	Harvest cells from ON growth on BAP, resuspend, add proteinase K and 1% Gold agarose containing 1% SDS	ESP	*Xba*1, *Bln*I, or *Spe*1
Klebsiella sp.	Harvest cells from ON growth on BAP, resuspend, add 1% Gold agarose containing 1% SDS	ESP	*Xba*1
Acinetobacter sp.	Harvest cells from ON growth on BAP, resuspend, add 1% Gold agarose containing 1% SDS	ESP	*Sma*I, *Apa*1
Pseudomonas aeruginosa	Harvest cells from ON growth on BAP, resuspend, add proteinase K and 1% Gold agarose containing 1% SDS	ESP	*Spe*1[c]
Mycobacterium tuberculosis	Harvest cells from 2 to 3 week 7H9 broth with 10% ADC, freeze and thaw pelleted cells, resuspend, and add 1% Gold agarose	ESP	*Ase*I, *Spe*I, or *Xba*I

[a] ON = overnight, BAP = blood agar plate, LB = Luria broth, SDS = sodium dodecyl sulfate, ADC = acid-albumin-dextrose-catalase.
[b] EC = EC buffer, ESP = Proteinase K buffer.
[c] Running buffer containing 200 uM thiourea minimizes degradation of DNA during the electrophoresis.

Note: References for the pathogen-specific PFGE procedures include: Arbeit et al. (22) (*E. coli*); Bannerman et al. (2) (*S. aureus*); Barrett et al. (23) (*E. coli*); D'Agata et al. (24) (multiple); Donabedian et al. (25) (*Enterococcus*); Fawley and Wilcox (26) (*C. difficile*); Goering and Winter (27) (multiple); Gouby et al. (28) (*A. baumannii*); Hansen et al. (29) (*Klebsiella*); Hughes et al. (30) (multiple); Kato et al. (31) (*C. difficile*); Klaassen et al. (32) (*C. difficile*); Kristjánsson et al. (33) (*C. difficile*); Macfarlane et al. (34) (*S. aureus*); McDougal et al. (19) (*S. aureus*); Murray et al. [35] (*Enterococcus*); Reed et al. (5) (*S. aureus*); Sader et al. (36) (*P. aeruginosa*); Samore et al. (37) (*C. difficile*); Seifert and Gerner-Smidt (38) (*Acinetobacter*); Singh et al. (39) (*M. tuberculosis*); Tenover et al. (40) (multiple); van Embden et al. (41) (*M. tuberculosis*).

for a list of pathogens and associated references). PFGE is capable of determining whether epidemiologically linked isolates are genetically related or not, likely to represent a common source, or whether they have unique and unrelated genomic profiles. By establishing this genetic relationship, infection control practitioners are able to make evidence-based decisions to implement intervention measures to break the transmission chain. The results of PFGE are nearly reproducible between laboratories because protocols are becoming increasingly standardized due to common equipment and analytical and interpretation software. This standardization of PFGE methodology has benefited from the PulseNet program at CDC which hosts a large database of PFGE types of foodborne pathogens. An additional advantage of PFGE is that its discriminatory ability is based on differences identified by the restriction and separation of DNA from the entire bacterial genome. This feature is a potential benefit over other methods that rely on changes in more limited targets because it allows for the identification of genetic variability throughout the genome. While the advantages of PFGE are well-defined, it is also generally considered to be a labor-intensive procedure still requiring 48–72 hours to produce results in the hands of staff with technical expertise. Thus the availability of PFGE is typically still limited to large reference laboratories.

PFGE Background

PFGE has been used for molecular typing of pathogens due to its discrete ability to separate relatively large DNA fragments (1000 kbp) from small ones (~50 kbp) which are otherwise not possible by traditional electrophoresis methods. This methodology, first described by Schwartz and Cantor (1), makes use of alternating electric fields to separate DNA in an enclosed system. Since its initial development, a number of variations of PFGE have been developed, the most common of which is "contour-clamped homogeneous electric field" (CHEF). In a CHEF unit, 24 electrodes oriented around a hexagonal contour allows programmed switching of current between alternate electrodes causing DNA to migrate in a zig-zag motion at 120-degree angles, which facilitates enhanced separation of larger DNA fragments from the smaller ones relative to the unidirectional electric field.

The basic steps begin with harvesting cells grown from a single bacterial colony. The harvested cells are suspended in a buffer to standardize the concentration of cells. The cell suspensions are mixed with molten agarose and dispensed into plastic plug molds. The solidified plugs containing bacterial cells are incubated in specific enzymes and detergents to lyse the cells *in situ* to minimize the chromosomal shearing. The plugs are washed several times to eliminate any residual cellular debris. A section of the plug is subjected to a strain-specific rare-cutting restriction endonuclease. The digested plug is loaded onto an agarose gel and the restricted fragments are electrophoresed under the alternating electric fields. Larger fragments move slowly due to additional time they need to recoil in an alternative electrical field compared to the smaller fragments that move relatively faster through the agarose matrix. The gel is then stained with a fluorescent intercalating agent such as ethidium bromide and imaged using a digital photodocumentation system. DNA migration profiles derived from the restriction fragments are normalized to in-gel size standards at the computer-assisted analysis stage and compared to one another or other profiles in a PFGE database.

General Protocol

The following provides an in-depth description of the individual steps of PFGE (Figure 9.1). The protocol outlined below has been adapted from previously described methods (2–4). It should be considered as the starting point and a general guide for the typing of a number of nosocomial organisms. The methods of preparing genomic DNA for restriction digestion share many common steps and laboratory resources. However, pathogen-specific

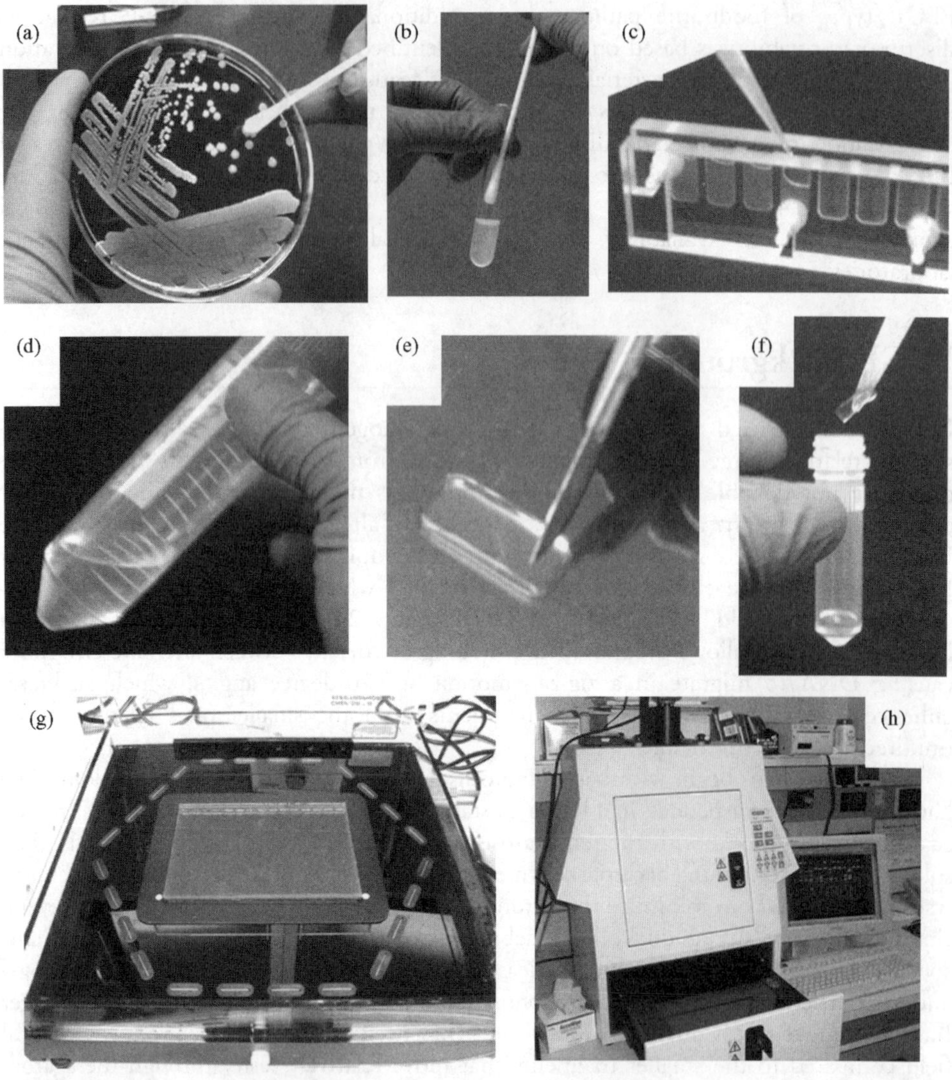

FIGURE 9.1 Basic steps used to carry out PFGE analysis. (A) Harvest cells with a swab. (B) Optimize the cells in suspension. (C) Pipet cells combined with melted agar into wells of a plug mold. (D) Lyse the cells within the plug using detergents. (E) Cut a slice of the plug for analysis. (F) Subject the DNA in the slice to restriction enzyme. (G) Load the plugs in a gel and electrophorese in a CHEF unit. (H) Image the DNA patterns using a digital gel documentation system. The specific PFGE steps are described in greater detail in the text.

modifications can be made to this protocol to address the variations associated with individual organisms (Table 9.1).

GROWTH AND HARVESTING OF CELLS

In order to prepare for PFGE, it is important to begin with an isolate that has been subcultured from a single colony to ensure the purity of the strain. A single colony of the isolate to be typed is inoculated to a 5% sheep blood agar plate and incubated overnight at 35°C in ambient conditions. Several colonies from the plate are harvested with a sterile cotton swab and suspended in a 5-ml culture tube containing 2 ml of cell suspension buffer (0.1 M Tris Cl, 0.15 M NaCl, 0.1 M EDTA; Figures 9.1A and 9.1B). The cell suspension is adjusted until its turbidity level reaches 20% transmittance using a Vitek colorimeter (bioMerieux, Durham, NC) or an equivalent reader. In general, the optimal density of cells is approximately 1×10^9 cells/ml. While preparing for PFGE analysis, it is also important to work up reference strains as well, because they will serve as an added quality control to evaluate the efficacy of the plug preparation, restriction digestion and serve as a comparative standard during analysis. Frequently used reference strains include *Staphylococcus aureus* NCTC 8325 digested with *Sma*I (5) and *Salmonella enterica* ser. Braenderup H9812 digested with *Xba*I (6).

PLUG PREPARATION

Following the normalization of cell concentrations, a 400-μl aliquot of the cell suspension is transferred to a 2-ml microcentrifuge tube and mixed with 10–20 μl of a cell-lysing enzyme (Table 9.1). The suspension is next combined with 400 μl of melted 1% Seakem Gold agarose (Lonza # 50150) prepared in TE buffer [10 mM Tris HCl, 1 mM EDTA (pH 8.0)], and the mixture is quickly dispensed into one or more wells of a plug mold (Bio-Rad Laboratories, Hercules, CA; Figure 9.1C). The plugs are allowed to solidify at 4°C for 10 minutes. Each plug is transferred to a labeled 50-ml conical tube containing 5 ml of EC lysis buffer [6 mM Tris Cl, 1.0 M NaCl, 0.1 M EDTA, 0.5% Brij 58, 0.2% deoxycholate, 0.5% Sarkosyl (pH 7.5); Figure 9.1D]. The plugs are incubated at 37°C in a shaking water bath for at least 2 hours. Following the initial lysis, the EC buffer is decanted off and replaced with 5 ml of ESP buffer [10 mM Tris Cl, 1.0 mM EDTA, 1% sodium dodecyl sulfate (SDS), 1 mg/ml Proteinase K (pH 8.0)]. Incubation proceeds overnight at 50°C in a shaking water bath. The cellular debris in the plugs is washed from the plugs by four successive gentle washes in 10 ml TE buffer for 30 minutes each at room temperature. Freshly washed plugs can proceed to the digestion step or be stored in TE buffer at 4°C.

RESTRICTION DIGESTION

To digest the plugs, an adequate amount of 1× concentration of restriction enzyme buffer is prepared such that is 200 μl per digest. For each reaction, 200 μl of the 1× restriction buffer is added to a labeled, 2-ml microcentrifuge tube. An approximate 3-mm × 5-mm piece of the plug (cut using a scalpel or single-edged razor blade) is added to the tube, and the plug is preincubated in the restriction buffer at the optimum enzyme activity temperature (Figures 9.1E and 9.1F). After 15–30 minutes, the buffer is carefully removed with a pipet to avoid damaging the plug and 200 μl of 1× restriction buffer containing 20–50 units of the desired restriction enzyme (Table 9.1) is added and the restriction reaction is allowed to proceed for at least 2 hours. To ensure proper restriction, make sure that the plug slice is completely covered in the restriction buffer. It is important to note that the remainder of a plug can be stored and later digested with other enzymes as needed to improve discrimination among isolates. This may be important if the PFGE patterns from two or more isolates are indistinguishable using the first enzyme and there is epidemiological evidence that may suggest that the isolates may not be directly linked to one another. The digestion with the second enzyme will help to verify whether or not the strains are truly indistinguishable.

PREPARING AND LOADING THE AGAROSE GEL

As the digestion nears completion, prepare a 1% agarose gel (14 × 12.5 cm) using Seakem Gold agarose in a 0.5 × concentration of TBE buffer (0.89 M Tris, 0.89 M boric acid, 20 mM EDTA pH 8.0). The volume of agarose will depend on the size of the gel being cast. Assemble the casting stand with the running platform inside and tighten the screws. Place the assembly on a level surface and adjust the sides of the casting stand until it is level. Pour the molten agarose into the casting stand and position the comb. Allow the gel to solidify for approximately 1 hour before removing the comb. Position the digested plugs in the wells of the gel against the front wall of the well and top of the wells by pipetting molten agarose into the wells to seal the plugs into position. When placing the plugs into the gel, it is important to space multiple reference strain plugs across the lanes of each gel (e.g., in lanes 1, 5, 10, and 15 of a 15-well gel) to function as global standards during the normalization step of the analysis.

ELECTROPHORESIS

Once the gel has solidified, electrophoresis is carried out in a pulsed-field unit such as the CHEF DR-II or DR-III system from BioRad. To prepare for the run, 2 liters of 0.5× TBE is added to the chamber and continually circulated using a pump system through a chiller module to cool the buffer to 14°C. The gel is placed into the running frame inside the electrophoresis chamber containing the chilled buffer (Figure 9.1G) and the electrophesis unit is programmed for an initial and a final switch time (in seconds), length of run (in hours), and voltage (per centimeter of the gel) based on organism specific running conditions (Table 9.2). For example, the parameters for running a methicillin-resistant *Staphylococcus aureus* include an initial switch time of 5 seconds and a final switch of 40 seconds for 20 hours at 6 V/cm (5).

GEL IMAGING

Following completion of the run, the gel is transferred to a staining tray and covered with an ethidium bromide solution (1 μg/ml). The gel is typically stained for 30 minutes on a rotor with gentle agitation (ethidium bromide is a known mutagen and must be handled with gloves and disposed of properly). Next, the gel is destained in water for 15–30 minutes or longer, if needed, and visualized under ultraviolet light using a digital photodocumentation system to identify band patterns (Figure 9.1H). The gels are digitized and saved as image files such as an *.img or *.1sc files and are converted to a *.tif image for analysis in the fingerprint software.

TABLE 9.2 Representative interrelationships between PFGE switching parameters and the optimal DNA size separated[a]

DNA size range (kb)	Initial pulse time (seconds)	Final pulse time (seconds)	Run time (hours)
1–50	0.1	2.0	7
1–100	1.0	3.0	12
1–200	1.0	8.0	13
25–300	1.0	17.0	17
25–400	1.0	23.0	20
50–500	5.0	35.0	22
50–600	5.0	42.0	22
50–700	5.0	50.0	22
50–900	5.0	60.0	22
50–1000	5.0	66.0	22

[a] Electrophoresis conditions: 0.8–1.0% agarose, 0.5 × Tris-borate buffer, 120° reorientation angle, 6 V/cm, with standard non-linear switching as performed by the CHEF DRIII Pulsed Field Gel Electrophoresis System.
Source: Adapted with permission from Bio-Rad Laboratories, Hercules, CA.

FINGERPRINT AND CLUSTER ANALYSIS

Following the acquisition of the raw data, the gel images need to be analyzed. One of the most common software programs for the analysis of PFGE banding patterns is BioNumerics Software (Applied Maths, Kortrijk, Belgium). The following description is based on BioNumerics: If another software program is used, the program's instruction manual should be followed for the analysis. To process a gel image for analysis in BioNumerics, the file is imported into a selected database as a.tif image. In BioNumerics analysis, begin with Step 1: "Strips — Defining the lanes." The area of the gel to be analyzed is selected within the rectangle, and the lane finding search is carried out to define the individual lanes in the selected area. Adjustments can be made to parameters such as the lanes thickness, contrast, and its tone curve to improve analysis. Save the settings and proceed to Step 2: "Curves — Calculating the densitometric curves." In this step the gel image is optimized by a spectral analysis for background subtraction and noise filtering. After saving changes, proceed to Step 3: "Normalization — Adjusting lanes with respect to a reference." This is the most important step of the analysis because it adjusts the lanes proportionately to the reference strain (Figure 9.2). The reference system is set up during the analysis of the first gel entered into the database in which a reference strain containing bands of known molecular weights is established as the comparison for future gel analysis. For example, the known band sizes for a *Sma*I digest of *Staphylococcus aureus* NCTC 8325 are 674, 361, 324, 262, 257, 208, 175, 135, 117, 80, 76, 44, 36, 19, 16, and 9 kbp, and for the of *Xba*1 digested *Salmonella* ser. Braenderup H9812 the fragments are approximately 1135, 669, 453, 398, 337, 310, 244, 217, 139, 105, 78, 55, 33, 29, and 20.5 kbp. Subsequent gels that are entered into the selected database must be run with the same reference strain in multiple positions on the gel and by the same run parameters to facilitate inter-gel comparison of isolate profiles. By running subsequent gels under the same conditions, the lanes can be normalized to the reference system so that isolates can be compared to others in the database as if they were run

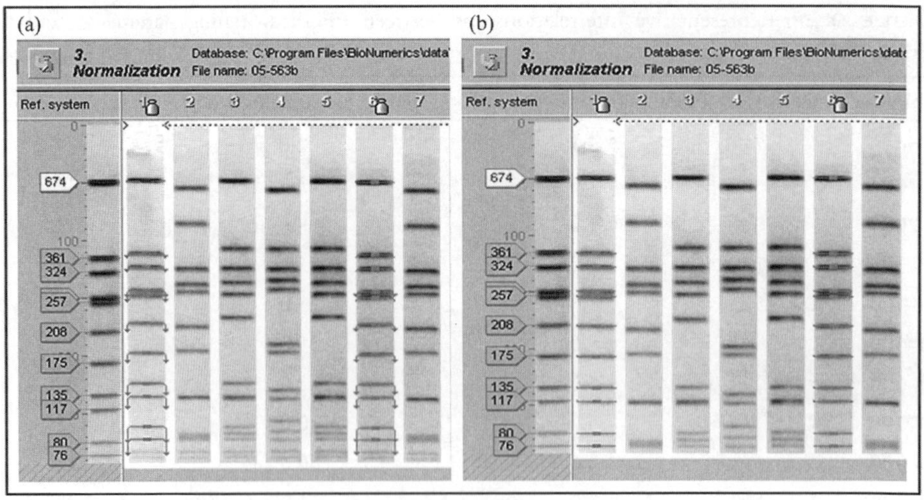

FIGURE 9.2 Normalization of PFGE patterns to the internal reference system during analysis in BioNumerics software. The marked fragments of the reference strain indicate the downward shift that all lanes will undergo to align with the internal reference system. (A) Prenormalization of *Sma*I digested MRSA PFGE patterns. (B) Normalized patterns.

at the same time. The normalized lanes are saved and the gel proceeds to Step 4: "Bands — Defining bands and quantification." The software will automatically search for the bands within each lane based on designated search criteria. However, the bands should be carefully reviewed to ensure proper identification of bands. The lanes of a processed gel are assigned

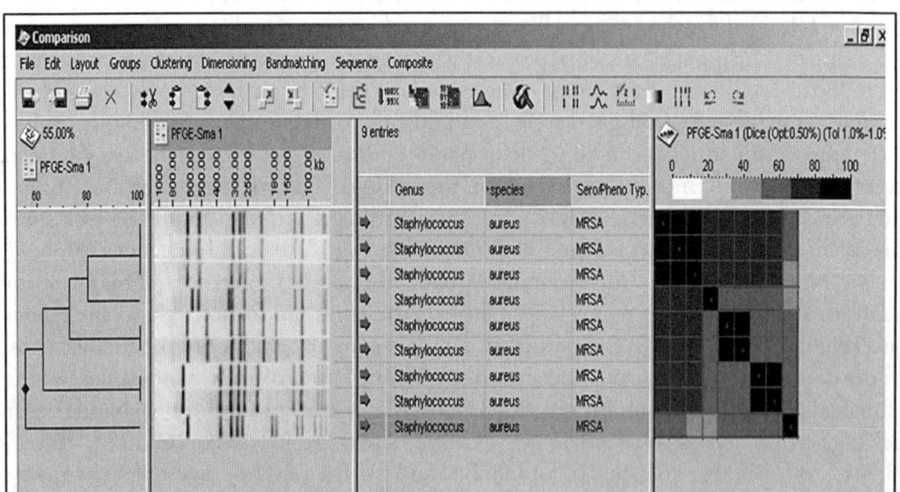

FIGURE 9.3 Dendrogram analysis of *Sma*I digested PFGE patterns of MRSA in BioNumerics software. The restricted DNA patterns were compared using the dice coefficient and unweighted pair group of arithmetic averages (UPGMA) method. The dendrogram shows the percent similarity on the far left, followed by the PFGE images and corresponding identification fields. The multi-shaded rectangles show the similarity matrix on the far right.

isolate-specific information by populating designated fields in the database, and the lanes are then linked to the corresponding information in the database. To carry out a comparison among isolates that are associated with a potential outbreak, the isolates to be included in the analysis are selected and compared to one another using one of a number of different comparison algorithms. In BioNumerics, for example, there are several different comparison methods and settings available; however, one of the most commonly used sets of algorithms is the Dice coefficient and unweighted pair group method using averages (UPGMA) analysis with a band position tolerance of 1.25% and an optimization of 0.5%. The results of the analyses are typically shown graphically in a dendrogram, which shows the percent similarity of the isolates (Figure 9.3).

Data Interpretation

Regardless of the method used, no aspect of epidemiological analysis is more important than proper interpretation of the data. With regard to PFGE, this issue was first addressed in 1995 with general guidelines proposed by Tenover et al. (7). The proposition acknowledged, as stated earlier, that chromosomal comparison is the most fundamental means of assessing isolate relatedness but that the chromosomal sequence of a bacterial isolate is not frozen in time and is subject to the increasing probability of (mutational) change because it persists in a given environment (e.g., hospital ward, transferred between patients). Thus, as a working paradigm, the guidelines proposed that at least some degree of genetic difference is consistent with a presumption of potential epidemiological relatedness. In terms of PFGE interpretation, as an operating hypothesis the guidelines proposed that isolates with identical patterns be considered to represent the same epidemiological type while related subtypes could logically differ by a single genetic event. The guidelines further proposed that isolates could still be possibly related though differing by two genetic events while three or more differences would most likely indicate a lack of relatedness. The vagueness of these guidelines was intentional because it is well known that epidemiological analysis, including molecular typing by PFGE as well as other methods, requires more data rather than less and thus is most accurate when all available clinical and epidemiological data are combined (8–10).

On this basis of the above guidelines, it is useful to reconsider the effect different mutational events may have on PFGE banding patterns. In simplest terms, one may visualize three general categories of genetic events for their potential to affect PFGE patterns: insertions, deletions, and rearrangements, visualized in Figure 9.4. Considering first events that do not affect a restriction-enzyme site, chromosomal insertions result in a restriction fragment of increased size which, when compared with its "original" in a related isolate, would be seen as a difference of two bands in a PFGE pattern. The converse would occur with chromosomal deletions, again resulting in a comparative two-band difference. Rearrangement of a chromosomal region not including restriction sites would be undetected by PFGE. Similar events, but including or affecting a restriction site, would result in a three-band difference for insertions or deletions where two chromosomal fragments suffering a deletion including an adjoining restriction site would become one larger fragment. The introduction of DNA containing a restriction site into a chromosomal region would result in the inverse effect where one restriction fragment now becomes two (again a three-band difference). Single base changes either destroying or producing a restriction site would have a similar effect. Finally, inversion of a chromosomal region containing a restriction site would essentially result in a lateral shift of restriction affecting adjoining fragments such that one

Event	PFGE Result	PFGE GEL
(NOT AFFECTING RESTRICTION SITE)		
insertion or deletion	2 band difference	
rearrangement (e.g., 180° inversion)	no detectable change	
(AFFECTING RESTRICTION SITE)		
insertion or deletion	3 band difference	
rearrangement (e.g., 180° inversion)	4 band difference	

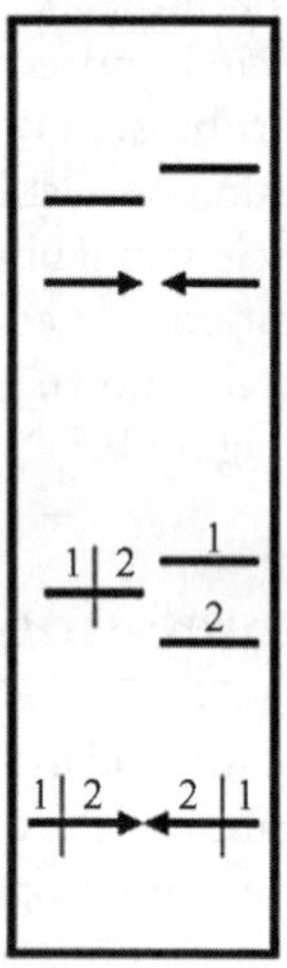

FIGURE 9.4 Summary of mutagenic events (insertions, deletions, rearrangements) and their influence on PFGE banding patterns. In some instances, PFGE bands are depicted as arrows or with numbers to aid in visualizing changes.

would become larger and the other smaller, resulting in PFGE patterns with a four-band difference when comparing the two isolates. More than one genetic event would result in multiples of these outcomes. Thus, clinical isolates with up to four differences in PFGE banding pattern could result from a single genetic event and be considered related subtypes. However, this is far from unambiguous since a four-band difference could also result from more than one genetic event (e.g., two different insertions not affecting a restriction site). Since the simplest genetic event (i.e., a single base change affecting a restriction site) would result in a three-band difference, some have taken this measure as a working rule (i.e., the "three-band rule") for defining probable relatedness where isolates differing at no more than three PFGE band positions are considered to be likely related subtypes. While not addressed by the above guidelines, single-band differences in PFGE patterns may also occur, potentially due to the carriage of large (>50 kb) plasmids or comigration of similarly sized restriction fragments. In this regard, it is important to note that, as a general rule, electrophoretic procedures (including PFGE) have difficulty discriminating DNA fragments differing in size by <10%. Thus, the above genetic events will only be visualized by PFGE if the difference in sizes of the resulting DNA fragments is large enough to be detected.

In considering the interpretation of PFGE patterns, it is important to note that epidemiological analysis is highly context-driven. Interactions between the bacterial pathogen, host (i.e., the patient), and environment all have the potential to influence the process (11). For example, all organisms are not equal with regard to inherent genomic variability. Some organisms, such as *Helicobacter pylori*, are so genomically diverse that PFGE analysis is unable to establish clear lines of relatedness (12). Conversely, highly problematic community-associated methicillin-resistant *Staphylococcus aureus* (CA-MRSA) strain

USA 300 is so genomically stable (clonal) that epidemiologically unrelated isolates may give indistinguishable PFGE patterns (13). Thus, the proper use of PFGE patterns in epidemiological analysis requires knowledge and consideration of the pathogen being analyzed. In general terms, the greater the genomic stability of the organism or the longer a particular bacterial strain has been present in a given environment, the more significance one should place on small differences in the highly uniform PFGE patterns commonly observed. In such instances, considering isolates with more than one or two band differences as related may risk the inclusion of unrelated isolates into an outbreak scenario that may confuse identification of transmission routes and source (14).

While PFGE patterns must clearly be examined by visual inspection, computer-assisted analysis and documentation are essential for anything more than a few isolates as well as for database storage and retrieval. Over the years a number of programs have been commercially developed for this purpose; however, BioNumerics and GelCompar (Applied Maths) clearly have the largest installed user base. The basic procedural steps for PFGE analysis with BioNumerics is described in the subsection "Fingerprint and Cluster Analysis." It is important to note that all computer-assisted programs of this nature are obviously associated with expense and a challenging learning curve. The algorithms used by such programs have been reviewed elsewhere (15–17). Despite the value of computer-assisted analysis, specific band identification must always be confirmed visually. For example, computer analysis is not as accurate as the human eye in identifying minor pattern differences, especially in instances where band comigration may have occurred. While computer-assisted analysis may employ a variety of clustering algorithms and correlation coefficients to assess relatedness, the UPGMA coupled with the Dice coefficient are a commonly used combination. In comparison to visual analysis, a clustered Dice coefficient of around 0.85 (i.e., 85% similar) is generally comparable to a "three-band rule" difference as discussed above. Thus, for isolates with moderate genomic divergence, one often sees studies employing >80% similarity, determined by computer analysis, as the breakpoint for relatedness clustering.

In the past, the PFGE nomenclature of localized outbreaks has often used arbitrary terminology, identifying a major epidemic pattern alphabetically (e.g., A, B, C) with a numerical designation for related subtypes (e.g., A1, A2, B1, B2). However, computer-assisted databases are now capable of comparing isolates from local outbreaks to previously identified local or more widespread patterns. This is especially the case with *S. aureus* where pulsotypes of the most common epidemic MRSA strains have been identified (18–20). Thus, computer-assisted analysis may serve the valuable purpose of allowing the nomenclature of isolates from local outbreaks to reflect previously reported more generally disseminated (epidemic) strains.

Troubleshooting

There are a number of factors and laboratory practices that contribute to the quality of PFGE gels. General considerations include the appropriate preparation of reagents, use of clean glassware, ultrapurified water, wearing gloves throughout much of the procedure, and evaluating the overall integrity of the PFGE equipment. In addition to these general factors, poor gels may be the result of inadequate lysis of the cells in the plugs, insufficient washing of the plugs, or incomplete restriction digestion of the DNA. To resolve incomplete lysis of the cells, which minimizes the amount of DNA released, increase the length of the lysis time or increase the concentration of lysing enzymes used. Thorough washing of the plugs is necessary to eliminate residual proteinase activity that will inhibit restriction enzyme digest. Increasing the number and length of washes may resolve the contrast of the DNA fragments.

The presence of ghost or shadow bands is typically the result of incomplete restriction enzyme digestion. This is resolved by ensuring that the plug slice is adequately covered in restriction enzyme and incubated appropriately at the optimal temperature. Similarly, too much DNA in the plugs can result in incomplete digestion or DNA bands that are thick or potentially overlap another band. This could be improved by optimizing the number of cells in the starting suspension to approximately 1×10^9 cells/ml. Gels that show uneven staining or lanes that do not run straight could be due to an unlevel gel or electrophoresis chamber. Prior to pouring the gel, ensure that the casting tray is level and that the gel is placed flat within the running frame of the electrophoresis chamber. Damaged or thin electrodes or an insufficient amount of running buffer may also account for lanes that are not straight. Occasionally there are isolates, particularly some strains of *C. difficile* and *P. aeruginosa*, that appear as a smear in the lane due to DNA degradation during the electrophoresis. A possible resolution to these untypable isolates is to add thiourea to the $0.5 \times$ TBE running buffer, which often minimizes the smearing to resolve an interpretable profile.

Conclusions and Future Directions

This chapter has attempted to provide an in-depth look at PFGE typing methods for nosocomial pathogens. Improvements of PFGE typing methodology will continue to evolve, including some degree of automation. Additionally, in the present genomic era, the selection of more efficient and appropriate enzymes will be possible. The use of *in silico* virtual restriction digestion of bacterial genomes will allow for the comparison of a wide selection of enzymes to identify those that will provide the optimal number of cuts and sized fragments to facilitate efficient analysis.

It appears that PFGE will remain the primary typing method in molecular epidemiology laboratories within the healthcare settings due to the ease of use and modest equipment needs. As more laboratories begin to use DNA sequence-based pathogen identification, the availability of DNA sequencers may allow for additional subtyping methods to be utilized. However, having a visual overview of isolate chromosomal relatedness may provide information and insight not as readily available by methods such as the sequence-based approaches. For example, as noted earlier, one of the most problematic infectious disease issues today is the pathogenicity and spread of CA-MRSA such as USA 300. This had led to worldwide emphasis on the early detection of MRSA in populations, especially including hospitalized patients. However, it is becoming increasingly clear that such organisms may apparently lose their methicillin/oxacillin resistance while fully retaining their pathogenicity armamentarium (21). As shown in Figure 9.5, PFGE is uniquely capable of visually demonstrating the interrelationship between such MRSA and methicillin-susceptible isolates, a potentially important capability in terms of infection control and disease prevention. Thus, despite its years of use, PFGE would appear to have staying power remaining as the current "gold standard" for the epidemiological analysis of a number of important bacterial pathogens, not totally replaced in the immediate years ahead but serving alongside or as a potential adjunct to newer, more sequence-based methods. Nevertheless, PFGE is not as a stand-alone method in an overall epidemiologic investigation that, by including all available molecular, clinical, and epidemiological data, has the greatest change of achieving a reliable and clinically useful answer.

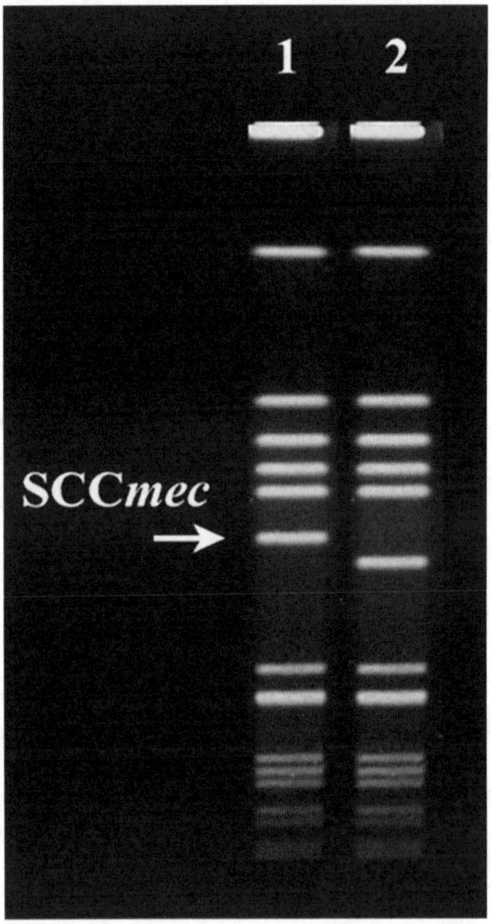

FIGURE 9.5 PFGE analysis of *Sma*I-digested chromosomal DNA from methicillin-resistant (lane 1) and methicillin-susceptible (lane 2) *S. aureus* USA300 isolates differing in the presence or absence of the methicillin-resistance encoding staphylococcal chromosomal cassette SCC*mec*.

REFERENCES

1. Schwartz DC, Cantor CR. Separation of yeast chromosomesized DNAs by pulsed field gradient gel electrophoresis. *Cell* 1984;**37**:67–75.
2. Bannerman TL, Hancock GA, Tenover FC, Miller JM. Pulsed-field gel electrophoresis as a replacement for bacteriophage typing of *Staphylococcus aureus*. *J Clin Microbiol* 1995;**33**:551–555.
3. Maslow JN, Mulligan ME, Arbeit RD. Molecular epidemiology: Application of contemporary techniques to the typing of microorganisms. *Clin Infect Dis* 1993;**17**:153–162.
4. Ribot RM, Fitzgerald C, Kubota K, Swaminathan B, Barrett TJ. Rapid pulsed-field gel electrophoresis protocol for subtyping of *Campylobacter jejuni*. *J Clin Microbiol* 2001;**39**:1889–1894.
5. Reed KD, Stemper ME, Shukla SK. Pulsed-field gel electrophoresis of MRSA. *Methods Mol Biol;* 2007;**391**:59–69.

6. Hunter SB, Vauterin P, Lambert-Fair MA, Van Duyne MS, Kubota K, Graves L, Wrigley D, Barrett T, Ribot E. Establishment of a universal size standard strain for use with the PulseNet standardized pulsed-field gel electrophoresis protocols: Converting the national databases to the new size standard. *J Clin Microbiol* 2005;**43**:1045–1050.
7. Tenover FC, Arbeit RD, Goering RV, Mickelsen PA, Murray BE, Persing DH, Swaminathan B. Interpreting chromosomal DNA restriction patterns produced by pulsed-field gel electrophoresis: Criteria for bacterial strain typing. *J Clin Microbiol* 1995;**33**:2233–2239.
8. Goering RV. The molecular epidemiology of nosocomial infection: An overview of principles, application, and interpretation. In Specter S, Bendinelli M, Friedman H. (eds.), *Rapid Detection of Infectious Agents*. Plenum Press, New York, 1998, pp. 131–157.
9. Goering RV. The molecular epidemiology of nosocomial infection: past, present, and future. *Rev Med Microbiol* 2000;**11**:145–152.
10. Van Belkum A, Tassios PT, Dijkshoorn L, Haeggman S, Cookson B, Fry NK, Fussing V, Green J, Feil E, Gerner-Smidt P, Brisse S, Struelens M. Guidelines for the validation and application of typing methods for use in bacterial epidemiology. *Clin Microbiol Infect* 2007;**13**(Suppl3): 1–46.
11. Van Belkum A, De Jonckheere J, Quint WGV. Genotyping *Naegleria* spp. and *Naegleria fowleri* isolates by interrepeat polymerase chain reaction. *J Clin Microbiol* 1992;**30**:2595–2598.
12. Taylor DN, Wachsmuth IK, Shangkuan YH, Schmidt EV, Barrett TJ, Schrader JS, Scherach CS, McGee HB, Feldman RA, Brenner DJ. Salmonellosis associated with marijuana: A multistate outbreak traced by plasmid fingerprinting. *N Engl J Med* 1982;**306**:1249–1253.
13. Tenover FC, McDougal LK, Goering RV, Killgore G, Projan SJ, Patel JB, Dunman PM. Characterization of a strain of community-associated methicillin-resistant *Staphylococcus aureus* widely disseminated in the United States. *J Clin Microbiol* 2006;**44**:108–118.
14. Gerner-Smidt P, Kincaid J, Kubota K, Hise K, Hunter SB, Fair MA, Norton D, Woo-Ming A, Kurzynski T, Sotir MJ, Head M, Holt K, Swaminathan B. Molecular surveillance of shiga toxigenic *Escherichia coli* O157 by PulseNet USA. *J Food Prot* 2005;**68**:1926–1931.
15. Heersma HF, Kremer K, Van Soolingen D, Hauman J. Setting up intra- and inter-laboratory databases of electrophoretic profiles, In Dijkshoorn L, Towner KJ, Struelens M. (eds.), *New Approaches for the generation and analysis of Microbial Typing Data*. Elsevier, Amsterdam, 2001, pp 47–75.
16. van Ooyen A. Theoretical aspects of pattern analysis, In Dijkshoorn L, Towner KJ, Struelens M. (eds.), *New Approaches for the Generation and Analysis of Microbial Typing Data*. Elsevier, Amsterdam, 2001, pp. 31–45.
17. Vauterin L, Vauterin P. Integraded databasing and analysis, In Stackebrandt E. (eds.), *Molecular Identification, Systematics, and Population Structure of Prokaryotes*. Springer, Berlin, 2006, pp. 141–217.
18. Larsen AR, Bocher S, Stegger M, Goering R, Pallesen LV, Skov R. Epidemiology of European community-associated methicillin-resistant *Staphylococcus aureus* clonal complex 80 type IV strains isolated in Denmark from 1993 to 2004. *J Clin Microbiol* 2008;**46**:62–68.
19. McDougal LK, Steward CD, Killgore GE, Chaitram JM, McAllister SK, Tenover FC. Pulsed-field gel electrophoresis typing of oxacillin-resistant *Staphylococcus aureus* isolates from the United States: Establishing a national database. *J Clin Microbiol* 2003;**41**:5113–5120.
20. Murchan S, Kaufmann ME, Deplano A, De Ryck R, Struelens M, Zinn CE, Fussing V, Salmenlinna S, Vuopio-Varkila J, El Solh N, Cuny C, Witte W, Tassios PT, Legakis N, Van Leeuwen W, Van Belkum A, Vindel A, Laconcha I, Garaizar J, Haeggman S, Olsson-Liljequist B, Ransjo U, Coombes G, Cookson B. Harmonization of pulsed-field gel electrophoresis protocols for epidemiological typing of strains of methicillin-resistant *Staphylococcus aureus*: A single approach developed by consensus in 10 European laboratories and its application for tracing the spread of related strains. *J Clin Microbiol* 2003;**41**:1574–1585.

21. Hulten KG, Kaplan SL, Gonzalez BE, Hammerman WA, Lamberth LB, Versalovic J, Mason EO Jr. Three-year surveillance of community onset health care-associated *Staphylococcus aureus* infections in children. *Pediatr Infect Dis J* 2006;**25**:349–353.

22. Arbeit RD, Arthur M, Dunn R, Kim C, Selander RK, Goldstein R. Resolution of recent evolutionary divergence among *Escherichia coli* from related lineages: The application of pulsed-field electrophoresis to molecular epidemiology. *J Infect Dis* 1990;**161**:230–235.

23. Barrett TJ, Lior H, Green JH, Khakhria R, Wells JG, Bell BP, Greene KD, Lewis J, Griffin PM. Laboratory investigation of a multistate food-borne outbreak of *Escherichia coli* O157:H7 by using pulsed-field gel electrophoresis and phage typing. *J Clin Microbiol* 1994;**32**:3013–3017.

24. D'Agata EM, Gerrits MM, Tang YW, Samore M, Kusters JG. Comparison of pulsed-field gel electrophoresis and amplified fragment-length polymorphism for epidemiological investigations of common nosocomial pathogens. *Infect Control Hosp Epidemiol* 2001;**22**:550–554.

25. Donabedian SM, Chow JW, Boyce JM, McCabe RE, Markowitz SM, Coudron PE, Kuritza A, Pierson CL, Zervos MJ. Molecular typing of ampicillin-resistant, non-beta-lactamase-producing *Enterococcus faecium* isolates from diverse geographic areas. *J Clin Microbiol* 1992;**30**:2757–2761.

26. Fawley WN, Wilcox MH. Pulsed-field gel electrophoresis can yield DNA fingerprints of degradation-susceptible *Clostridium difficile* strains. *J Clin Microbiol* 2002;**40**:3546–3547.

27. Goering RV, Winters MA. Rapid method for the epidemiological evaluation of Gram-positive cocci by field inversion gel electrophoresis. *J Clin Microbiol* 1992;**30**:577–580.

28. Gouby A, Carles-Nurit M-J, Bouziges N, Bourg G, Mesnard R, Bouvet PJ. Use of pulsed-field gel electrophoresis for investigation of hospital outbreaks of *Acinetobacter baumannii*. *J Clin Microbiol* 1992;**30**:1588–1591.

29. Hansen DS, Skov R, Benedí JV, Sperling V, Kolmos HJ. *Klebsiella* typing: Pulsed-field gel electrophoresis (PFGE) in comparison with O:K-serotyping. *Clin Microbiol Infect.* 2002;**8**:397–404.

30. Hughes VM, Stevenson K, Sharp JM. Improved preparation of high molecular weight DNA for pulsed-field gel electrophoresis from mycobacteria. *J Microbiol Methods* 2001;**44**:209–215.

31. Kato H, Kato N, Watanabe K, Ueno K, Ushijima H, Hashira S, Abe T. Application of typing by pulsed-field gel electrophoresis to the study of *Clostridium difficile* in a neonatal intensive care unit. *J Clin Microbiol* 1994;**32**:2067–2070.

32. Klaassen CH, van Haren HA, Horrevorts AM. Molecular fingerprinting of *Clostridium difficile* isolates: Pulsed-field gel electrophoresis versus amplified fragment length polymorphism. *J Clin Microbiol* 2002;**40**:101–104.

33. Kristjánsson M, Samore MH, Gerding DN, DeGirolami PC, Bettin KM, Karchmer AW, Arbeit RD. Comparison of restriction endonuclease analysis, ribotyping, and pulsed-field gel electrophoresis for molecular differentiation of *Clostridium difficile* strains. *J Clin Microbiol* 1994;**32**:1963–1969.

34. Macfarlane L, Walker J, Borrow R, Oppenheim BA, Fox AJ. Improved recognition of MRSA case clusters by the application of molecular subtyping using pulsed-field gel electrophoresis. *J Hosp Infect* 1999;**41**:29–37.

35. Murray BE, Singh KV, Heath JD, Sharma BR, Weinstock GM. Comparison of genomic DNAs of different enterococcal isolates using restriction endonucleases with infrequent recognition sites. *J Clin Microbiol* 1990;**28**:2059–2063.

36. Sader HS, Pignatari AC, Leme IL, Burattini MN, Tancresi R, Hollis RJ, Jones RN. Epidemiologic typing of multiple drug resistant *Pseudomonas aeruginosa* isolated from an outbreak in an intensive care unit. *Diagn Microbiol Infect Dis* 1993;**17**:13–18.

37. Samore M, Killgore G, Johnson S, Goodman R, Shim J, Venkataraman L, Sambol S, DeGirolami P, Tenover F, Arbeit R, Gerding D. Multicenter typing comparison of sporadic and outbreak

Clostridium difficile isolates from geographically diverse hospitals. *J Infect Dis* 1997; **176**:1233–1238.

38. Seifert H, Gerner-Smidt P. Comparison of ribotyping and pulsedfield gel electrophoresis for molecular typing of *Acinetobacter isolates*. *J Clin Microbiol* 1995;**33**:1402.
39. Singh SP, Salamon H, Lahti CJ, Farid-Moyer M, Small PM. Use of pulsed-field gel electrophoresis for molecular epidemiologic and population genetic studies of *Mycobacterium tuberculosis*. *J. Clin. Microbiol.* 1999;**37**:1927–1931.
40. Tenover FC, Arbeit RD, Archer G, Biddie J, Byrne S, Goering R, Hancock G, Hebert GA, Hill B, Hollis R, Jarvis WR, Kreiswirth B, Eisner W, Maslow J, McDougal LK, Miller JM, Mulligan M, Pfaller MA. Comparison of traditional and molecular methods of typing isolates of *Staphylococcus aureus*. *J Clin Microbiol* 1994;**32**:407–415.
41. van Embden JDA, Cave MD, Crawford JT, Dale JW, Eisenach KD, Gicquel B, Hermans P, Martin C, McAdam R, Shinnick TM, Small PM. Strain identification of *Mycobacterium tuberculosis* by DNA fingerprinting: Recommendations for a standardized methodology. *J Clin Microbiol* 1993;**31**:406–409.

Part THREE

Application of Techniques to Characterize Predominant Nosocomial Pathogens

CHAPTER TEN

Staphylococcus aureus

VANTHIDA HUANG AND SAMANTHA J. EELLS

Introduction

Staphylococcus aureus has been recognized as a major human and animal pathogen for over 100 years when first described by Sir Alexander Ogston (1–4). Staphylococci are facultative anaerobes in the *Staphylococcus* genus, which was formerly classified in the *Micrococcus* genus; micrococci tend to form clusters similar in appearance to grapes when viewed at high magnification. *Staphylococcus aureus* is a nonmotile, non-spore-forming, coagulase-positive organism that differentiates it from *S. epidermidis*. Staphylococci form a fairly large colony that is smooth, opaque, and creamy yellow to golden in color. It is often hemolytic on blood agar, whereas *S. epidermidis* is nonhemolytic. This organism can survive in the most hostile environmental conditions.

Polymorphonuclear granulocyte killing is impaired due to its golden pigmentation that promotes virulence via its antioxidant activity (5). *Staphylococcus aureus* is characterized by rapid growth in the blood agar and other nonselective media (6–8), and the *S. aureus* pathogen can be identified phenotypically by coagulase tests and agglutination tests (9). Other methods are occasionally utilized to identify *S. aureus* from blood cultures that include mannitol fermentation, presence of thermostable deoxyribonuclease, and multiplex polymerase chain reaction (PCR) (10, 11).

While staphylococci are versatile pathogens, they are naturally susceptible to all classes of antimicrobial; however, resistance has evolved with these agents. The resistance is acquired via horizontal transfer of genes from external sources, which has facilitated the expansion to

Molecular Techniques for the Study of Hospital-Acquired Infection, First Edition. Edited by Steven L. Foley, Anne Y. Chen, Shabbir Simjee, and Marcus J. Zervos.

the hospital environment. Chromosomal mutations and antimicrobial selection play an important role in this transfer.

Staphylococcus aureus asymptomatically colonizes the skin and mucosa of humans and animals, which in turn can produce a variety of diseases. *Staphylococcus aureus* is part of the normal human flora, and it is estimated that 30% of humans are nasal carriers (12, 13). The development of disease will depend on a variety of host factors that predispose an individual to infections since *S. aureus* is transmitted by direct contact. The risk of infections is greater in *S. aureus* carriers, and they are the major source of transmission. These diseases encompass a spectrum of severity from relatively benign skin infections (boils, folliculitis, and furunculosis) to life-threatening conditions (pneumonia, endocarditis, bacteremia, and septicemia) (14–16). Overall, *S. aureus* is the leading cause of hospital-acquired infections as identified by the National Healthcare Safety Network (NHSN) (17). Furthermore, the prevalence of *S. aureus* infections continues to increase worldwide and is now being complicated by multidrug resistance to the standards of therapy.

History *Staphylococcus aureus* as Nosocomial Pathogen

Staphylococcus aureus was once regarded as one of the most devastating human pathogen in the preantibiotic era as mortality was 80% (18, 19). Two years after the introduction of penicillin for medical use, the first case of penicillin-resistant *S. aureus* strains were observed in the community. Similarly, just 2 years after the introduction of methicillin, the first case of methicillin-resistant *S. aureus* (MRSA) was reported in Europe in the 1960s (20). At the same time, the rate of penicillin-resistant *S. aureus* has increased to 60%. In the 1970s, reports of MRSA outbreaks throughout the hospitals increased in the United States and worldwide (21). By the 1980s, these strains of MRSA became endemic, which led to the worldwide pandemic of MRSA in the hospitals that continues to increase to the present time.

Healthcare-associated MRSA (HA-MRSA) infections often result from hospitalization of patients with certain risk factors that include recent prior hospital admission, longer length of stay, and previous surgery. The most frequent types of MRSA infections encountered in healthcare settings are those associated with skin and soft tissue (SST), surgery, use of indwelling devices, pneumonia, bacteremia, and sepsis. In recent years, *S. aureus* has become the overall leading pathogen in the healthcare-associated infections as illustrated in the NHSN; this is especially true of the multidrug-resistant strains (17). Overall, *S. aureus* is the leading cause of such infections with skin and soft tissue (SSTIs), ventilator-associated pneumonia (VAP), and central line-associated bloodstream infection (CLABSI) (22, 23).

Molecular Epidemiology of *Staphylococcus aureus* in the Hospital Setting

Multiple molecular typing techniques have been used to identify and monitor the spread and patterns of *S. aureus* strains. Multilocus sequence typing (MLST) provides a uniform nomenclature for describing MRSA sequence types (ST) assigned with reference to the MLST database (URL: http://www.mlst.net) (24). *Staphylococcus aureus* protein A (*spa*) locus is another way to strain type MRSA by analyzing the repeats in the staphylococcal protein A gene. A *spa* type is assigned using a reference database

(URL: http://spaserver.ridom.de/) (25). The use of multiple-locus variable-number tandem-repeat assay (MLVA) has been used as an additional means of describing *S. aureus* strains (26). The MLVA assay uses targeted variable-number tandem repeats in the *clfA*, *clfB*, *sdrCDE*, *spa*, and *sspA* loci and gel electrophoresis to analyze the banding patterns of the strain. Pulsed-field gel electrophoresis (PFGE) is considered the most powerful technique for identification of *S. aureus* strains. In the United States, PFGE is used by the Center for Disease Control and Prevention (CDC) to assess the USA strain type of *S. aureus* isolates. Each USA strain type is described by a similar PFGE pattern, antibiogram, *mec* type, and the presence or absence of the Panton–Valentine leukocidin (PVL) gene. Each of the USA strain types has a corresponding MLST and *spa* type (27).

STRAIN TYPING

The healthcare-associated MRSA strains include USA100, USA200, and USA500. The most common strain type of HA-MRSA is the USA100 strain (27, 28). It is important to note that community-associated MRSA (CA-MRSA) strains appear to have become predominant in the healthcare setting (29, 30). Methicillin-resistant *S. aureus* strains contain the *mecA* gene, which encodes an altered penicillin-binding protein 2a (PBP2a) that causes decreased binding affinity to ß-lactam antimicrobials. The *mecA* gene is carried on a mobile genetic element called the staphylococcal cassette chromosome *mec* (SCC*mec*). Staphylococcal cassette chromosome *mec* is integrated into the chromosomal DNA of MRSA isolates, causing oxacillin resistance. All MRSA isolates carry the *mecA* gene (31). The use of PCR techniques to determine the SCC*mec* type can help distinguish strains of MRSA as healthcare or community origin (32). The most common HA-MRSA *mec* type is type II. Healthcare-associated MRSA SCC*mec* types also include types I and III (31). Staphylococcal cassette chromosome *mec* type II, commonly found in HA-MRSA strains, is characterized by its larger size and genetic material conferring resistance non-ß-lactam antimicrobials (33). Staphylococcal cassette chromosome *mec* type II/III containing HA-MRSA isolates replicate more slowly *in vitro* when compared with methicillin-susceptible *S. aureus* (MSSA) strains (33).

TOXINS AND VIRULENCE

Healthcare-associated MRSA strains are classically resistant to many non-ß-lactam antimicrobials (34–36). These isolates do not generally express the toxins that are often found in CA-MRSA strains such as the PVL toxin. Panton–Valentine leukocidin is a pore-forming toxin causing lysis of several mammalian cell lines. It is thought to be responsible for certain novel clinical features of severe CA-MRSA disease, although the role of PVL virulence remains controversial (37, 38).

Toxin genes have been shown to be associated with HA-MRSA isolates when compared to CA-MRSA isolates among the known toxin genes present in *S. aureus* strains. One investigation found that seven genes were significantly more likely to be found among HA-MRSA strains, and six different genes were significantly more likely to be found among CA-MRSA strains (39). The exotoxin genes significantly associated with HA-MRSA isolates include *sed, seg, sei, sej, sem, sen,* and *seo.* The implication of these virulent toxin genes and their expressed toxins in the pathogenesis of *S. aureus* infections is not currently well understood.

The Brazilian epidemic clonal complex (BECC, PFGE type A_1) caused an epidemic in the 1990s at Joao Barros Barreto University Hospital in Belem, Brazil (40). This clone accounted for 38% of *S. aureus* isolates at that time and up to 79% of isolates by 1998. The Brazilian strains were found to produce more significant biofilm than MSSA or MRSA strains in an *in vitro* experiment (41). This clone is more likely to invade these cells because it has a higher adhesion to polystyrene and bronchial epithelial cells. This study suggests that this clone is more successful because it has enhanced ability to bind, persist, and invade the host.

Pathogenesis

Persons may have asymptomatic colonization with *S. aureus* (both methicillin-susceptible and -resistant) in the community and healthcare settings before developing infections. The main reservoir of *S. aureus* resides in the anterior nares. Approximately 20% of individuals are persistently colonized, while 30% are intermittently colonized (42–44). Graham and colleagues recently completed a large population-based survey in the United States and concluded that most subjects are nasally colonized with *S. aureus* (28.6%) with 1.5% of subjects colonized with MRSA (44). There are various other sites where persons may be colonized with *S. aureus* including the axillae, groin, gastrointestinal tract, perineal, and throat (45–47). Colonization provides a reservoir for the bacteria to be introduced when the host defenses become breached. Colonizers of *S. aureus* have increased risk for subsequent infection (15, 48, 49). Furthermore, transmission among individuals is common in both community and healthcare settings via direct contact with colonizers. Colonized individuals will most likely be infected by the strains with which they are colonized (49–51). Davis and colleagues demonstrated that individuals who colonized with MRSA are 10 times more likely to become infected with the colonized strain than individuals who harbor MSSA (52). Hospitalized individuals and other high risk groups tend to display higher rates of colonization than the general population. The development of nosocomial *S. aureus* bacteremia, dialysis-associated infections, or postoperative staphylococcal surgical site infections by nasal *S. aureus* carriers is more likely than in noncarriers (53–58).

The pathogenesis of *S. aureus* is not completely understood; however, there is a diverse arsenal of components and products that *S. aureus* contributes to the pathogenesis of infections. These components and products can act either alone or cohesively due to their overlapping roles. *Staphylococcus aureus* has a remarkable set of virulence factors, considering that it is a commensal pathogen that can colonize many parts of one's body. Infections are typically initiated via breach of the skin barrier or any mucosal tissue, thereby allowing the organism access to the blood or adjacent tissue. The severity of the infection will depend on the individual host's defenses as well as the virulence of the pathogen. Mucin appears to be a critical host surface that is colonized in a process that involves interactions between staphylococcal proteins and mucin carbohydrate (59, 60). This helps explain why the highest number of *S. aureus* carriers are colonized in the nares.

Emerging Issues in Antimicrobial Resistance in *Staphylococcus aureus*

The emergence of antimicrobial resistance continues to be a major crisis globally (61). Alarmingly, there has been a decline in the research and development of new antimicrobial agents to fight this growing problem (62). Subsequently, antimicrobial resistance results in frequent treatment failures with severe outcomes as well as dramatic increases in total healthcare costs (63, 64). *Staphylococcus aureus*, especially MRSA, is one of the many significant pathogens that cause nosocomial infections that are often referred to as "ESKAPE" (*Enterococcus faecium, Staphylococcus aureus, Klebsiella pneumonia, Acinetobacter baumannii, Pseudomonas aeruginosa*, and *Enterobacter* species) (65, 66). According to the recent report from the NHSN, these pathogens cause nearly half of the infections in the intensive care unit with *S. aureus* infections leading the way (17). In addition to its prevalence in causing nosocomial infections, *S. aureus* is increasingly prominent in the community settings (39).

GLYCOPEPTIDES

Vancomycin and teicoplanin are antimicrobials in the glycopeptide class that are widely used for the treatment of Gram-positive pathogens (67, 68). Originally, the role of vancomycin role was mainly preserved for patients with staphylococcal infections who were allergic or intolerant to other classes of antibiotics. In recent decades, vancomycin became the gold standard in the treatment of MRSA while it continued to emerge as a problematic pathogen. With such a prominent role, vancomycin use has dramatically increased for the treatment of serious infection due to MRSA. With the increased utilization, resistance to glycopeptides has emerged as a major challenge for clinicians (69).

The effectiveness of glycopeptides against *S. aureus* has decreased over the last two decades as cases of reduced susceptibility have been reported worldwide (68, 69). In 1996, the first case of vancomycin-intermediate *S. aureus* (VISA) was reported in Japan (70, 71). Since then, other cases of VISA infections have been reported worldwide (72–74). These VISA strains are generally found in patients who have been exposed to long-term vancomycin therapy with antibiotic minimum inhibitory concentrations (MICs) of 4–8 μg/ml based on the current Clinical and Laboratory Standards Institute (CLSI) breakpoints (75). There are several methods used to define vancomycin MIC which are approved by CLSI such as broth or agar dilution, Etest, or commercial tests (Vitek 2 or Microscan). However, there are many inconsistencies among these methods in determining vancomycin MICs. Therefore, it has been suggested that the broth dilution MIC method performed according to CLSI should be used to define VISA (75). Fortunately, the reports of VISA have been rare after the breakpoint was decreased from 4 μg/ml to 2 μg/ml in 2006 (76).

Following the reports of VISA, Hiramatsu and colleagues reported the first case of heterogeneous vancomycin-intermediate *S. aureus* (hVISA) from a 64-year-old patient with pneumonia who failed vancomycin therapy, and the isolate was designated as Mu3 (ATCC 700698) (77). The first reports of clinical *S. aureus* isolates with reduced susceptibility to teicoplanin were in Europe; however, this isolate was still susceptible to vancomycin (78–80). Heterogeneous VISA is defined as an *S. aureus* isolate with vancomycin MIC within the susceptible range when tested by routine methods but has a subpopulation of daughter cells that are vancomycin-intermediate or -resistant (81–83).

Heterogeneous VISA, identified among clinical isolates of MRSA, has varied worldwide. Rybak and colleagues reported hVISA to be 8.3% in suburban Detroit, Michigan from 2003 to 2007, which demonstrates a 2.2% increase from 1986 to 1993 (84). Similarly, Lalani and colleagues found 8% (7/89) of MRSA isolates from a prospective trial from patients with *S. aureus* bacteremia and endocarditis (85). The most recent study in Nebraska reported an incidence of hVISA at 1.2% over a 9-year period using three separate methods (86). The prevalence of hVISA globally is not known and is most likely underestimated due to the lack of standardized methodologies in the detection. It has been postulated that the lack of standardization for detection of hVISA by standard susceptibility testing methods is due to the use of a low inoculum (76). The population analysis profile (PAP) is still the gold standard in identifying hVISA, however, this is a very labor-intensive process for the standard microbiology laboratory (87).

Heterogeneous VISA is believed to be the precursor in the development of vancomycin-intermediate *S. aureus* (VISA) (82). In this case, vancomycin exhibits selective pressure that leads the entire population to become fully VISA, which is believed to be due to the adaptive features of actual mechanism of the resistance (82, 83).

Not long after reports of VISA and hVISA, there was a case report of vancomycin-resistant *S. aureus* (VRSA) in 2002 from Detroit, Michigan with an MIC of 1024 μg/ml (88). Then within 2 months, a second case of VRSA was reported in Pennsylvania with an MIC of 32 μg/ml (89). Two years after the report of the Pennsylvania case, a third case was reported in New York which had an MIC of 64 μg/ml (90). As of this writing, there have been 11 cases of VRSA reported worldwide, with the majority of the cases coming from Michigan (91–97).

Understanding the mechanism of resistance to vancomycin in *S. aureus* is still not well understood. However, phenotypic distinctions have been noted among hVISA, VISA, and VRSA. There are several different phenotypic changes seen with VISA and hVISA. These changes include increased cell wall thickness, reduced autolysis, and decreased activity of the accessory gene regulator (*agr*) (92). The cell wall thickness is a major contributor to the mechanism of resistance. The cell wall thickness is due to increased peptidoglycan; as a result, vancomycin molecules become trapped in the layers, thereby preventing the drug from reaching its target site (81, 91, 92). Furthermore, there are a number of studies that have demonstrated a reversion of glycopeptide resistance in hVISA/VISA clinical isolates (82, 98). A reversion phenomenon suggests that the hVISA/VISA phenotype is unstable and impairs the fitness of the organism to maintain a decrease in susceptibility unless under continued selective pressure with vancomycin (82, 98).

Vancomycin-resistant *S. aureus* demonstrated a transfer of *vanA* gene cluster (Tn1546) from *Enterococcus* species to MRSA *in vivo* which has been reported *in vitro* previously (99–101). There are two known outcomes as a result from the transfer of the *vanA* gene from enterococci to MRSA: (1) replication of the actual enterococcal *vanA* plasmid in the new staphylococcal host after plasmid transfer by conjugation and (2) transposition of the Tn1546 element to a staphylococcal plasmid with subsequent loss of the enterococcal plasmid (91, 100). The interesting part of the investigation was that one of the nine VRSA isolates evaluated required vancomycin for growth. It was postulated that *Enterococci* has the ability to transfer *vanA* genes to MRSA and was unique to the VRSA strains found in Michigan (102).

OXAZOLIDINONES

Linezolid, an oxazolidinone, is active against Gram-positive pathogens including MRSA and vancomycin-resistant enterococci (VRE) (103). Linezolid use is considered the last-line treatment and is mainly reserved for severe infections that fail vancomycin therapy. Though development of resistance to linezolid is still extremely rare in staphylococci, cases of resistance among *S. aureus* including MRSA have been reported (103–106). Linezolid resistance has been described previously to be associated with mutation (G2576T) in the central loop of the domain V region of the 23S rRNA gene (105–107). Recently, Garcia and colleagues reported an outbreak of linezolid-resistant *S. aureus* (LRSA) in six patients in the intensive care unit (ICU) in Spain. This strain possesses a chloramphenicol-florfenicol resistance (*cfr*)-mediated resistance (108). It appears that these patients had a short exposure to treatment prior to developing *cfr*-mediated resistance.

LIPOPEPTIDE

Daptomycin is a lipopeptide antibiotic that was approved by the US Food and Drug Administration (FDA) for the treatment of complicated skin and soft structure infections (SSSIs) implicated by *S. aureus*, including MRSA, in 2006. It is a rapidly bactericidal antimicrobial with a unique mechanism of action that involves calcium-dependent binding to the bacterial plasma membrane and disruption of membrane function (109). Daptomycin role in the treatment of MRSA is also a last line of therapy. Though resistance to daptomycin is still extremely rare, cases reported of resistance and failed therapy has been described worldwide (110). Spontaneous resistance is not common since daptomycin-resistant breakpoint has not been established (111). Resistance mutations of daptomycin involving *mprF*, *yyG*, *rpoB*, and *rpoC* in *S. aureus* have been described (111). Further work needs to be done to elucidate the mechanism of daptomycin resistance.

Nosocomial Infections Due to Multidrug-Resistant *Staphylococcus aureus*

Staphyloccus aureus is the second leading nosocomial pathogen in the ICU according to the most recent surveillance data by NHSN (17). Antimicrobial resistance has a major impact on development of multidrug resistance to the currently viable classes. Infections caused by these multidrug-resistant *S. aureus* species have a huge impact on patients' outcomes as well as costs (63).

NOSOCOMIAL INFECTIONS DUE TO VANCOMYCIN NONSUSCEPTIBLE *Staphylococcus aureus*

Vancomycin has remained the agent of choice in the treatment of Gram-positive bacterial infections, including MRSA in both the community and healthcare settings (68, 69). Therefore, the use of vancomycin has increased parallel to the dramatic rise in MRSA infections worldwide. Furthermore, the usefulness of glycopeptides has invariably diminished due to the development of resistance by MRSA. Therefore, serious MRSA infections are not responding to vancomycin, despite showing susceptibility using standard routine tests in the microbiology laboratory. The emergence of hVISA, VISA, and VRSA has been challenging for clinician as well as microbiologist in their attempt to define and evaluate the susceptibility of vancomycin against MRSA.

The true incidence of hVISA cases remains unclear primarily due to the variation in detection methodology. Recent reports by Rybak and Lalani estimate that the prevalence of hVISA has been increasing and is currently about 8% (84, 85). What is clear is that staphylococcal infections due to hVISA are spreading via nosocomial outbreaks, and these infections continue to fail therapy with vancomycin and other antimicrobials such as daptomycin and linezolid. Risk factors associated for hVISA/VISA infection are thought to include prior MRSA infection or colonization as well as exposure to vancomycin (94, 112, 113). Also of concern are patients who have a comorbid disease (diabetes, renal failure, etc.) or high bacterial load infection (endocarditis) which leads to prolonged treatment duration resulting in treatment failure (114, 115).

In addition to increased reporting of hVISA/VISA, there has been significant interest regarding MIC tolerance and "creep" (116, 117). The changes in the MICs of vancomycin will directly impact the rates of hVISA. There has been two large-scale attempts to globally investigate the issue of MIC creep; one was able to demonstrate an increase in MIC while the other did not. A smaller-scale study by Steinkraus and colleagues found a modest increase vancomycin MICs (116).

VIRULENCE IN COMMUNITY-ASSOCIATED *Staphylococcus aureus* CROSSOVER TO HOSPITAL SETTING

We are in the midst of a CA-MRSA epidemic across the United States in recent years. This clone causes very invasive infections as well as increasing mortality (118). The rapid introduction of the CA-MRSA into the hospital has blurred the distinction between CA-MRSA and HA-MRSA. The predominant clone is USA300, which comprises about 80% of CA-MRSA versus 43% in HA-MRSA (119). A retrospective study demonstrated that CA-MRSA caused an increase in hospital onset of bacteremia from 24% to 49% between 2000 and 2006 (118). Furthermore, the community onset HA-MRSA does not have the classical risk factors of traditional MRSA, because patients appear to be less sick. Thus the USA300 clone is a very important cause of nosocomial bloodstream infections (120).

SMALL-COLONY VARIANTS OF *Staphylococcus aureus*

Small-colony variants of *S. aureus* (SCVs) are strains that produce slow-growing subpopulations that phenotypically differ from the parent strains (121). Small-colony variants of *S. aureus* are naturally occurring pathogens that are very fastidious with decreased hemolytic, pigmentation, and coagulase activity (121). Small-colony variants of *S. aureus* are characterized by a large reduction of growth rate, very small colonies morphologically, and an unusual biochemical basis (92). Evidence suggests that another key characteristic is that SCVs are considered to be intracellular pathogens; therefore, they will be persistent whereas traditionally *S. aureus* is not (122). Clinically, SCVs are associated with persistent, recurring, and relapse infections, particularly in bone and joint infections (osteomyelitis), respiratory tract infections (cystic fibrosis), and bacteremia (122–124). There is a limited availability of antimicrobial options for the treatment of SCVs alone or in combination due to the atypical growth of cells. Vancomycin activity will be reduced in SCVs as compared to parental *S. aureus* strains (92, 125). An antimicrobial with intracellular penetration or one effective against slow-growing bacterial such as rifampin is the optimal choice (121). However, rifampin is not a monotherapeutic antimicrobial due to rapid resistance (121). Sendi and colleagues proposed a successful combination of fluoroquinolones plus rifampin against SCVs (122).

Summary

Staphylococcus aureus has become increasingly problematic in the last few decades with the emergence of multidrug resistance, especially to glycopeptides, but now the resistance has spread into our community. It is one of the leading nosocomial pathogens causing invasive infections of the skin and skin structure, bloodstream, bones and joints, heart, and lungs. Resistance and reduced susceptibility is rapidly increasing, especially with vancomycin as a workhorse against MRSA. Heteroresistance among VISA is significantly important due to their increased prevalence. The prevalence of hVISA is probably underestimated due to the lack of detection methods. With the decrease in breakpoint for *S. aureus* against vancomycin, the rate of VISA and VRSA will continue to rise with time. Creep of vancomycin MICs is of great concern because the use of glycopeptide increases with the rise in multidrug-resistant *S. aureus*. Resistance with the alternate agents such as daptomycin and linezolid are still rare; however, it is emerging as their use increases.

Multidrug-resistant *S. aureus* infections are spreading rapidly worldwide. *Staphyloccus aureus* is no longer confined to the healthcare setting as community pathogens emerge. The future clinical implications for *S. aureus* are identifying, treating, and monitoring the spread of a variety of staphylococcal clones worldwide.

REFERENCES

1. Ogston A. Micrococcus poisoning. *J Anat Physiol* 1882;**17**(Pt 1):24–58.
2. Shinefield HR, Ruff NL. Staphylococcal infections: A historical perspective. *Infect Dis Clin North Am* 2009;**23**(1):1–15.
3. Tang YW, Stratton CW. *Staphylococcus aureus*: An old pathogen with new weapons. *Clin Lab Med* 2010;**30**(1):179–208.
4. Classics in infectious diseases. "On abscesses". Alexander Ogston (1844–1929). *Rev Infect Dis 1984;***6**(1):122–128.
5. Liu GY, Essex A, Buchanan JT, et al. *Staphylococcus aureus* golden pigment impairs neutrophil killing and promotes virulence through its antioxidant activity. *J Exp Med* 2005;**202**(2) 209–215.
6. Mandell GL, Bennett JE, Dolin R. *Mandell, Douglas, and Bennett's Principles and Practice of Infectious Diseases*, 7th ed. Churchill Livingstone, Philadelphia, 2010.
7. Murray PR, Baron EJ, Jorgensen JH, et al. *Manual of Clinical Microbiology*, 9th ed. American Society of Microbiology, Washington DC, 2007.
8. Murray PR, Rosenthal KS, Pfaller MA. *Medical Microbiology*, 12th ed. Mosby Elsevier, Philadelphia, 2009.
9. Kwok AY, Chow AW. Phylogenetic study of *Staphylococcus* and *Macrococcus* species based on partial hsp60 gene sequences. *Int J Syst Evol Microbiol* 2003;**53**(Pt 1):87–92.
10. Ratner HB, Stratton CW. Thermonuclease test for same-day identification of *Staphylococcus aureus* in blood cultures. *J Clin Microbiol* 1985;**21**(6):995–996.
11. Tang YW, Kilic A, Yang Q, et al. StaphyPlex system for rapid and simultaneous identification of antibiotic resistance determinants and Panton–Valentine leukocidin detection of staphylococci from positive blood cultures. *J Clin Microbiol* 2007;**45**(6):1867–1873.
12. Kluytmans J, van Belkum A, Verbrugh H. Nasal carriage of *Staphylococcus aureus*: Epidemiology, underlying mechanisms, and associated risks. *Clin Microbiol Rev* 1997; **10**(3):505–520.
13. Gorwitz RJ, Kruszon-Moran D, McAllister SK, et al. Changes in the prevalence of nasal colonization with *Staphylococcus aureus* in the United States, 2001–2004. *J Infect Dis* 2008; **197**(9):1226–1234.
14. Lowy FD. *Staphylococcus aureus* infections. *N Engl J Med* 1998;**339**(8):520–32.

15. Gordon RJ, Lowy FD. Pathogenesis of methicillin-resistant *Staphylococcus aureus* infection. *Clin Infect Dis* 2008;**46**(Suppl 5):S350–S359.
16. Enright MC. The evolution of a resistant pathogen--the case of MRSA. *Curr Opin Pharmacol* 2003;**3**(5):474–479.
17. Hidron AI, Edwards JR, Patel J, et al. NHSN annual update: Antimicrobial-resistant pathogens associated with healthcare-associated infections: annual summary of data reported to the National Healthcare Safety Network at the Centers for Disease Control and Prevention, 2006–2007. *Infect Control Hosp Epidemiol* 2008;**29**(11):996–1011.
18. Smith IM, Vickers AB. Natural history of 338 treated and untreated patients with staphylococcal septicaemia (1936–1955). *Lancet* 1960;**1**(7138):1318–1322.
19. Skinner D, Keefer CS. Significance of bacteremia caused by *Staphylococcus aureus*: A study of one hundred and twenty-two cases and a review of the literature concerned with experimental infection in animals. *Arch Intern Med* 1941;**68**(5):851–875.
20. Jessen O, Rosendal K, Bulow, et al. Changing staphylococci and staphylococcal infections. A ten-year study of bacteria and cases of bacteremia. *N Engl J Med* 1969;**281**(12):627–635.
21. Peacock JE Jr, Marsik FJ, Wenzel RP. Methicillin-resistant *Staphylococcus aureus*: Introduction and spread within a hospital. *Ann Intern Med* 1980;**93**(4):526–32.
22. Shorr AF, Tabak YP, Killian AD, et al. Healthcare-associated bloodstream infection: A distinct entity? Insights from a large U. S. database. *Crit Care Med* 2006;**34**(10):2588–2595.
23. Zilberberg MD, Shorr AF, Micek ST, et al. Epidemiology and outcomes of hospitalizations with complicated skin and skin-structure infections: Implications of healthcare-associated infection risk factors. *Infect Control Hosp Epidemiol* 2009;**30**(12):1203–1210.
24. Enright MC, Day NP, Davies CE, et al. Multilocus sequence typing for characterization of methicillin-resistant and methicillin-susceptible clones of *Staphylococcus aureus*. *J Clin Microbiol* 2000;**38**(3):1008–1015.
25. Ruppitsch W, Indra A, Stoger A, et al. Classifying spa types in complexes improves interpretation of typing results for methicillin-resistant *Staphylococcus aureus*. *J Clin Microbiol* 2006; **44**(7):2442–8.
26. Tenover FC, Vaughn RR, McDougal LK, et al. Multiple-locus variable-number tandem-repeat assay analysis of methicillin-resistant *Staphylococcus aureus* strains. *J Clin Microbiol* 2007; **45**(7):2215–2219.
27. McDougal LK, Steward CD, Killgore GE, et al. Pulsed-field gel electrophoresis typing of oxacillin-resistant *Staphylococcus aureus* isolates from the United States: establishing a national database. *J Clin Microbiol* 2003;**41**(11):5113–5120.
28. Diep BA, Carleton HA, Chang RF, et al F. Roles of 34 virulence genes in the evolution of hospital- and community-associated strains of methicillin-resistant *Staphylococcus aureus*. *J Infect Dis* 2006;**193**(11):1495–1503.
29. Maree C, Daum RS, Boyle-Vavra S, et al. Community-associated methicillin-resistant *Staphylococcus aureus* strains causing healthcare-associated infections. *Emerg Infect Dis* 2007;**13**:236–242.
30. Seybold U, Kourbatova EV, Johnson JG, et al. Emergence of community-associated methicillin-resistant *Staphylococcus aureus* USA300 genotype as a major cause of health care-associated blood stream infections. *Clin Infect Dis* 2006;**42**(5):647–656.
31. Daum RS, Ito T, Hiramatsu K, et al. A novel methicillin-resistance cassette in community-acquired methicillin-resistant *Staphylococcus aureus* isolates of diverse genetic backgrounds. *J Infect Dis* 2002;**186**(9):1344–1347.
32. Carleton HA, Diep BA, Charlebois ED, et al. Community-adapted methicillin-resistant *Staphylococcus aureus* (MRSA): population dynamics of an expanding community reservoir of MRSA. *J Infect Dis* 2004;**190**(10):1730–1738.

33. Okuma K, Iwakawa K, Turnidge JD, et al. Dissemination of new methicillin-resistant *Staphylococcus aureus* clones in the community. *J Clin Microbiol* 2002;**40**(11):4289–4294.

34. Deresinski S. Methicillin-resistant *Staphylococcus aureus*: An evolutionary, epidemiologic, and therapeutic odyssey. *Clin Infect Dis* 2005;**40**(4):562–573.

35. Eguia JM, Chambers HF. Community-acquired methicillin-resistant *Staphylococcus aureus*: Epidemiology and potential virulence factors. *Curr Infect Dis Rep* 2003;**5**(6):459–466.

36. Weber JT. Community-associated methicillin-resistant *Staphylococcus aureus*. *Clin Infect Dis* 2005;**41**(Suppl 4):S269–S272.

37. Voyich JM, Otto M, Mathema B, et al. Is Panton–Valentine leukocidin the major virulence determinant in community-associated methicillin-resistant *Staphylococcus aureus* disease? *J Infect Dis* 2006;**194**(12):1761–1770.

38. Boyle-Vavra S, Daum RS. Community-acquired methicillin-resistant *Staphylococcus aureus*: The role of Panton-Valentine leukocidin. *Lab Invest* 2007;**87**(1):3–9.

39. Naimi TS, LeDell KH, Como-Sabetti K, et al. Comparison of community- and health care-associated methicillin-resistant *Staphylococcus aureus* infection. *JAMA* 2003; **290**(22):2976–2984.

40. Teixeira LA, Resende CA, Ormonde LR, et al. Geographic spread of epidemic multiresistant *Staphylococcus aureus* clone in Brazil. *J Clin Microbiol* 1995;**33**(9):2400–2404.

41. Amaral MM, Coelho LR, Flores RP, et al. The predominant variant of the Brazilian epidemic clonal complex of methicillin-resistant *Staphylococcus aureus* has an enhanced ability to produce biofilm and to adhere to and invade airway epithelial cells. *J Infect Dis* 2005;**192**(5):801–810.

42. Kluytmans J, van Belkum A, Verbrugh H. Nasal carriage of *Staphylococcus aureus*: Epidemiology, underlying mechanisms, and associated risks. *Clin Microbiol Rev* 1997;**10**(3):505–520.

43. Williams RE. Healthy carriage of *Staphylococcus aureus*: Its prevalence and importance. *Bacteriol Rev* 1963;**27**:56–71.

44. Graham PL 3rd, Lin SX, Larson EL. A U.S. population-based survey of *Staphylococcus aureus* colonization. *Ann Intern Med* 2006;**144**(5):318–325.

45. Boe J, Solberg CO, Vogelsang TM, et al. Perineal carriers of staphylococci. *Br Med J* 1964; **2**(5404):280–281.

46. Boyce JM, Havill NL, Maria B. Frequency and possible infection control implications of gastrointestinal colonization with methicillin-resistant *Staphylococcus aureus*. *J Clin Microbiol* 2005;**43**(12):5992–5995.

47. Nilsson P, Ripa T. *Staphylococcus aureus* throat colonization is more frequent than colonization in the anterior nares. *J Clin Microbiol* 2006;**44**(9):3334–3339.

48. Wertheim HF, Melles DC, Vos MC, et al. The role of nasal carriage in *Staphylococcus aureus* infections. *Lancet Infect Dis* 2005;**5**(12):751–762.

49. McConeghy KW, Mikolich DJ, LaPlante KL. Agents for the decolonization of methicillin-resistant *Staphylococcus aureus*. *Pharmacotherapy* 2009;**29**(3):263–280.

50. William RE, Jevons MP, Shooter RA, et al. Nasal staphylococci and sepsis in hospital patients. *Br Med J* 1959;**2**(5153):658–662.

51. Simor AE, Daneman N. *Staphylococcus aureus* decolonization as a prevention strategy. *Infect Dis Clin North Am* 2009;**23**(1):133–151.

52. Davis KA, Stewart JJ, Crouch HK, et al. Methicillin-resistant *Staphylococcus aureus* (MRSA) nares colonization at hospital admission and its effect on subsequent MRSA infection. *Clin Infect Dis* 2004;**39**(6):776–782.

53. Wertheim HF, Vos MC, Ott A, et al. Risk and outcome of nosocomial *Staphylococcus aureus* bacteraemia in nasal carriers versus non-carriers. *Lancet* 2004; 21–27; **364**(9435): 703–705.

54. Von Eiff C, Becker K, Machka K. Nasal carriage as a source of *Staphylococcus aureus* bacteremia. Study Group. *N Engl J Med* 2001;**344**(1):11–16.
55. Luzar MA, Coles GA, Faller B, et al. Ambulatory peritoneal dialysis. *N Engl J Med* 1990; **322**(8):505–509.
56. Wenzel RP, Perl TM. The significance of nasal carriage of *Staphylococcus aureus* and the incidence of postoperative wound infection. *J Hosp Infect* 1995;**31**(1):13–24.
57. Kalmeijer MD, van Nieuwland-Bollen E, Bogaers-Hofman D, et al. Nasal carriage of *Staphylococcus aureus* is a major risk factor for surgical-site infections in orthopedic surgery. *Infect Control Hosp Epidemiol* 2000;**21**(5):319–323.
58. Kluytmans JA, Mouton JW, Ijzerman EP, et al. Nasal carriage of *Staphylococcus aureus* as a major risk factor for wound infections after cardiac surgery. *J Infect Dis* 1995;**171** (1):216–219.
59. Shuter J, Hatcher VB, Lowy FD. *Staphylococcus aureus* binding to human nasal mucin. *Infect Immun* 1996;**64**(1):310–318.
60. Elek SD, Conen PE. The virulence of *Staphylococcus pyogenes* for man; A study of the problems of wound infection. *Br J Exp Pathol* 1957;**38**(6):573–586.
61. Spellberg B, Guidos R, Gilbert D, et al. The epidemic of antibiotic-resistant infections: A call to action for the medical community from the Infectious Diseases Society of America. *Clin Infect Dis* 2008;**46**(2):155–164.
62. Boucher HW, Talbot GH, Bradley JS, et al. Bad bugs, no drugs: No ESKAPE! An update from the Infectious Diseases Society of America. *Clin Infect Dis* 2009;**48**(1):1–12.
63. Cosgrove SE, Qi Y, Kaye KS, et al. The impact of methicillin resistance in *Staphylococcus aureus* bacteremia on patient outcomes: Mortality, length of stay, and hospital charges. *Infect Control Hosp Epidemiol* 2005;**26**(2):166–174.
64. Filice GA, Nyman JA, Lexau C, et al. Excess costs and utilization associated with methicillin resistance for patients with *Staphylococcus aureus* infection. *Infect Control Hosp Epidemiol* 2010;**31**(4):365–373.
65. Rice LB. Federal funding for the study of antimicrobial resistance in nosocomial pathogens: no ESKAPE. *J Infect Dis* 2008;**197**(8):1079–1081.
66. Rice LB. Progress and challenges in implementing the research on ESKAPE pathogens. *Infect Control Hosp Epidemiol* 2010;**31**(Suppl 1):S7–S10.
67. Cavalcanti AB, Goncalves AR, Almeida CS, et al. Teicoplanin versus vancomycin for proven or suspected infection. *Cochrane Database Syst Rev* 2010;**16**(6):CD007022.
68. Levine DP. Vancomycin: A history. *Clin Infect Dis* 2006;**42**(Suppl 1):S5–S12.
69. Levine DP. Vancomycin: Understanding its past and preserving its future. *South Med J* 2008;**101** (3):284–291.
70. Centers for Disease Control and Prevention (CDC). Reduced susceptibility of *Staphylococcus aureus* to vancomycin—Japan, 1996. *Morb Mortal Wkly Rep* 1997;**46**(27):624–626.
71. Hiramatsu K, Hanaki H, Ino T, et al. Methicillin-resistant *Staphylococcus aureus* clinical strain with reduced vancomycin susceptibility. *J Antimicrob Chemother* 1997;**40**(1):135–136.
72. Smith TL, Pearson ML, Wilcox KR, et al. Emergence of vancomycin resistance in *Staphylococcus aureus*. Glycopeptide-Intermediate *Staphylococcus aureus* Working Group. *N Engl J Med* 1999; **340**(7):493–501.
73. Ploy MC, Grelaud C, Martin C, et al. First clinical isolate of vancomycin-intermediate *Staphylococcus aureus* in a French hospital. *Lancet* 1998;**351**:1212.
74. Kim MN, Pai CH, Woo JH, et al. Vancomycin-intermediate *Staphylococcus aureus* in Korea. *J Clin Microbiol* 2000;**38**(10):3879–3881.

75. Clinical and Laboratory Standards Institute (CLSI). Performance standards for antimicrobial susceptibility testing. CLSI Document M100-S18. Clinical and Laboratory Standards Institute, Wayne, PA, 2008.
76. Tenover FC, Moellering R.C. Jr. The rationale for revising the Clinical and Laboratory Standards Institute vancomycin minimal inhibitory concentration interpretive criteria for *Staphylococcus aureus. Clin Infect Dis* 2007;**44**(9):1208–1215.
77. Hiramatsu K, Aritaka N, Hanaki H, et al. Dissemination in Japanese hospitals of strains of *Staphylococcus aureus* heterogeneously resistant to vancomycin. *Lancet* 1997; **350**(9092):1670–1673.
78. Kaatz GW, Seo SM, Dorman NJ, et al. Emergence of teicoplanin resistance during therapy of *Staphylococcus aureus* endocarditis. *J Infect Dis* 1990;**162**(1):103–108.
79. Manquat G, Croize J, Stahl JP, et al. Failure of teicoplanin treatment associated with an increase in MIC during therapy of *Staphylococcus aureus* septicaemia. *J Antimicrob Chemother* 1992; **29**(6):731–732.
80. Mainardi JL, Shlaes DM, Goering RV, et al. Decreased teicoplanin susceptibility of methicillin-resistant strains of *Staphylococcus aureus. J Infect Dis* 1995;**171**(6):1646–1650.
81. Hiramatsu K. Vancomycin-resistant *Staphylococcus aureus*: A new model of antibiotic resistance. *Lancet Infect Dis* 2001;**1**(3):147–155.
82. Liu C, Chambers. *Staphylococcus aureus* with heterogeneous resistance to vancomycin: epidemiology, clinical significance, and critical assessment of diagnostic methods. *Antimicrob Agents Chemother* 2003;**47**(10):3040–3045.
83. Rong SL, Leonard SN. Heterogeneous vancomycin resistance in *Staphylococcus aureus*: A review of epidemiology, diagnosis, and clinical significance. *Ann Pharmcother* 2010; **44**(5);844–850.
84. Rybak MJ, Leonard SN, Rossi KL, et al. Characterization of vancomycin-heteroresistant *Staphylococcus aureus* from the metropolitan area of Detroit, Michigan, over a 22-year period (1986 to 2007). *J Clin Microbiol* 2008;**46**(9):2950–2954.
85. Lalani T, Federspiel JJ, Boucher HW, et al. Associations between the genotypes of *Staphylococcus aureus* bloodstream isolates and clinical characteristics and outcomes of bacteremic patients. *J Clin Microbiol* 2008;**46**(9);2890–2896.
86. Pitz AM, Yu F, Hermsen ED, et al. Vancomycin susceptibility trends and prevalence of heterogeneous vancomycin-intermediate *Staphylococcus aureus* (hVISA) in clinical methicillin-resistant *S. aureus* (MRSA) isolates. *J Clin Microbiol* 2011;**49**(1):269–274.
87. Wootton M, Howe RA, Hillman R, et al. A modified population analysis profile (PAP) method to detect hetero-resistance to vancomycin in *Staphylococcus aureus* in a UK hospital. *J Antimicrob Chemother* 2001;**47**(4):399–403.
88. Centers for Disease Control and Prevention (CDC). *Staphylococcus aureus* resistant to vancomycin—United States, 2002. *Morb Mortal Wkly Rep* 2002;**51**(6):565–567.
89. Centers for Disease Control and Prevention (CDC). Vancomycin-resistant *Staphylococcus aureus*—Pennsylvania, 2002. *Morb Mortal Wkly Rep* 2002;**51**(40):902.
90. Centers for Disease Control and Prevention (CDC). Vancomycin-resistant *Staphylococcus aureus*—New York, 2004. *Morb Mortal Wkly Rep* 2004;**53**(15):322–323.
91. Nannini E, Murray BE, Arias CA. Resistance or decreased susceptibility to glycopeptides, daptomycin, and linezolid in methicillin-resistant *Staphylococcus aureus. Curr Opin Pharmacol* 2010;**10**(5):516–521.
92. Howden BP, Davies JK, Johnson PD, et al. Reduced vancomycin susceptibility in *Staphylococcus aureus,* including vancomycin-intermediate and heterogeneous vancomycin-intermediate strains: Resistance mechanisms, laboratory detection, and clinical implications. *Clin Microbiol Rev* 2010;**23**(1):99–139.

93. Aligholi M, Emaneini M, Jabalameli F, et al. Emergence of high-level vancomycin-resistant *Staphylococcus aureus* in the Imam Khomeini Hospital in Tehran. *Med Princ Pract* 2008;**17**(5):432–434.
94. Foucault ML, Courvalin P, Grillot-Courvalin C. Fitness cost of VanA-type vancomycin resistance in methicillin-resistant *Staphylococcus aureus*. *Antimicrob Agents Chemother* 2009;**53**(6):2354–2359.
95. Moubareck C, Meziane-Cherif D, Courvalin P, et al. VanA-type *Staphylococcus aureus* strain VRSA-7 is partially dependent on vancomycin for growth. *Antimicrob Agents Chemother* 2009;**53**(9):3657–3663.
96. Saha B, Singh AK, Ghosh A, et al. Identification and characterization of a vancomycin-resistant *Staphylococcus aureus* isolated from Kolkata (South Asia). *J Med Microbiol* 2008;**57**(Pt 1):72–79.
97. Sievert DM, Rudrik JT, Patel JB, et al. Vancomycin-resistant *Staphylococcus aureus* in the United States, 2002–2006. *Clin Infect Dis* 2008;**46**(5):668–674.
98. Boyle-Vavra S, Berke SK, Lee JC, et al. Reversion of the glycopeptide resistance phenotype in *Staphylococcus aureus* clinical isolates. *Antimicrob Agents Chemother* 2000;**44**(2):272–277.
99. Weigel LM, Clewell DB, Gill SR, et al. Genetic analysis of a high-level vancomycin-resistant isolate of *Staphylococcus aureus*. *Science* 2003;**302**(5650):1569–1571.
100. Perichon B, Courvalin P. VanA-type vancomycin-resistant *Staphylococcus aureus*. *Antimicrob Agents Chemother* 2009;**53**(11):4580–4587.
101. Noble WC, Virani Z, Cree RG. Co-transfer of vancomycin and other resistance genes from *Enterococcus faecalis* NCTC 12201 to *Staphylococcus aureus*. *FEMS Microbiol Lett* 1992;**93**(2):195–198.
102. Zhu W, Clark NC, Mcdougal LK, et al. Vancomycin-resistant *Staphylococcus aureus* isolates associated with Inc18-like vanA plasmids in Michigan. *Antimicrob Agents Chemother* 2008;**52**(2):452–457.
103. Di Paolo A, Malacarne P, Guidotti E, et al. Pharmacological issues of linezolid: an updated critical review. *Clin Pharmacokinet* 2010;**49**(7):439–447.
104. Tsiodras S, Gold HS, Sakoulas G, et al. Linezolid resistance in a clinical isolate of *Staphylococcus aureus*. *Lancet* 2001;**358**(9277):207–208.
105. Meka VG, Pillai SK, Sakoulas G, et al. Linezolid resistance in sequential *Staphylococcus aureus* isolates associated with a T2500A mutation in the 23S rRNA gene and loss of a single copy of rRNA. *J Infect Dis* 2004;**190**(2):311–317.
106. Ikeda-Dantsuji Y, Hanaki H, Sakai F, et al. Linezolid-resistant *Staphylococcus aureus* isolated from 2006 through 2008 at six hospitals in Japan. *J Infect Chemother* 2011;**17**(1):45–51.
107. Prystowsky J, Siddiqui F, Chosay J, et al. Resistance to linezolid: Characterization of mutations in rRNA and comparison of their occurrences in vancomycin-resistant enterococci. *Antimicrob Agents Chemother* 2001;**45**(7):2154–2156.
108. Sanchez Garcia M, De la Torre MA, Morales G, et al. Clinical outbreak of linezolid-resistant *Staphylococcus aureus* in an intensive care unit. *JAMA* 2010;**303**(22):2260–2264.
109. Kosmidis C, Levine DP. Daptomycin: pharmacology and clinical use. *Expert Opin Pharmacother* 2010;**11**(4):615–625.
110. Tenover FC, Sinner SW, Segal RE, et al. Characterisation of a *Staphylococcus aureus* strain with progressive loss of susceptibility to vancomycin and daptomycin during therapy. *Int J Antimicrob Agents* 2009;**33**(6):564–568.
111. Boucher HW, Sakoulas G. Perspectives on daptomycin resistance, with emphasis on resistance in *Staphylococcus aureus*. *Clin Infect Dis* 2007;**45**(5):601–608.

112. Fridkin SK, Hageman J, McDougal LK, et al. Epidemiological and microbiological characterization of infections caused by *Staphylococcus aureus* with reduced susceptibility to vancomycin, United States, 1997–2001. *Clin Infect Dis* 2003;**36**(4):429–439.

113. Howden BP, Johnson PD, Ward PB, et al. Isolates with low-level vancomycin resistance associated with persistent methicillin-resistant *Staphylococcus aureus* bacteremia. *Antimicrob Agents Chemother* 2006;**50**(9):3039–3047.

114. Hidayat LK, Hsu DI, Quist R, High-dose vancomycin therapy for methicillin-resistant *Staphylococcus aureus* infections: Efficacy and toxicity. *Arch Intern Med* 2006; **166**(19):2138–2144.

115. Lodise TP, Miller CD, Graves J, et al. Predictors of high vancomycin MIC values among patients with methicillin-resistant *Staphylococcus aureus* bacteraemia. *J Antimicrob Chemother* 2008; **62**(5):1138–1141.

116. Steinkraus G, White R, Friedrich L. Vancomycin MIC creep in non-vancomycin-intermediate *Staphylococcus aureus* (VISA), vancomycin-susceptible clinical methicillin-resistant *S. aureus* (MRSA) blood isolates from 2001–05. *J Antimicrob Chemother* 2007;**60**(4):788–794.

117. Wang G, Hindler JF, Ward KW, et al. Increased vancomycin MICs for *Staphylococcus aureus* clinical isolates from a university hospital during a 5-year period. *J Clin Microbiol* 2006; **44**(1):3883–3886.

118. Popovich KJ, Weinstein RA, Hota B. Are community-associated methicillin-resistant *Staphylococcus aureus* (MRSA) strains replacing traditional nosocomial MRSA strains? *Clin Infect Dis* 2008;**46**(6):787–794.

119. Liu C, Graber CJ, Karr M, et al. A population-based study of the incidence and molecular epidemiology of methicillin-resistant *Staphylococcus aureus* disease in San Francisco, 2004–2005. *Clin Infect Dis* 2008;**46**(11):1637–1646.

120. Vidal PM, Trindade PA, Garcia TO, et al. Differences between "classical" risk factors for infections caused by methicillin-resistant *Staphylococcus aureus* (MRSA) and risk factors for nosocomial bloodstream infections caused by multiple clones of the staphylococcal cassette chromosome *mec* type IV MRSA strain. *Infect Control Hosp Epidemiol* 2009;**30**(2):139–145.

121. Vaudaux P, Kelley WL, Lew DP. *Staphylococcus aureus* small colony variants: Difficult to diagnose and difficult to treat. *Clin Infect Dis* 2006;**43**(8):968–970.

122. Sendi P, Rohrbach M, Graber P, et al. *Staphylococcus aureus* small colony variants in prosthetic joint infection. *Clin Infect Dis* 2006;**43**(8):961–967.

123. Kahl B, Herrmann M, Everding AS, et al. Persistent infection with small colony variant strains of *Staphylococcus aureus* in patients with cystic fibrosis. *J Infect Dis* 1998;**177**(4):1023–1029.

124. Proctor RA, von Eiff C, Kahl BC, et al. Small colony variants: A pathogenic form of bacteria that facilitates persistent and recurrent infections. *Nat Rev Microbiol* 2006;**4**(4):295–305.

125. Tsuji BT, von Eiff C, Kelchlin PA, et al. Attenuated vancomycin bactericidal activity against *Staphylococcus aureus* hemB mutants expressing the small-colony-variant phenotype. *Antimicrob Agents Chemother* 2008;**52**(4):1533–1537.

CHAPTER ELEVEN

Escherichia coli

JOHANN D. D. PITOUT

Introduction

Escherichia coli inhabits the human gastrointestinal tract and makes up the majority of aerobic Gram-negative bacteria of the intestinal tract. It is a non-spore-forming rod and is motile by means of peritrichous flagella. These bacteria are facultative anaerobic; that is, they grow aerobically as well as anaerobically, although they prefer to grow aerobically. The majority of isolates are lactose fermenters, and the appearance of colonies on MacConkey agar includes smooth, glossy, and translucent colonies that are rose pink in color (1). Most isolates of *E. coli* ferment carbohydrates effectively, leading to the production of acid and gas although some isolates can produce acid without gas. *Escherichia coli* is also characterized by (a) the ability to reduce nitrates to nitrites and (b) indole production with a positive methyl-red reaction while the Voges–Proskauer test is negative. *Escherichia coli* isolates do not hydrolyze urea or produce hydrogen sulfide, and phenylalanine deaminase activity is absent. *Escherichia coli* cannot use citrate as the sole source of carbon and will not grow in the presence of potassium cyanide (2).

Conventional approaches (e.g., sugar fermentation) in combination with growth on selective or differential media, colonial characteristics, and cell morphology on a Gram stain are still valid and sufficient to identify *E. coli* (1, 2). Commercially available methods that use rapid chromogenic enzyme substrates, such as the API or automated systems, have gained popularity among clinical laboratories to routinely identify *E. coli* (2).

Escherichia coli can be subdivided into serogroups, serotypes, and biotypes (3). Two of the compounds present on the surface of *E. coli* form the basis for the serologic classification

Molecular Techniques for the Study of Hospital-Acquired Infection, First Edition. Edited by Steven L. Foley, Anne Y. Chen, Shabbir Simjee, and Marcus J. Zervos.

system: (a) heat-stable somatic O antigen of LPS and (b) heat-labile flagella H antigen. The O antigen identifies the serogroup of an isolate while the H antigen identifies the serotype. The biotype is determined by the biochemical profile (i.e., sugar fermentation, etc.). If an *E. coli* isolate contains a capsule, a capsular or K antigen can also be used for classification purposes. K antigens are often associated with invasive *E. coli* disease, and isolates with K1 antigen commonly cause systemic diseases, in infants (4).

While most isolates of *E. coli* reside harmlessly in the lumen of human colons and fail to cause disease in healthy individuals, different virulent types do exist that have the ability to cause specific types of illness in normal hosts and those with compromised defense mechanisms (5). The development and the severity of the infection depend strongly on both the virulence of the bacteria and the state of the host's defense mechanisms (6). The virulent types differ from commensal organisms in that they produce specific virulence factors that may be encoded by bacteriophages, on plasmids, or on stretches of chromosomal DNA known as pathogenicity islands (3, 7).

Escherichia coli is an important cause of urinary tract infections (UTIs), enteric infections, and systemic infections in humans (3). These systemic infections include bacteremia, nosocomial pneumonia, cholecystitis, cholangitis, peritonitis, cellulitis, osteomyelitis, and infectious arthritis while *E. coli* is a leading cause of neonatal meningitis. Isolates that are responsible for extra-intestinal infections often originate from within the gastrointestinal tract. The most important virulence factors associated with the pathogenesis of UTIs are the O-K serotypes, hemolysins, iron-sequestration systems, and the presence of adhesins for uroepithelial cells (Type 1 and P fimbrae) (8).

Escherichia coli as a Nosocomial Pathogen

Healthcare-associated infections often result from the use of indwelling devices such as endotracheal tubes, intravenous lines, or urinary catheters, or they follow surgery or other invasive procedures (9). The most frequent types of healthcare-associated infections are pneumonia, surgical site, urinary tract, and bloodstream types of infections (10).

During recent years Enterobacteriaceae, including species such as *E. coli*, have become less prevalent than Gram-positive cocci (i.e., staphylococci and enterococci) as causes of nosocomial infections. This is mostly due to the increased use of invasive devices in intensive care units. This was illustrated in a recent article from the National Noscommial Infections Surveillance system that compared the bacterial isolates associated with nosocomial infections isolated in 1975 to those isolates in 2003 (11). However, *E. coli* still remains an important cause of nosocomial-acquired infections, especially of urinary tract infections, bloodstream infections, surgical site infections, pneumonia, and Gram-negative sepsis (11).

Escherichia coli ranks second as the most common cause of nosocomial-acquired bloodstream infections and is most often responsible for septic shock caused by Gram-negative bacteria (12–18). These bloodstream infections usually arise as a complication of focal infections of the urinary (especially due to indwelling urinary catheters) or gastrointestinal tracts. Occasionally, *E. coli* may be responsible for primary bacteremia without a definable source. *Escherichia coli* is also a major cause of invasive infections, including sepsis and meningitis in the neonatal period (19). The overall mortality rate from *E. coli* bacteremia is approximately 20% (20).

Escherichia coli is the leading pathogen responsible for nosocomial-acquired urinary tract infections (UTIs), being implicated in 26% of all nosocomial UTIs (21). Recognized major risk factors for nosocomial-acquired UTIs include urinary catheterization and obstruction to urine flow.

The lungs are another common site of nosocomial-acquired infections due to *E. coli*, although it can sometimes be difficult to discriminate between *E. coli* colonizing the upper airways and *E. coli* causing pulmonary infections (11). *Escherichia coli* is also an important cause of surgical infections, especially those infections associated with intraabdominal surgery or trauma (11). Nosocomial central nervous system infections due to *E. coli* occur mainly in the neonatal period or in neurosurgical patients undergoing procedures that penetrate the central nervous system (22).

Techniques for Typing *Escherichia coli* in the Hospital Setting

The various bacterial traits of *E. coli*, routinely analyzed in molecular epidemiological studies, range from subgenic DNA sequence (the most basic), through genes, operons, and pathogenicity islands (intermediate), to clones, clonal groups, and phylogenetic groups (the most complex) (23). Each level is important and informative; each requires distinctive typing methods. The investigation of the basic and intermediate traits of *E. coli* in molecular epidemiological studies involves mostly the analysis of virulence associated genes or their flanking regions and include techniques such as restriction fragment-length polymorphism (RFLP) analysis, direct DNA sequencing, probe hybridization, and PCR detection (24). However, these techniques are not often used to investigate nosocomial outbreaks caused by *E. coli*.

The most complex level (i.e., determining clones, clonal groups, and phylogenetic groups) is commonly identified at the molecular level by using typing methods that scan the entire genome (24). These include techniques such as pulsed field gel electrophoresis (PFGE) analysis, ribotyping, PCR-based fingerprinting, multilocus enzyme electrophoresis (MLEE), and multilocus sequence typing (MLST). These techniques are often used to type *E. coli* involved in nosocomail outbreaks; however, MLEE and MLST are not particularly amenable to widespread, large-scale use.

In ribotyping, ribosomal DNA probes are used for Southern hybridization with total DNA that has been restricted with a conventional endonuclease such as *Hin*dIII and electrophoretically size-separated (25). PCR-based methods are more useful for identifying broader clonal groups and include (a) random amplified polymorphic DNA (RAPD) analysis, which uses random or arbitrary primers, and (b) repetitive element PCR, which uses primers targeting various known genomic repeat elements and generates distinctive banding patterns that reflect the spacing of suitable primer sites in the genome of the particular isolate (26, 27). For any of these methods, in addition to simple "same-versus-different" comparisons, genomic profiles can be subjected to cluster analysis to define quantitative similarity relationships among isolates (24). Isolates can also be sorted readily into the four major phylogenetic groups of *E. coli* (A, B1, B2, and D), as originally defined by MLEE (28), by using a simple multiplex PCR-based method (29).

PFGE is considered as the gold standard and the most discriminating for typing of medically important bacteria, including *E. coli* (30). This method is based on the specific digestion (or cutting), using a restriction enzyme such as *Xba*I, of bacterial DNA into fragments of varying sizes, followed by the separation of these DNA fragments into fingerprints by gel electrophoresis. This involves electrophoretic separation of total bacterial DNA that has been digested. Clones consist of bacteria that originate from the same parent, and PFGE is excellent for identifying different clones responsible for recent or ongoing outbreaks (31). Identity of two isolates by PFGE analysis implies that they represent the same strain, or clone. Unfortunately, PFGE is labor-intensive and time-consuming and only delivers the best results when performed by a person or persons with extensive technical experience in this method.

Bacterial barcodes, a type of repetitive-element PCR (rep-PCR), is a rapid, automated, PCR-based, commercial typing system that can easily be performed by a bench technologist with some molecular experience (32). Rep-PCR was described in 1993 as a rapid method for strain typing that relies on amplification of the sequences between various repetitive elements interspersed throughout the genome (27). Kits containing standard primers and PCR master mix reagents are marketed by BioMérieux, Inc. Gel electrophoresis has been replaced by separation in a microfluidics chamber, and digitized gel images are generated and compared by using proprietary computer software. Although this method is limited by the requirement of significant expenditure for reagents and equipment, it has two major advantages (33). First, results are generated more rapidly than for either PFGE or MLST. A batch of 12 samples is easily performed within a single day. Second, standardized, digitized gel images are stored for comparison between runs and between laboratories. This technique has the potential to tract resistant bacteria in a real-time basis.

Enterobacterial repetitive intergenic consensus (ERIC) sequences found in *E. coli* and *Salmonella* are used in another PCR-based strain typing assay (34). This method is also a type of rep-PCR typing method (but is not commercialized and is called ERIC PCR) that amplifies the DNA located between repetitive sequence elements that are variably spaced around the bacterial genome, producing DNA fragments of varying sizes. The fragments are separated using gel electrophoresis, and the result is a unique DNA fingerprint (genotype) for each isolate. The ERIC2 version has been modified several times to give the best results for typing *E. coli* when using noncommercialized rep-PCR typing methods (34). This method is relatively fast and cost-effective and provides a simple method to group similar isolates into clonal groups. This technique also has the potential to tract resistant bacteria in a real-time basis.

MLST is a portable, universal, and definitive sequence-based typing method that examines the nucleotide sequences of multiple loci of housekeeping genes (35). MLST will identify different allelic profiles by sequencing seven housekeeping genes. This makes it the most suitable typing method for comparing data generated independently from different laboratories and ideal for tracking antimicrobial resistant bacteria on a worldwide basis (35). Unfortunately, MLST is expensive, time-consuming, and not really suitable to track resistant clones in the rapid real-time fashion.

Emerging Issues in Antimicrobial Resistance in *Escherichia coli*

The emergence of antimicrobial resistant bacteria ranks among the most important contemporary healthcare issues to date (36). The consequences of antimicrobial resistance have resulted in treatment failures with adverse outcomes for patients and dramatic cost implications for healthcare systems (37). The Enterobacteriaceae, most notably *E. coli*, are among the most important causes of serious nosocomial and community-onset bacterial infections in humans, and resistance to antimicrobial agents in these species has become an increasingly relevant problem (38).

NEWER BETA-LACTAMASES

Beta-lactam antibiotics are a major drug class used to treat serious infections caused by *E. coli*, and resistance to these agents will continue to challenge clinical therapeutic choices (39). In *E. coli*, β-lactamase production remains the most important contributing factor to β-lactam resistance. Beta-lactamases are bacterial enzymes that inactivate β-lactam antibiotics by hydrolysis, which results in ineffective compounds (39). Most importantly within the *E. coli* is the increasing recognition of isolates producing the so-called "newer β-lactamases" that consist of plasmid-mediated AmpC ß-lactamases or cephamycinases (e.g., CMY types), extended-spectrum β-lactamases (e.g., CTX-M types), and carbapenem-hydrolyzing enzymes (CHEs) (e.g., the class A or KPC types (40). The class B CHEs, also referred to as the metallo-β-lactamases, are relatively rare among *E. coli* (41). The production of newer β-lactamases results in broad-spectrum resistance to most of the β-lactam antibiotics.

The most well known of the newer types of β-lactamases was described for the first time in 1983 and referred to as "extended spectrum ß-lactamases" (ESBLs), which have the ability to hydrolyze the penicillins, cephalosporins, and monobactams but not the cephamycins and carbapenems (42). ESBLs are inhibited by "classical" β-lactamase inhibitors such as clavulanic acid, sulbactam, and tazobactam. Although ESBLs have been identified in a range of Enterobacteriaceae, they are most often present in *E. coli* and *K. pneumoniae*. These bacteria are major causes of hospital-acquired infections on a worldwide basis. The majority of ESBLs identified in clinical isolates to date have been of the SHV or TEM types that have evolved from parent enzymes such as TEM-1, TEM-2, and SHV-1 (42). CTX-M β-lactamases, which classically cause resistance to cefotaxime but remain sensitive to ceftazidime, have originated from the environmental *Kluyvera* spp, and recently gained prominence with reports of clinical isolates producing these enzymes from Europe, Africa, Asia, and South and North America (43). Organisms producing ESBLs are clinically relevant and remain an important cause for failure of therapy with cephalosporins (42). ESBLs are often encoded by genes located on very large plasmids that also carry genes for resistance to other antimicrobial agents such as the aminoglycosides, trimethoprim, sulfonamides, tetracyclines, and chloramphenicol. Thus, very broad antimicrobial resistance extending to multiple classes is a frequent characteristic of ESBL-producing organisms (42).

Escherichia coli possesses a chromosomal gene that encodes for an AmpC β-lactamase. Usually, low amounts of β-lactamases are produced because the AmpC gene is regulated by a weak promoter and a strong attenuator (44). Surveys of resistance mechanisms in cephamycin-resistant isolates have identified promoter or attenuator mutations, which results in the up-regulation of AmpC ß-lactamase production (45). Occasionally, cephamycin-resistant strains produce plasmid-mediated β-lactamases such as CMY-2 derived from bacteria with chromosomally encoded AmpC cephalosporinases (46). These enzymes are derivatives of the chromosomally encoded AmpC cephalosporinases of bacteria such as *Enterobacter, Citrobacter feundii, Morganella morganii, Aeromonas* spp., and *Hafnia alvei* (46). These β-lactamases at high levels hydrolyze penicillins, most cephalosporins, cephamycins, and monobactams but not cefepime and carbapenems. AmpC enzymes are not inhibited by "classical" β-lactamase inhibitors such as clavulanic acid, sulbactam, and tazobactam, although different inhibitors such as boronic acid and cloxacillin have shown good activity (47). The genes are also typically encoded on large plasmids containing additional antimicrobial resistance genes, leaving few therapeutic options. Just like ESBL-producing bacteria, organisms with plasmid-mediated AmpC enzymes are mostly responsible for nosocomial outbreaks on a worldwide basis (46).

Pseudomonas aeruginosa that produces metallo-β-lactamases (MBLs) was first reported from Japan in 1991 and since then have been described from various parts of the world (48). MBLs are mostly associated with this species and are relatively rare among Enterobacteriaceae (49). However, VIM and IMP types of MBLs have been described from various countries in Europe, Asia, South America, and Australia in the following members of the Enterobacteriaceae: *Klebsiella* spp., *E. coli*, *Shigella flexneri*, *S. marcescens*, *M. morganii*, *P. mirablis*, *Proteus vulgaris*, *Providencia rettgeri*, and *Citrobacter* spp. (41). MBLs have the ability to hydrolyze a wide variety of β-lactam agents such as penicillins, cephalosporins, and carbapenems but not the monobactams (i.e., aztreonam) (49). These enzymes require zinc for their catalytic activity and are inhibited by metal chelators such as EDTA. The dissemination of acquired MBLs in members of the family Enterobacteriaceae is regarded as an emerging clinical threat.

The most recent of the "newer" β-lactamases belongs to class A CHEs and is named the KPC types (so far four variants have been described) (50). KPC-1 was reported in the late 1990s from a *K. pneumoniae* isolated in North Carolina. These enzymes provide resistance to the carbapenems, cephalosporins, and monobactams and are inhibited by "classical" β-lactamase inhibitors such clavulanic acid, sulbactam, and tazobactam. KPC-2 and -3 have been shown to be widespread in enterobacterial species including *Klebsiella* spp., *E. coli*, and *Enterobacter* spp. from Brooklyn, New York, and in several areas in Pennsylvania and other states in the United States (51–53). KPC are also present in European countries, South America, Asia, and the Middle East (especially Israel) (50). The genes responsible for the production of KPC enzymes are often located on transferable plasmids, thereby explaining their spread among clinically relevant pathogens. KPC-producing *K. pneumoniae* have the ability to spread within healthcare facilities, causing substantial mortality associated with bacteraemia (51). Although KPC β-lactamases are relatively rare in *E. coli* at this moment in time, the discovery of these enzymes represents an additional significant threat in the evolving world of β-lactamase-mediated resistance in bacteria.

PLASMID-MEDIATED QUINOLONE RESISTANCE

The fluoroquinolones are another group of antimicrobial agents often used to treat infections caused by Enterobacteriaceace, including *E. coli*. Resistance to these agents have traditionally been associated with chromosomal mutations (54); but recently, plasmid-mediated quinolone resistance (PMQR), due to the production of pentapeptide repeat proteins, has been described in clinical isolates of Enterobacteriaceae from different parts of the world (55). These proteins named QnrA, QnrB, and QnrS block the action of fluoroquinolones on bacterial topoisomerases and are associated with class 1 integrons. Qnr B and QnrS share 40% and 59% amino acid identity, respectively, with QnrA. Qnr determinants confer resistance to nalidixic acid and reduced susceptibility to the fluoroquinolones (i.e., norfloxacin, ciprofloxacin, levofloxacin) (56). It has been shown that the Qnr determinants originate from the aquatic species of bacteria, such as *Shewanella algae* and *Vibrio splendidus,* being the progenitors of *qnrA*-and *qnrS*-like genes (57, 58).

A different mechanism of transferable quinolone resistance that involved the enzymatic inactivation of certain quinolones was first reported in 2006 (59). This is due to a variant of an aminoglycoside-modifying enzyme *aac(6′)-Ib* and is named *aac(6′)-Ib-cr*. The parent enzyme and its variant provide resistance to the following aminoglycosides: kanamycin, tobramycin, and amikacin. The variant enzyme *aac(6′)-Ib-cr* has the additional ability to hydrolyze fluoroquinolones with an unprotected amino nitrogen on the piperazine ring such as norfloxacin and ciprofloxacin (59). As with Qnr determinants, *aac(6′)-Ib-cr* confer resistance to nalidixic acid and reduced susceptibility to the fluoroquinolones with a piperazine ring (56).

A third type of PMQR determinant has only recently been identified in *E. coli* isolated in Japan and Belgium (60, 61). The *qepA* gene encodes for a protein that acts as an efflux pump; that is, hydrophilic quinolones such as norfloxacin and ciprofloxacin are "pumped out" of the bacterial cell, causing resistance (i.e., 32- to 64-fold increase in MIC) to these agents.

A recent surveillance study investigated the prevalence of PMQR determinants in 2004 and 2007 among clinical isolates of Enterobacteriaceae in Canada; 12/201 (6%) of *E. coli* were positive for *aac(6′)-Ib-cr* in 2004 while 53/398 (13%) were positive in 2007; 3/398 (0.7%) were positive for *qnrS* and 1 isolate for both *aac(6′)-Ib-cr* and *qnrS*. This study showed that *E. coli* with *aac(6′)-Ib-cr* is emerging as an important cause of fluoroquinolone resistance in the community and hospital settings that is mostly due to the influx of CTX-M-15 producing isolates (62).

Nosocomial-Acquired Infections Due to Mulitidrug-Resistant *Escherichia coli*

Recent surveillance studies in the United States and Europe show that the predominant Gram-negative pathogens responsible for nosocomial infections are *E. coli, K. pneumoniae, Enterobacter species, Serratia species, P. aeruginosa*, and *Acinetobacter baumannii* (11, 63–65). Antibiotic resistance in nosocomial isolates of each of these pathogens, including *E. coli*, has considerable clinical impact and many strains of these species have become multidrug-resistant—that is, are consistently resistant to three or more classes of antibiotic (65–67). Many of the infections caused by Gram-negative bacteria are opportunistic and thus are particularly relevant to the growing population of patients with cancer and AIDS who are immunosuppressed.

EXTENDED-SPECTRUM-BETA-LACTAMASES

Organisms producing ESBLs are clinically relevant and remain an important cause for failure of therapy with cephalosporins. Enterobacteriaceae (mostly *Klebsiella* spp. and *E. coli*) that produce SHV and TEM types of ESBLs have traditionally been responsible for serious nosocomial infections (42). During the 1990s there was a growing number of reports of TEM- and SHV-derived ESBLs, particularly in association with nosocomial outbreaks, from many parts of the world (68). A variety of units were affected, including chronic care facilities, neonatology, neurosurgery, pediatrics, and obstetrics. However, most outbreaks were reported from intensive care units (ICUs) (42). Although ESBL-producing *E. coli, Salmonella enterica* serovar Typhimurium, *Citrobacter diversus*, and *Klebsiella oxytoca* caused some outbreaks, by far the most common producer species was *K. pneumoniae* (42, 69, 70). Many outbreaks were caused by patient-to-patient spread of particular clones, but one in a pediatric oncology unit in the United Kingdom was the result of plasmid transfer between unrelated strains of the same species, with some dissemination to different species (71). One US study conducted in 1997 found that 4.7% of hospital isolates of *E. coli* and 9.5% of *Proteus mirabilis* isolates were ESBL producers, compared with 44% of *K. pneumoniae* (72).

Specific risk factors for acquisition of ESBL-producing Enterobacteriaceae identified during the 1990s included length of hospital stay, severity of illness, time in the intensive care unit (ICU), intubations and mechanical ventilation, urinary or arterial catheterization, and previous exposure to antibiotics (42). The majority of the patients infected with ESBL-producing *E. coli* have been admitted to ICUs, but infections can also occur in almost any other area of the hospital.

A study from Israel has shown that nosocomial bacteremia caused by ESBL-producing Enterobacteriaceae (most often *E. coli*), as compared to non-ESBL producers, was associated with severe adverse outcomes (including higher mortality), increased length of stay in the hospital, delay in appropriate therapy, delay in discharge to chronic care, and significantly higher costs (37). A Spanish study shows that inadequate initial therapy and an unidentified source of the primary infection were predictors of mortality in nosocomial bloodstream infections caused by ESBL-producing *E. coli* (73).

In 2000 *E. coli* that produces CTX-M enzymes increased in prevalence among ESBL-producing bacteria and have become the most prevalent type of ESBLs described during the last 5 years, especially from certain European, Asian, and South and North American countries (43). ESBL-producing *K. pneumoniae* still remain an important issue, but it is evident that the epidemiology of *E. coli* that produces CTX-M enzymes is very different from those that produce TEM- and SHV-derived ESBLs. CTX-M enzymes are not limited to nosocomial infections caused by *Klebsiella* spp. *Escherichia coli* is most often responsible for producing these types of β-lactamases and are considered to be community and nosocomial ESBL-producing pathogens (74). Surveys from several countries worldwide have illustrated an alarming trend of associated resistance to other classes of antimicrobial agents among CTX-M-producing organisms isolated from hospital and community sites (75). These surveys show co-resistance to trimethoprim-sulfamethoxazole, tetracycline, gentamicin, and ciprofloxacin (as many as 70% of isolates were resistant to ciprofloxacin).

A Canadian study describes the molecular epidemiology of CTX-M-producing *E. coli* in a large well-defined geographical region over a 6-year period. This study showed a predominance of clonally related CTX-M-14 producers during the first 4 years of the study period associated with community outbreaks followed by a substantial increase of CTX-M-15 that occurred during the last 18 months. This increase was mostly due to two similar CTX-M-15-producing clones in the community, which were introduced into the hospital and nursing home sectors (76). A different study from Canada investigated the prevalence of antimicrobial resistance during 2005–2006 among clinical isolates from ICUs (65). They documented that ESBL-producing *E. coli* are more common than ESBL-producing *Klebsiella* spp. in Canadian ICUs.

Carriage of Enterobacteriaceae in the lower gastrointestinal tract is an important factor in the subsequent development of clinical infection. A Spanish study demonstrated a significant increase in fecal carriage of ESBL-producing *E. coli* between 1991 and 2003 in Spain (77). Carriage rates in hospital- and community-based patients rose from 0.3% and 0.7%, respectively, in 1991 to 11.8% and 5.5%, respectively, in 2003 ($P < 0.001$). They also screened samples from 108 healthy volunteers, 4 (3.7%) of whom were found to carry ESBL-producing Enterobacteriaceae by 2003, compared with none in 1991.

It is evident today that ESBL-producing *Klebsiella* spp. and *E. coli* are major players in the world of antimicrobial resistance. A report from the Infectious Diseases Society of America (IDSA) recently published listed ESBL-producing *Klebsiella* spp. and *E. coli* as one of the six priority drug-resistant microbes to which new therapies are urgently needed (36).

PLASMID-MEDIATED AmpC-BETA-LACTAMASES

Just like ESBL-producing bacteria, organisms with plasmid-mediated AmpC enzymes have mostly been responsible for nosocomial outbreaks on a worldwide basis during the late 1980s and 1990s, although the risk factors associated with infection are not as well defined as those associated with ESBL-producing bacteria (46). However, analysis of these outbreaks show that increased length of hospital stay, severity of illness, admission to an ICU, and previous exposure to antibiotics are associated with infection with plasmid-mediated cephamycinase-producing Enterobacteriaceae (40, 78). In a study reported from Korea, patients infected by plasmid-mediated AmpC-producing organisms had clinical features and outcomes similar to those of patients infected with TEM- or SHV-related ESBL producers (79).

The SENTRY Antimicrobial Surveillance Program in the United States found plasmid-mediated AmpC β-lactamases in 2% of 1429 *E. coli* isolates from 30 centers; with CMY-2, FOX-5, and DHA-1 being identified (80). A UK study found acquired cephamycinases in 49% of cefoxitin-resistant *E. coli* and 55% of cefoxitin-resistant *Klebsiella* spp. (81). Another recent survey of 752 isolates of *E. coli* and klebsiellae collected in the United States between 1992 and 2000 revealed that 8.5% of *K. pneumoniae*, 6.9% of *K. oxytoca*, and 4% *of E. coli* isolates carried plasmid-mediated AmpC (82). In the survey from the United Kingdom using isolates collected in London and Southeast England during 2004, AmpC was the mechanism responsible for cephalosporin resistance in 41/574 *E. coli* (7.1%) (83).

It seems that CMY-2 is the most common plasmid-mediated cephamycinase reported in Enterobacteriaceae from different areas of the world. Jacoby and colleagues found plasmid-mediated AmpC-type resistance in 7 of 75 of ceftazidime-resistant *E. coli* from 25 US states; 2 of these isolates produced CMY-2 (82). Mulvey and colleagues studied 232 cefoxitin-resistant *E. coli* from 12 different hospitals in Canada and found that 25 (11%) strains contained CMY-2 and that 51 (22%) had different promoter and attenuator mutations (84). Recent hospital surveys from Asia, North America, and Europe have shown that the DHA types of cephamycinases are mostly present in *Klebsiella* spp. from Asia, CMY types are present in *E. coli* from Asia, North America, and Europe, and FOX types are present in *Klebsiella* spp. from North America and Europe (81, 82, 84–86).

Summary

Escherichia coli still remains an important cause of nosocomial-acquired infections, especially of urinary tract, bloodstream, surgical site infections, pneumonia, and Gram-negative sepsis. Resistance to antimicrobial agents such as cephalosporins and fluroquinolones in *E. coli* has become an increasingly relevant problem. Most importantly within the *E. coli* is the increasing recognition of isolates producing the so-called "newer β-lactamases" that consist of plasmid-mediated AmpC ß-lactamases (e.g., CMY types), extended-spectrum β-lactamases (e.g., CTX-M types), and carbapenem-hydrolyzing enzymes (CHEs) (e.g., the class A or KPC types). It is clear that the epidemiology of ESBL-producing Enterobacteriaceae is becoming more complex with increasingly blurred limits between hospitals and the community. *Escherichia coli* producing CTX-M β-lactamases (especially CTX-M-15) seem to be present in the community and hospital settings with different behavior than *Klebsiella* spp. that produce TEM- and SHV-derived ESBLs. These bacteria have become widely prevalent in the community setting in certain areas of the world, and they are most likely being imported into the hospital setting.

The spread of Enterobacteriaceae that produce newer β-lactamases and PMQR will have important future implications for the empiric treatment of hospital and community-associated infections. These multiresistant bacteria merit close monitoring with worldwide multicenter surveillance studies. There is an urgent need for internationally funded efforts to track and monitor the worldwide spread of Enterobacteriaceae that produce newer β-lactamases within the hospital and community settings.

REFERENCES

1. Forbes BA, Sahm DF, Weissfeld AS. *Bailey & Scott's Diagnostic Microbiology,* 12th ed. Mosby Elsevier, St. Louis, 2007, pp. xviii, 1031.
2. Koneman EW, Winn WC. *Koneman's Color Atlas and Textbook of Diagnostic Microbiology,* 6th ed. Lippincott Williams & Wilkins, Philadelphia, 2006, pp. xxxi, 30, 1535, 79 leaves of plates.
3. Mandell GL, et al. *Mandell, Douglas, and Bennett's Principles and Practice of Infectious Diseases,* 6th ed. Churchill Livingstone, New York, 2005.
4. Wilfert CM. *E. coli* meningitis: K1 antigen and virulence. *Annu Rev Med* 1978;**29**:129–136.
5. Eisenstein BI, Jones GW. The spectrum of infections and pathogenic mechanisms of *Escherichia coli. Adv Intern Med* 1988;**33**:231–252.
6. Kaper JB, Nataro JP, Mobley HL. Pathogenic *Escherichia coli. Nat Rev Microbiol* 2004; **2**(2):123–140.
7. Hacker J, Kaper JB. Pathogenicity islands and the evolution of microbes. *Annu Rev Microbiol* 2000;**54**:641–679.
8. Bergsten G, Wullt B, Svanborg C. *Escherichia coli,* fimbriae, bacterial persistence and host response induction in the human urinary tract. *Int J Med Microbiol* 2005;**295**(6–7):487–502.
9. Wenzel RP. Health care-associated infections: Major issues in the early years of the 21st century. *Clin Infect Dis* 2007;**45**(Suppl1):S85–8.
10. Gasink LB, Lautenbach E. Prevention and treatment of health care-acquired infections. *Med Clin North Am* 2008;**92**(2):295–313, viii.
11. Gaynes R, Edwards JR. Overview of nosocomial infections caused by Gram-negative bacilli. *Clin Infect Dis* 2005;**41**(6):848–854.
12. Berkley JA, et al. Bacteremia among children admitted to a rural hospital in Kenya. *N Engl J Med* 2005;**352**(1):39–47.
13. Uslan DZ, et al. Age- and sex-associated trends in bloodstream infection: A population-based study in Olmsted County Minnesota. *Arch Intern Med* 2007;**167**(8):834–839.
14. Laupland KB, et al. Burden of community-onset bloodstream infection: A population-based assessment. *Epidemiol Infect* 2007;**135**(6):1037–1042.
15. Skogberg K, et al. Increase in bloodstream infections in Finland, 1995–2002. *Epidemiol Infect* 2007;**136**(1):1–7.
16. Schonheyder HC. Two thousands seven hundred and thirty nine episodes of bacteremia in the county of Northern Jutland 1996–1998. Presentation of a regional clinical database. *Ugeskr Laeger* 2000;**162**(20):2886–2891.
17. Madsen KM, et al. Secular trends in incidence and mortality of bacteraemia in a Danish county 1981–1994. *Apmis,* 1999;**107**(3):346–52.
18. Diekema DJ, et al. Epidemiology and outcome of nosocomial and community-onset bloodstream infection. *J Clin Microbiol* 2003;**41**(8):3655–3660.
19. Bonacorsi S, Bingen E. Molecular epidemiology of *Escherichia coli* causing neonatal meningitis. *Int J Med Microbiol* 2005;**295**(6–7)373–381.

20. Lode H. Management of serious nosocomial bacterial infections: Do current therapeutic options meet the need? *Clin Microbiol Infect* 2005;**11**(10):778–787.

21. Jacobsen SM, et al. Complicated catheter-associated urinary tract infections due to *Escherichia coli* and *Proteus mirabilis. Clin Microbiol Rev* 2008;**21**(1):26–59.

22. Klastersky J, et al. Post neurosurgery Gram-negative bacillary meningitis. *J Infect* 1981;**3** (1Suppl):45–51.

23. Boyd EF, Hartl DL. Chromosomal regions specific to pathogenic isolates of *Escherichia coli* have a phylogenetically clustered distribution. *J Bacteriol* 1998;**180**(5):1159–1165.

24. Johnson JR, Russo TA. Molecular epidemiology of extraintestinal pathogenic (uropathogenic) *Escherichia coli. Int J Med Microbiol* 2005;**295**(6–7):383–404.

25. Stull TL, LiPuma JJ, Edlind TD. A broad-spectrum probe for molecular epidemiology of bacteria: Ribosomal RNA. *J Infect Dis* 1988;**157**(2):280–286.

26. Versalovic J, et al. Use of the polymerase chain reaction for physical mapping of *Escherichia coli* genes. *J Bacteriol* 1991;**173**(17):5253–5255.

27. Woods JP, et al. Use of arbitrarily primed polymerase chain reaction analysis to type disease and carrier strains of *Neisseria meningitidis* isolated during a university outbreak. *J Infect Dis* 1994;**169**(6):1384–1389.

28. Herzer PJ, et al. Phylogenetic distribution of branched RNA-linked multicopy single-stranded DNA among natural isolates of *Escherichia coli. J Bacteriol* 1990;**172**(11):6175–6181.

29. Clermont O, Bonacorsi S, Bingen E. Rapid and simple determination of the *Escherichia coli* phylogenetic group. *Appl Environ Microbiol* 2000;**66**(10):4555–4558.

30. Tenover FC. Rapid detection and identification of bacterial pathogens using novel molecular technologies: Infection control and beyond. *Clin Infect Dis* 2007;**44**(3):418–423.

31. Tenover FC, et al. Interpreting chromosomal DNA restriction patterns produced by pulsed-field gel electrophoresis: Criteria for bacterial strain typing. *J Clin Microbiol* 1995;**33** (9):2233–2239.

32. Foley SL, et al. Evaluation of molecular typing methods for *Escherichia coli* O157:H7 isolates from cattle, food, and humans. *J Food Prot* 2004;**67**(4):651–657.

33. Harrington SM, et al. Genotypic analysis of invasive *Streptococcus pneumoniae* from Mali, Africa, by semiautomated repetitive-element PCR and pulsed-field gel electrophoresis. *J Clin Microbiol* 2007;**45**(3):707–714.

34. Johnson JR, O'Bryan TT. Improved repetitive-element PCR fingerprinting for resolving pathogenic and nonpathogenic phylogenetic groups within *Escherichia coli. Clin Diagn Lab Immunol* 2000;**7**(2):265–273.

35. Maiden MC. Multilocus sequence typing of bacteria. *Annu Rev Microbiol* 2006;**60**:561–588.

36. Talbot GH, et al. Bad bugs need drugs: An update on the development pipeline from the Antimicrobial Availability Task Force of the Infectious Diseases Society of America. *Clin Infect Dis* 2006;**42**(5):657–668.

37. Schwaber MJ, et al. Clinical and economic impact of bacteremia with extended- spectrum-beta-lactamase-producing Enterobacteriaceae. *Antimicrob Agents Chemother* 2006;**50** (4):1257–1262.

38. Chopra I, et al. Treatment of health-care-associated infections caused by Gram-negative bacteria: A consensus statement. *Lancet Infect Dis* 2008;**8**(2):133–139.

39. Livermore DM, Woodford N. The beta-lactamase threat in Enterobacteriaceae, *Pseudomonas and Acinetobacter. Trends Microbiol* 2006;**14**(9):413–420.

40. Jacoby GA, Munoz-Price LS. The new beta-lactamases. *N Engl J Med* 2005;**352**(4):380–391.

41. Queenan AM, Bush K. Carbapenemases: The versatile beta-lactamases. *Clin Microbiol Rev* 2007;**20**(3):440–458, table of contents.

42. Paterson DL, Bonomo RA. Extended-spectrum beta-lactamases: A clinical update. *Clin Microbiol Rev* 2005;**18**(4):657–686.
43. Canton R, Coque TM. The CTX-M beta-lactamase pandemic. *Curr Opin Microbiol* 2006; **9**(5):466–475.
44. Olsson O, Bergstrom S, Normark S. Identification of a novel ampC beta-lactamase promoter in a clinical isolate of *Escherichia coli. EMBO J*, 1982;**1**(11):1411–1416.
45. Forward KR, et al. Molecular mechanisms of cefoxitin resistance in *Escherichia coli* from the Toronto area hospitals. *Diagn Microbiol Infect Dis* 2001;**41**(1–2):57–63.
46. Philippon A, Arlet G, Jacoby GA. Plasmid-determined AmpC-type beta-lactamases. *Antimicrob Agents Chemother* 2002;**46**(1):1–11.
47. Doi Y, Paterson DL. Detection of plasmid-mediated class C beta-lactamases. *Int J Infect Dis* 2007;**11**(3):191–197.
48. Poirel L, Pitout JD, Nordmann P. Carbapenemases: Molecular diversity and clinical consequences. *Future Microbiol* 2007;**2**(5):501–512.
49. Walsh TR, et al. Metallo-beta-lactamases: The quiet before the storm? *Clin Microbiol Rev* 2005;**18**(2):306–325.
50. Walther-Rasmussen J, Hoiby N. Class A carbapenemases. *J Antimicrob Chemother* 2007;**60** (3):470–482.
51. Bratu S, et al. Rapid spread of carbapenem-resistant *Klebsiella pneumoniae* in New York City: A new threat to our antibiotic armamentarium. *Arch Intern Med* 2005;**165** (12):1430–1435.
52. Deshpande LM, et al. Emergence of serine carbapenemases (KPC and SME) among clinical strains of Enterobacteriaceae isolated in the United States Medical Centers: Report from the MYSTIC Program (1999–2005). *Diagn Microbiol Infect Dis* 2006;**56**(4):367–372.
53. Pope J, et al. KPC type beta-lactamase, rural Pennsylvania. *Emerg Infect Dis* 2006;**12** (10):1613–1614.
54. Jacoby GA. Mechanisms of resistance to quinolones. *Clin Infect Dis* 2005;**41**(Suppl2): S120–S126.
55. Nordmann P, Poirel L. Emergence of plasmid-mediated resistance to quinolones in Enterobacteriaceae. *J Antimicrob Chemother* 2005;**56**(3):463–469.
56. Robicsek A, Jacoby GA, Hooper DC. The worldwide emergence of plasmid-mediated quinolone resistance. *Lancet Infect Dis* 2006;**6**(10):629–640.
57. Cattoir V, et al. *Vibrio splendidus* as the source of plasmid-mediated QnrS-like quinolone resistance determinants. *Antimicrob Agents Chemother* 2007;**51**(7):2650–2651.
58. Poirel L, et al. Origin of plasmid-mediated quinolone resistance determinant QnrA. *Antimicrob Agents Chemother* 2005;**49**(8):3523–3525.
59. Robicsek A, et al. Fluoroquinolone-modifying enzyme: A new adaptation of a common aminoglycoside acetyltransferase. *Nat Med* 2006;**12**(1):83–88.
60. Perichon B, Courvalin P, Galimand M. Transferable resistance to aminoglycosides by methylation of G1405 in 16S rRNA and to hydrophilic fluoroquinolones by QepA-mediated efflux in *Escherichia coli. Antimicrob Agents Chemother* 2007;**51**(7):2464–2469.
61. Yamane K, et al. New plasmid-mediated fluoroquinolone efflux pump, QepA, found in an *Escherichia coli* clinical isolate. *Antimicrob Agents Chemother* 2007;**51**(9):3354–3360.
62. Pitout JD, et al. Surveillance for plasmid-mediated quinolone resistance determinants in Enterobacteriaceae within the Calgary Health Region Canada: The emergence of aac(6')-Ib-cr. *J Antimicrob Chemother* 2008;**61**(5):999–1002.
63. Erb A, et al. Prevalence of antibiotic resistance in *Escherichia coli*: Overview of geographical, temporal, and methodological variations. *Eur J Clin Microbiol Infect Dis* 2007;**26**(2):83–90.

64. Loivukene K, et al. Surveillance of antimicrobial resistance of invasive pathogens: The Estonian experience. *Euro Surveill* 2006;**11**(2):47–49.

65. Zhanel GG, et al. Antimicrobial-resistant pathogens in intensive care units in Canada: results of the Canadian National Intensive Care Unit (CAN-ICU) study, 2005–2006. *Antimicrob Agents Chemother* 2008;**52**(4):1430–1437.

66. Paterson DL. Resistance in Gram-negative bacteria: Enterobacteriaceae. *Am J Infect Control* 2006;**34**(5Suppl 1): S20–S28; discussion S64–S73.

67. Siegel JD, et al. Management of multidrug-resistant organisms in health care settings 2006. *Am J Infect Control* 2007;**35**(10Suppl 2): S165–S193.

68. Denton M. Enterobacteriaceae. *Int J Antimicrob Agents* 2007;**29**(Suppl3):S9–S22.

69. Palucha A, Mikiewicz B, Gniadkowski M. Diversification of *Escherichia coli* expressing an SHV-type extended-spectrum beta-lactamase (ESBL) during a hospital outbreak: Emergence of an ESBL-hyperproducing strain resistant to expanded-spectrum cephalosporins. *Antimicrob Agents Chemother* 1999;**43**(2):393–396.

70. Venezia RA, et al. Molecular epidemiology of an SHV-5 extended-spectrum beta-lactamase in enterobacteriaceae isolated from infants in a neonatal intensive care unit. *Clin Infect Dis* 1995;**21** (4):915–923.

71. Hibbert-Rogers LC, et al. Molecular epidemiology of ceftazidime resistant Enterobacteriaceae from patients on a paediatric oncology ward. *J Antimicrob Chemother* 1995;**36**(1):65–82.

72. Saurina G, et al. Antimicrobial resistance in Enterobacteriaceae in Brooklyn, NY: epidemiology and relation to antibiotic usage patterns. *J Antimicrob Chemother* 2000;**45**(6): 895–898.

73. Tumbarello M, et al. Predictors of mortality in patients with bloodstream infections caused by extended-spectrum-beta-lactamase-producing Enterobacteriaceae: Importance of inadequate initial antimicrobial treatment. *Antimicrob Agents Chemother* 2007;**51**(6):1987–1994.

74. Pitout JD, et al. Emergence of Enterobacteriaceae producing extended-spectrum beta-lactamases (ESBLs) in the community. *J Antimicrob Chemother* 2005;**56**(1):52–59.

75. Pitout JD, Laupland KB. Extended-spectrum beta-lactamase-producing Enterobacteriaceae: An emerging public-health concern. *Lancet Infect Dis* 2008;**8**(3):159–166.

76. Pitout JD, et al. Molecular epidemiology of CTX-M-producing *Escherichia coli* in the Calgary Health Region: emergence of CTX-M-15-producing isolates. *Antimicrob Agents Chemother* 2007;**51**(4):1281–1286.

77. Valverde A, et al. Dramatic increase in prevalence of fecal carriage of extended-spectrum beta-lactamase-producing Enterobacteriaceae during nonoutbreak situations in Spain. *J Clin Microbiol* 2004;**42**(10):4769–4775.

78. Hanson ND. AmpC beta-lactamases: What do we need to know for the future? *J Antimicrob Chemother* 2003;**52**(1):2–4.

79. Pai H, et al. Epidemiology and clinical features of bloodstream infections caused by AmpC-type-beta-lactamase-producing *Klebsiella pneumoniae. Antimicrob Agents Chemother* 2004;**48** (10):3720–3728.

80. Deshpande LM, et al. Occurrence of plasmidic AmpC type beta-lactamase-mediated resistance in *Escherichia coli*: Report from the SENTRY Antimicrobial Surveillance Program (North America, 2004). *Int J Antimicrob Agents* 2006;**28**(6):578–581.

81. Woodford N, et al. Wide geographic spread of diverse acquired AmpC beta-lactamases among *Escherichia coli* and *Klebsiella* spp. in the UK and Ireland. *J Antimicrob Chemother* 2007;**59** (1):102–105.

82. Alvarez M, et al. Epidemiology of conjugative plasmid-mediated AmpC beta-lactamases in the United States. *Antimicrob Agents Chemother* 2004;**48**(2):533–537.

83. Potz NA, et al. Prevalence and mechanisms of cephalosporin resistance in Enterobacteriaceae in London and South-East England. *J Antimicrob Chemother* 2006;**58**(2):320–326.
84. Mulvey MR, et al. Molecular characterization of cefoxitin-resistant *Escherichia coli* from Canadian hospitals. *Antimicrob Agents Chemother* 2005;**49**(1):358–365.
85. Li Y, et al. Prevalence of plasmid-mediated AmpC beta-lactamases in a Chinese university hospital from 2003 to 2005: First report of CMY-2-Type AmpC beta-lactamase resistance in China. *J Clin Microbiol* 2008;**46**(4):1317–1321.
86. Moland ES, et al. Prevalence of newer beta-lactamases in Gram-negative clinical isolates collected in the United States from 2001 to 2002. J Clin Microbiol 2006;**44**(9):3318–3324.

CHAPTER TWELVE

Fungal Infections

JOSE A. VAZQUEZ

Introduction

Fungi are important and common pathogens that cause severe and fatal infections in the immunocompromised host (1). In the past two decades, the incidence of invasive fungal infections has increased dramatically. During the same time, significant changes with regard to epidemiology, diagnosis, and treatment of fungal infections has also taken place (1).

Candida species remain the most common fungal pathogen among immunocompromised patients. However, recent epidemiologic studies show marked changes in the species of *Candida*, causing invasive infections. In addition to invasive fungal infections due to *Candida*, infections due to molds have also increased in frequency. Of the pathogenic molds, *Aspergillus* remains the most common pathogen identified in a compromised host, followed by *Fusarium* spp., *Scedosporium apiospermum* (*Pseudallescheria boydii*), and the *Zygomycetes* (1).

Recent studies evaluating the epidemiology of fungal infections have required that these organisms be characterized to a subspecies level when necessary, in order to better delineate modes of transmission among healthcare workers, the environment, and the involved patients. A great deal of research has been expended in the development of strain delineation (typing) techniques for fungi, especially for the study of *Candida* spp. However, many other fungi have also been evaluated, including *Aspergillus* spp., *Cryptococcus* spp., *Trichosporon asahii*, *Fusarium* spp., and, more recently, *Histoplasma encapsulatum* (2).

For many years, alloenzymes have been used as strain typing markers for all fungi. In recent years, attention has been focused on the DNA molecule as a source of informative

Molecular Techniques for the Study of Hospital-Acquired Infection, First Edition. Edited by Steven L. Foley, Anne Y. Chen, Shabbir Simjee, and Marcus J. Zervos.

polymorphisms. Because each strain's DNA sequence is theoretically unique, this sequence information can be utilized for any study of genetic diversity and relatedness between organisms. Overall, because of the use of newer molecular techniques, DNA-based strain delineation (typing or profiling) techniques have provided the investigators with the most useful technology to DNA "fingerprint" just about any fungi and, thus, are currently the most commonly utilized methodology (2).

Candida Species

Candida species are ubiquitous fungi and the most common fungal pathogens affecting humans (3). The growing problem of mucosal and systemic candidiasis reflects the enormous increase in the pool of patients at risk and the increased opportunity for *Candida* species to invade tissues normally resistant to invasion. *Candida* species are true opportunistic pathogens that exploit recent technological advances to gain access to the vascular circulation and deep tissues. *Candida*, in particular, affects high-risk patients who are either immunocompromised or critically ill.

Candida albicans is an important opportunist pathogen because of its ability to infect seriously ill, hospitalized patients (3–7). *Candida* species account for approximately 15% of all hospital-acquired infections and more than 80% of all nosocomial fungal infections (8–11). Serious and disseminated infections due to *Candida* have been well-described among burn patients, low-birth-weight infants, recipients of parenteral nutrition, persons with invasive blood pressure monitoring transducer devices, persons undergoing hemodialysis and long-term ambulatory peritoneal dialysis, and postoperative patients (3, 5, 7). Other risk factors for *Candida* colonization and infection include (a) immunocompromised hospitalized patients treated with broad-spectrum antibiotics, glucocorticoids, or cytotoxic chemotherapy and (b) patients with indwelling catheters or other prosthetic devices (3, 5, 10).

EPIDEMIOLOGY

The increased prevalence of local and systemic disease caused by *Candida* species has resulted in numerous clinical syndromes, the expression of which primarily depends on the host's immune status. *Candida* species produce a wide spectrum of diseases, ranging from superficial infections to invasive diseases such as hepatosplenic candidiasis (HSC), *Candida* peritonitis, and systemic candidiasis (3, 6). Management of serious and life-threatening invasive candidiasis remains severely hampered by delays in diagnosis because of a lack of reliable diagnostic methods that would allow the earlier detection and identification of fungemia and tissue invasion by the different *Candida* species.

Clinical and autopsy studies have confirmed the marked increase in the incidence of disseminated candidiasis, reflecting a parallel increase in the occurrence of candidemia (4, 11). This increase is multifactorial in origin and reflects increased recognition as well as a growing population of patients at risk (i.e., patients undergoing complex surgical procedures and those with indwelling vascular devices). The increase in disseminated candidiasis also reflects the improved survival of patients with underlying neoplasms, collagen vascular disease, and immunosuppression.

Candidiasis causes more fatalities than any other systemic mycosis (3, 6). In the febrile neutropenic patient who dies of sepsis, there is a 20–40% chance of finding evidence of invasive candidiasis at autopsy. Bodey described 21% of fatal infections in leukemic patients as the result of invasive fungal disease, in contrast with 13% and 6% of fatal infections in patients with lymphoma and solid tumors, respectively (4). Systemic candidiasis was described in 20–30% of patients undergoing bone marrow transplantation. In some university centers, *Candida* species are currently the second most common blood culture isolate. In a recent report from the National Healthcare Safety Network (NHSN), *Candida* species were the third (11.8%) most commonly isolated pathogens from blood cultures in 463 hospitals involved in the network. Only coagulase-negative *Staphylococcus* (34.1%) and *Enterococcus* spp. (16%) were more commonly recovered from line-related bloodstream infections (11).

Candidemia and disseminated candidiasis mortality rates have not improved markedly over the past decade and remain in the 30–40% range (3, 6). More than a decade ago, investigators reported the enormous economic impact of systemic candidiasis in hospitalized patients. The development of candidemia continues to be associated with a considerable prolongation of the length of hospital stay (70 days versus 40 days in patients who are comparable, matched, and nonfungemic). Although mucocutaneous fungal infections, such as oral thrush and *Candida* esophagitis, are common in HIV-positive patients, candidemia and disseminated candidiasis are not.

MICROBIOLOGY

Candida species are dimorphic yeast that can form true hyphae and pseudohyphae, depending on the conditions (3, 6). *Candida* species are typically confined to human and animal reservoirs; however, they are frequently recovered from the hospital environment, including food, countertops, air-conditioning vents, floor surfaces, respirators, and health-care workers (3, 6, 12, 13). In addition, they are also considered to be normal commensals of diseased skin and on mucosal surfaces of the gastrointestinal, genitourinary, and respiratory tracts.

More than 165 species of *Candida* exist, but only a few are recognized as causing disease in humans (3, 6, 7). The medically significant *Candida* species are shown in Table 12.1. *Candida glabrata* and *Candida albicans* account for 70–80% of yeasts isolated from patients with invasive candidiasis (3, 6, 7). *Candida glabrata* has recently become important because of its increasing worldwide incidence as a cause of candidemia and candidiasis (3, 6, 7).

TABLE 12.1 Distribution of the common *Candida* species

Species	Isolation rate (%)
C albicans	50–60
C glabrata	15–20
C parapsilosis	10–20
C tropicalis	6–12
C krusei	1–3
C guilliermondii	
C lusitaniae	
C dubliniensis	

In addition, *C. glabrata* has also been found to be less susceptible to all antifungals, including azoles and polyenes (3, 6, 7). More recent *in vitro* surveys have revealed that approximately 10–20% of the *C. glabrata* isolates are resistant to fluconazole and 5% are resistant to either voriconazole or posaconazole (14). Two uncommon *Candida* species, *Candida lusitaniae* and *Candida guilliermondii*, are important because of their innate resistance to amphotericin B (3, 6, 7, 12, 14). Another uncommon but important *Candida* species is *Candida krusei*; although not as common as some of the other *Candida* species, it is clinically significant because of its intrinsic resistance to fluconazole and itraconazole and its decreased susceptibility to all other antifungals, including amphotericin B (3, 6, 7, 12, 14).

In the past, epidemiologic studies have been hampered by two important factors: (1) the fact that most patients dying in an ICU do not undergo an autopsy examination (autopsy studies that have been performed indicate that disseminated candidiasis is frequently not diagnosed and thus goes untreated before the patient's demise) and (2) the lack of a reliable, reproducible, and simple typing system for *Candida* spp. Until recently, this typing system has not been available. Prospective molecular epidemiologic studies by several different investigators on the two high-risk groups of patients, ICU and bone marrow transplant patients, have described the frequent exogenous acquisition of many *Candida* spp., including *C. albicans*, *C. parapsilosis*, *C. glabrata*, and *C. lusitaniae* based on cultures of identical strain types from patients, hospital surfaces, and hospital personnel that were geographically and temporally associated (7, 10, 12, 13), thus providing evidence that one of the principal mechanisms of transmission was indirect contact between patients. Ecological studies on these same patients by Vazquez et al., utilizing pulsed-field gel electrophoresis on these same *Candida* spp., revealed that many environmental surfaces were culture-positive for yeast and that the environmental and hand isolates that were recovered were identical to patient strains in numerous instances (13). In addition, the same study also revealed that about 40% of the patients that were culture-positive for yeast carried different *Candida* spp. at multiple body sites over a period of time. As expected, the most likely combination was *C. albicans* with C. *glabrata* approximately 40% of the time (13).

STRAIN DELINEATION OF *CANDIDA* SPECIES

Early on, typing systems were based on phenotypic differences within the same species using biotyping, enzyme profiles, susceptibility to killer toxins, resistance patterns to organic and inorganic chemicals, biochemical analysis, serological agglutination reactions, and immunoblotting techniques (13, 15–17). However, these techniques either were too difficult to perform, were not reproducible by different institutions, or did not provide the necessary strain delineation power to be useful in epidemiologic surveys or studies.

Because of these reasons, DNA-based strain delineation techniques have proven to be the most useful (Table 12.2). Molecular techniques, specifically polymerase chain reaction (PCR), has been used extensively in forensic sciences and has been applied to a broad range of organisms, including pathogenic bacteria and viruses. A wide variety of methods have been developed and adapted to detect genetic polymorphisms in fungi (13, 15–17). These techniques include restriction enzyme analysis (REA), REA with specific DNA probes or restriction fragment-length polymorphisms (RFLP), pulsed field gel electrophresis (PFGE), randomly amplifies polymorphic DNA (RAPD), multilocus enzyme electrophoresis (MLT), and multilocus sequence typing (MLT) (2, 17, 18). These methods vary in their resolution, strain delineation and have specific advantages and disadvantages that need to be taken into account when choosing a technique to investigate a particular problem.

TABLE 12.2 Overview of different strain delineation techniques used in *Candida* species

Typing methodology	Discriminatory power	Reproducibility	Ease of use	Species-specific	Interpretation
Biotyping	Poor	Poor	Easy	Yes	Difficult
Serotyping	Poor	Good	Easy	Yes	Moderate
Restriction enzyme analysis	Poor	Moderate	Easy	Yes	Difficult
RFLP with DNA probes	Moderate	Good	Moderate	Yes	Good
PFGE	Moderate	Good	Moderate	Yes	Good
PFGE with REA	Good	Good	Moderate	Yes	Good
Oligonucleotide fingerprinting	Good	Good	Moderate	Yes	Good
RAPD	Good	Good	Moderate	Yes	Good
MLST	Excellent	Good	Moderate	Yes	Good
MLEE	Moderate	Moderate	Difficult	Yes	Moderate

Restriction Enzyme Analysis Restriction enzyme analysis (REA) was one of the first molecular-based methods used to compare strains of *Candida* species (17–20) (Figure 12.1). This technique was used extensively in the early studies of *Candida* epidemiology. All *Candida* species can be differentiated using this methodology (17–20). These methods are based on the principle that isolates of the same strain type share the same DNA profile, while epidemiologically unrelated isolates will have distinctly different patterns. The technique is simple and relies on the extraction of DNA and the subsequent digestion of total genomic DNA with specific restriction enzymes (*Eco*RI, *Hin*F1, *Sma*I, *Msp*I). After digestion, the resulting DNA fragments are separated, depending on their size by electrophoresis on agarose gels. The gels are subsequently stained with ethidium bromide so the DNA fragments can be visualized. The resulting band patterns are then compared visually and subjectively differentiated. Using this technique because of the size of the *Candida* genome, the restriction patterns are frequently very complex and comprised of many bands, thus making the differentiation of strains very difficult. However, despite the fact that the technique is fast and simple, its lack of discriminatory capability has led to it being replaced by newer less subjective techniques.

Restriction Fragments-Length Polymorphisms Restriction fragment length polymorphisms (RFLPs) or restriction enzyme analysis and specific DNA probes are other techniques that have been frequently used to differentiate strains. These techniques combine the digestion of chromosomal DNA and species-specific DNA probes (1, 15, 18, 21). Every organism possesses unique nucleotide sequences that distinguish it from every other organism. A species-specific probe is used to identify those unique sequences such that they can be easily and rapidly identified. DNA is extracted from isolates and cleaved into fragments by restriction endonucleases; the fragments or bands are then separated by agarose gel electrophoresis, and RFLPs are detected by hybridization with a DNA probe generated from the species that is being evaluated. Different probes have been utilized in an attempt to

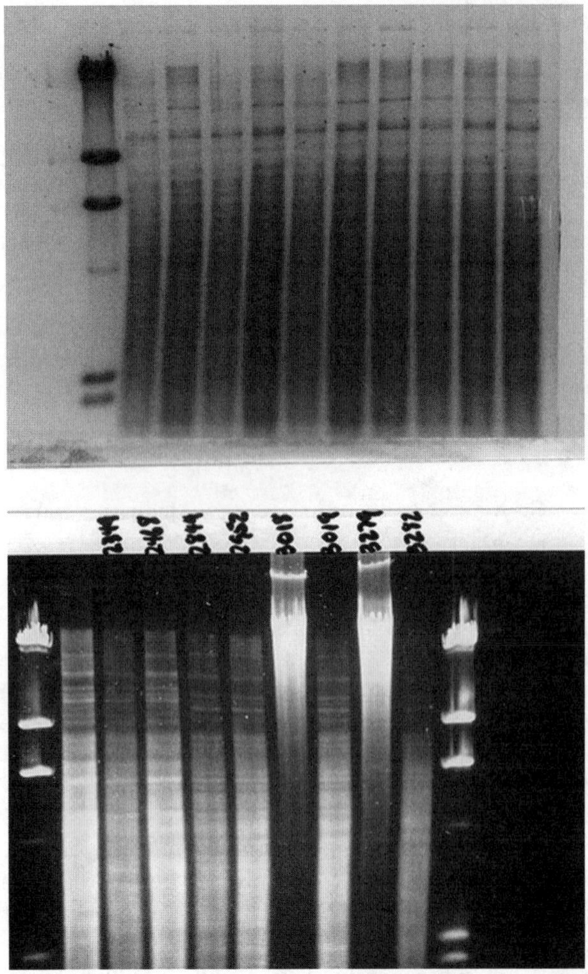

FIGURE 12.1 **Restriction enzyme analysis (REA) of *Candida albicans* on an agarose gel electrophoresis of purified DNA digested with MspI and stained with ethidium bromide.**

delineate strains of *Candida*. Some of the most commonly used probes include those generated from the actin gene, ribosomal DNA probes, mitochondrial DNA probes, and probes that hybridize with dispersed and repeated DNA segments from the *C. albicans* genome such as 27A and Ca3 (15, 18, 21). The probes to highly repeated DNA fragments appear to be able to delineate specific strains of *Candida* species. For epidemiologic studies, the probe to the actin gene has not been found to be useful for strain delineation. In general, however, these probes yield too few bands for a meaningful analysis. The most effective and most commonly used probes are the 27A and Ca3, both of which contain the repetitive elements (21). In contrast to the other probes, these probes yield strain-specific banding patterns composed of 10–20 bands of varying intensities. Their efficacy lies in the fact that some of these bands are highly pleomorphic and others are nonvariable. A more recently generated probe is the CARE-2 probe (22). However, the extreme variability of the bands generated decreases the efficacy of this probe for the strain delineation of different *Candida* species. The technique is simple and reproducible and produces DNA fingerprints that facilitate the comparison of strains. In addition, the DNA patterns obtained with species-specific probes are also amendable to computer-assisted analysis that can provide much more reliable and efficient quantitative comparison of large numbers of related strains. Although this method is reproducible, techniques that utilize Southern hybridization are time-consuming and labor-intensive; thus, this method is not suitable for the rapid analysis of large numbers of isolates.

Oligonucleotide fingerprinting uses probes that can be used to delineate strains from different species (15, 18, 23). The most frequently used probes correspond to microsatellite sequences, which are short repetitive sequences, scattered throughout the *Candida* genome. The technique uses short oligonucleotides that are labeled with radionucleotides and hybridized to restriction enzyme digested genomic DNA. The method generates multiple fingerprints from the same DNA specimen by performing sequential hybridizations with individual probes. The disadvantage of this method, as with other Southern hybridization techniques, is that it is labor-intensive and thus unsuitable for the analysis of large numbers of isolates.

Pulsed-Field Gel Electrophoresis Pulsed-field gel electrophoresis (PFGE) is one of the most commonly used techniques for the evaluation of strain differences in most *Candida* species (15, 16, 19, 20). PFGE was initially described in the mid-1980s as a method to evaluate chromosomes larger than 2 megabases (1, 13, 19, 20). The technique is based on the separation of large chromosome-sized DNA molecules through agarose gels using alternating electric fields, which allow for the separation of large DNA fragments that are too large to be electrophoresed with the conventional electrophoresis apparatus. This method can be used to discriminate between individual strains because the sizes of the individual chromosomes in different *Candida* strains vary widely, resulting in different fingerprints or patterns of chromosome-sized bands known as karyotypes (19, 20, 24). Countour-clamped homogeneous gel electrophoresis (CHEF) is a variation of PFGE that provides improved resolution of the large chromosomal DNA fragments (Figure 12.2). Because large chromosomal fragments are subject to breakage, the DNA extraction procedure is carried out with the yeast cells embedded in agarose gel plugs or inserts. The methodology is simple and the DNA

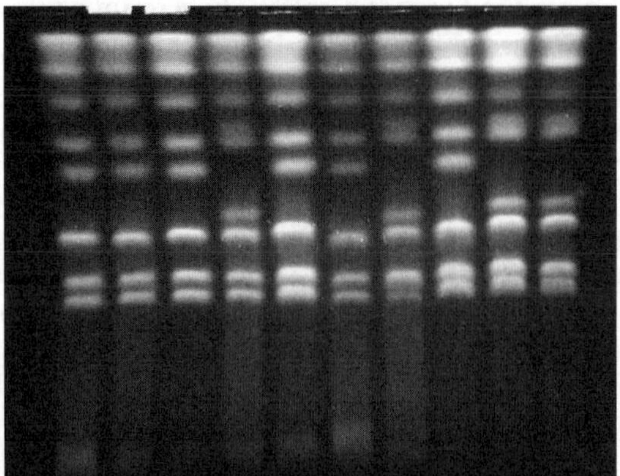

FIGURE 12.2 **Contour-clamped homogeneous electrophoresis (CHEF), a version of pulsed-field gel electrophoresis demonstrating two different genotypes of *C. albicans* recovered from one patient.**

inserts or plugs are stable over prolonged periods of time. In addition, the results are reproducible and the karyotypes are amendable to computer-assisted methods (13, 17–20). Numerous chromosomal bands are known to be conserved between strains of certain *Candida* species, whereas other chromosomal bands vary in size and, thus identify specific strains. CHEF has been applied successfully to many of the *Candida* species including *C. albicans, C. glabrata, C. parapsilosis, C. tropicalis, C. krusei*, and *C. kefyr* (13, 17–20). Although effective at strain delineation, some karyotypes can vary as a result of phenotypic switching seen in *C. albicans* and not because of a true strain difference. Furthermore, the equipment required is expensive, the sample is labor intensive, and the electrophresis times are frequently 48–72 hours in length. Because of this, PFGE is not suitable for the strain delineation of large numbers of specimens.

A variation on PFGE is PFGE with macrorestriction endonuclease fingerprint analysis. This methodology uses certain restriction endonucleases that cleave the large chromosomal bands into smaller sizes, thus increasing the numbers of bands that may be used to differentiate the strains. The restriction endonucleases used are enzymes that cleave the DNA infrequently (*Sfi*I and *Not*I) (25, 26). The pattern of fragments generated can also be used to discriminate between strains.

In studies comparing CHEF with REA of genomic DNA, CHEF appears to be a more sensitive molecular typing method for *Candida* species delineation (13, 19, 20). The use of PFGE and macrodigestion appears to be more sensitive for strain differentiation than PFGE alone. Limitations of PFGE such as being more time-consuming and more costly, however, make it difficult to utilize when large numbers of specimens are being analyzed.

Polymerse Chain Reaction Methodology Polymerse chain reaction (PCR), in addition to its application in the rapid identification of *Candida* species, has also been applied to the differentiation of distinct strains of *Candida* (16, 17, 25). Randomly amplified polymorphic DNA (RAPD) differs from conventional PCR in that it is based on the use of a single oligonucleotide (10–15 base pairs) of arbitrary sequence using low-stringency amplification reaction conditions (Figure 12.3). Because of the use of low annealing temperatures, primers may bind to many sites throughout the genome, thus allowing the amplification of products that vary in size. Once the optimum amplification conditions and primer sequences have been established empirically, these fragments, when separated by electrophoresis and stained with ethidium bromide, can produce strain-specific fingerprint patterns generating three to six bands. The differential patterns between strains occur as a result of nucleotide variations at the primer annealing sites (25). In addition, the patterns generated are amenable to computer-assisted analysis programs. Epidemiologic studies have demonstrated the ability of RAPD to cluster moderately related isolates together and is comparable to that of DNA fingerprinting with species-specific probes. Because the methodology is rapid and easy to perform, it has been used frequently in the molecular analysis of *Candida* epidemiology (15, 25, 27). Extreme care must be used to prevent variation in experimental conditions, because even subtle alterations in condition of assays such as a change in magnesium concentrations and temperatures can lead to the appearance or disappearance of bands, thus affecting methodology reproducibility. To minimize these variations, it is recommended that only strongly amplified bands be used for fingerprint analysis.

Multilocus Sequence Typing Multilocus sequence typing (MLST) is the most recent methodology used to attempt to improve the strain differentiation ability of PCR techniques (17, 28). This method utilizes known DNA sequences at multiple loci and has

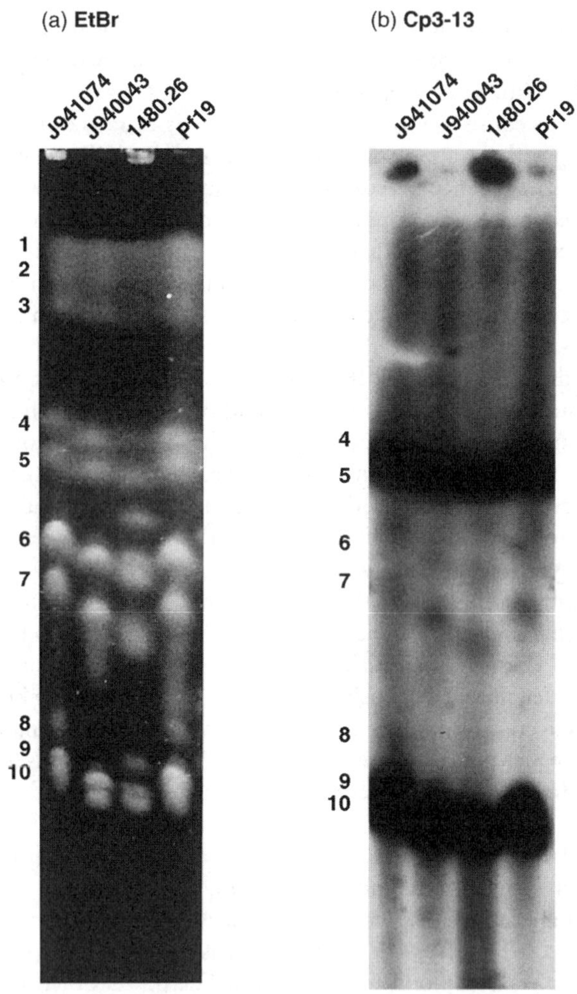

FIGURE 12.3 **Randomly amplified polymorphic DNA from *Candida parapsilosis* (A) and with species-specific DNA probe (B).**

greatly enhanced the study of epidemiology and evolutionary phylogenetics of many fugal pathogens. MLST schemes have now been published for the most common *Candida* species, including *C. albicans*, *C. glabrata*, *C. krusei*, *C. tropicalis*, and *C. dubliniensis*. In general, MLST generates patterns for similarities and differences between isolates from sequences determined, typically using six to eight independent chromosomal genes. MLST, initially described by Maiden and colleagues, offers several advantages over most earlier phenotypic and genotypic typing methods (28, 29). MLST sequencing data offer a higher level of reproducibility and minimal subjectivity in analysis compared with other technologies; the sequences can be stored in Internet databases, offering an unprecedented degree of accessibility. In addition, MLST is based on the same conceptual premise as multilocus enzyme electrophoresis, namely, allelic variation, which means that MLST provides information relevant to population genetic studies as well as to epidemiology (28, 29).

The choice of genes used for MLST can be made easily when full genomic information is available to help locate potential single nucleotide polymorphisms (SNP). The SNPs for most of the genes used for MLST with *Candida* species generate ratios (*dN*/*dS*) of nonsynonymous to synonymous amino acid changes in their encoded peptides of less than 1.0, the criterion for stabilizing selection.

The methodology consists of the following: DNA is extracted from the isolate, six-to eight PCRs are set up with the appropriate primer set, and the PCR products are purified and used for bidirectional sequence reactions. The sequencing chromatograms are checked visually and evaluated for heterozygous SNPs. Each sequence is compared with the reference database for the species. If it matches an existing sequence, it is assigned that sequence's allele number or genotype number. The set of six to eight allele/genotype numbers defines a strain type, numbered once again by reference to the database or by addition to it. The end of the product of the process is therefore the sequence type (ST) for haploid organisms or a diploid ST (DST) diploid organisms. If two organisms have different STs or DSTs, this is evidence that the strain types are different. In addition, the results from MLST are very amenable to computer-assisted methodology and the construction of dendograms. The drawbacks to MLST includes time and labor intensity which preclude its use in many hospital-based epidemiology laboratories. It is clear, however, that MLST has added significant contributions to the detailed understanding of the molecular epidemiology, transmission, and pyhlogenetics of *Candida* species.

A newer, recently published methodology utilizes the pyrosequence analysis of 20 nucleotides of internal transcribed spacer 2 (ITS-2) (30). This methodology uses the PCR amplification of the ITS2 region of *Candida* species. Afterwards, amplification products are subjected to pyrosequencing analysis using a PYROGOLD sequencing kit. This method has already been used effectively to discriminate between *Candida parapsilosis*, *C. metapsilosis*, and *C. orthopsilosis*, which are very closely related *Candida* species. This technique is simple, reliable, and reproducible and is conserved across multiple strains of *Candida*.

Multilocus Enzyme Electrophoresis Multilocus enzyme electrophoresis (MLEE) takes advantage of protein-derived differences among the different strains of *Candida*. MLEE has been used to fingerprint *C. albicans*, *C. tropicalis*, *C. lusitaniae*, *C. parapsilosis*, and *C. guilliermondii* (2, 15–17). In essence, MLEE can assess isoenzymes or alloenzymes using the codominant markers in diploids for each locus. The power of MLEE can discriminate among gene products of different alleles for a number of loci. The methodology uses multiple enzymes usually between 21 and 29 enzymes and evaluates the similarity coefficients between isolates. MLEE appears to be as good as RAPD with probes to delineate strains of *C. albicans* (31). The main drawback of this method is that it is relatively time-consuming, because one must combine the data form at least 10 enzymes that provide variability among isolates.

MOLECULAR EPIDEMIOLOGY OF CANDIDIASIS

Recent studies using molecular DNA typing methods have suggested a mechanism for the acquisition of nosocomial *Candida* from environmental and human sources. *Candida albicans* can be commonly cultured from environmental surfaces. In studies where environmental sampling was performed, *Candida* spp. were recovered from 25% to 50% of inanimate surfaces sampled. The role of the environment as a potential reservoir for *Candida* is suggested by studies showing isolation of identical strains of *C. albicans* from food prior to acquisition by patients (7, 13, 32). This suggests potential acquisition of the organism from hospital food, which must be an inadvertent transmitter of strains from the hands of healthcare workers. Furthermore, *Candida* strains have been cultured from inanimate surfaces in patient rooms before acquisition by the patients subsequently hospitalized in those rooms (3, 7, 10, 12, 13, 17). The surfaces harboring *Candida* spp. isolates were those in contact with the hands of personnel or patients. DNA typing techniques showed that strains found on these inanimate surfaces were identical to strains acquired by patients.

These findings are significant because organisms isolated from the inanimate hospital environment are generally thought to contribute negligibly to endemic nosocomial infection (32). For most other nosocomial organisms the environment becomes passively contaminated by organisms from patients. The above studies suggest that *C. albicans* can sometimes be transmitted directly or indirectly from contaminated environmental surfaces (12, 13). Although it appears possible to acquire *Candida* from the environment, it is probably less likely than the following mechanisms.

Current understanding of the pathogenesis of nosocomial *C. albicans* infections indicates that most organisms are acquired endogenously from the patient's own flora. Colonizing isolates in hospitalized patients has been well-described, with *C. albicans* recovered from urine, stool, vagina, and oropharynx. A study of bloodstream infections due to *C. albicans* has shown that 62% of patients had positive cultures from various anatomic sites before the onset of fungemia (32). However, the mechanism and extent to which hospitalization contributes to colonization has not been examined. Investigators have reported clusters or outbreaks of *Candida* infection in which patient-to-patient spread or acquisition from environmental sources was suspected. Twelve cases of *C. parapsilosis* fungemia were described in association with an infected blood pressure transducer in an ICU, and 15 cases of *C. parapsilosis* endophopthtalmitis occurred secondary to an infected irrigation solution, suggesting exogenous acquisition (33, 34). Another study implicated carriage on the hands of hospital personnel as a possible source of an outbreak (35). Eight cases of *C. tropicalis* mediastinitis after thoracic surgery were traced to an operating room nurse who had *C. tropicalis* isolated from both the oropharynx and hands (36). Unfortunately, molecular analysis of strains was not performed in these studies.

Two outbreaks were reported in neonatal ICUs (37, 38). Neonates with identical strains, as shown by DNA restriction enzyme analysis, were geographically and temporally related in one study. In another study, cultures in both personnel caring for infected infants and the environment in proximity to those infants yielded *Candida* (37). When handwashing techniques were improved using 70% isopropyl alcohol, the incidence of *C. albicans* infection decreased to pre-outbreak levels. In an outbreak of *C. albicans* in an adult ICU, the strain causing infection survived getter on hands and was more resistant to Hibiscrub (Imperial Chemical Industries, UK) than were control strains (39).

The most important mechanism for acquiring exogenous nosocomial strains and infection is through transient carriage on the hands of personnel after contact with infected patients. The epidemiology of nosocomial acquisition of *C. albicans*, therefore, may be similar to that of methicillin-resistant staphylococci, multidrug-resistant enterococci, and Gram-negative bacilli (1, 7, 10, 28, 40).

In a recent study of *C. albicans*, 27% had negative initial cultures and acquired the organisms after hospitalization (13). Risk factors for acquisition of *Candida* include prior antibiotics and lengthy hospitalization. Exposure to antibiotics is a well-described mechanism for colonization and infection with *Candida*. The isolation of identical strains of *C. albicans* in patients who were geographically and temporarily associated suggests that the major route of transmission is indirect contact between patients. The role of carriage by personnel in dissemination of *C. albicans* remains to be clarified. By use of DNA content as an epidemiologic marker of strain identity, these studies have shown that transmission of *C. albicans* probably occurs through indirect contact between patients by the hands of healthcare workers. That *C. albicans* is spread between hospital personnel also was suggested by isolation of *C. albicans* on environmental surfaces in contact with hands (13). Such surfaces included monitoring devices and handles, blood pressure cuffs, and tubing connected to patients.

Candida albicans is transmitted readily between patients in adjacent beds within ICUs. Proximity to a patient within infection or colonization increases the risk of acquisition. By use of DNA typing methods, patients with new acquisition of *Candida* have been found to have identical isolates to patients who are temporarily and geographically associated (10, 12–14, 33, 40–42). The source of the organism is likely to be the respiratory, gastrointestional, or genitourinary tracts of colonized patients because patients are often heavily colonized at these sites.

Prospective epidemiologic studies of *Candida* using longitudinal cultures and molecular typing have shown that patients generally carry the same strain type of *Candida* over time (1, 3, 10, 12, 13, 18). There is considerable strain diversity among individual patients, however. For nosocomial *C. albicans*, in one study, 73% of individuals were colonized with multiple strain types at different anatomic sites (13). Moreover, 39% of these patients with positive cultures for *C. albicans* had more than one *Candida* spp. identified during the course of admission.

Other studies have shown that patients may be colonized with more than one strain type (1, 5, 7, 12, 13). Phenotypic characterization is insufficient because *Candida* can switch phenotypes, and different phenotypes can coexist at the same site of infection (43, 44). Clinical infection occurs in a minority of hospitalized patients who are colonized with *Candida* spp. Colonizing strain types are identical to later strains, causing infections in most patients (12, 13, 42). These findings are also in agreement with epidemiologic studies of nosocomial bacterial infections.

Molecular DNA analysis has provided useful information in the study of nosocomial *Candida*. The most important inpatient hospital reservoir is colonized patients. Most patients are infected with strains they harbor. Findings from recent studies suggest that nosocomial *Candida* colonization is the result of exogenous acquisition of strains (10, 12, 17). Hospital personnel and the inanimate hospital environment may serve as a reservoir and source of acquired strains. The mechanism by which patients acquire *Candida* remains unproven, although most investigators agree that indirect contact transmission is the most likely route for exogenous nosocomial acquisition of strains. Environmental surfaces in contact with hands or patients also should be considered a source for some *Candida* organisms when infection control measures are designed. Further prospective studies using DNA typing methods for analysis of cultures and control strains are needed to clearly define the patient and the hospital reservoirs of infection, modes of transfer, and measures for preventing spread.

Aspergillus

The imperfect fungus *Aspergillus* is the most common airborne fungal pathogen in humans, causing invasive aspergillosis (45, 46). *Aspergillus* species are found worldwide and are ubiquitous in the environment. Aspergillosis encompasses a broad spectrum of diseases caused by members of the genus *Aspergillus*. The clinical manifestation and severity of the disease depend upon the immunologic state of the patient.

In the last decade, there have been significant advances in the diagnosis and treatment of invasive aspergillosis. However, invasive aspergillosis remains a major cause of morbidity and mortality in immunosuppressed patients (45–48). Lowered host resistance due to such factors as underlying debilitating disease, neutropenia, chemotherapy, immunosuppressive agents, antimicrobial agents, and steroids predisposes the patients to colonization, invasive disease, or both. Additionally, aspergillosis is occasionally seen as an opportunistic pathogen in patients with bronchiectasis, carcinoma, sarcoidosis, or tuberculosis.

EPIDEMIOLOGY

Aspergillus species are ubiquitous saprophytes found worldwide in nature. *Aspergillus* species are one of the most frequent organisms found in compost piles and readily isolated from the soil, air, water, and food. It is frequently isolated from hospital ventilation systems and hospital construction sites (45, 46). In addition, it may also be found in 1–16% of respiratory secretions in normal host. There are approximately 600 recognized species of *Aspergillus*, of which *A. fumigatus* is the most frequent cause of disease in humans, followed by *A. favus*, *A. niger*, and occasionally *A. terreus*, *A. nidulans*, *A. glaucus* (Table 12.3) (46–48). *Aspergilli* are molds that reproduce by means of spores termed conidia. Hyphae are septate and dichotomously branched.

Aspergillus is the second most common cause of fungal disease in hematopoietic stem cell transplant (HSCT) recipients, solid organ transplant recipients, and hematologic and oncologic malignancies (49, 50). In general, infection occurs in severely immunocompromised host, particularly in HSCT patients who develop graft versus host disease, patients who develop prolonged and profound neutropenia, or patients with neutrophil dysfunction due to corticosteroid therapy (49). Outbreaks in hospitals due to renovations, new constructions, and ventilation systems have been frequently reported (46–48). Similarly, patients with chronic granulomatous disease may present with invasive aspergillosis, because of the inability of their phagocytes to generate microbicidal substrates. Less frequently, patients with alcoholic cirrhosis, collagen vascular diseases, and post-influenza infection are also at risk to develop invasive aspergillosis and even nonimmunocompromised hosts may infrequently develop disseminated aspergillosis (45–48) (Table 12.4).

TABLE 12.3 Distribution of *Aspergillus* species

Aspergillus species	Isolation frequency (%)
A. fumigatus	66
A. flavus	14
A. niger	7
A, terreus	4
A. versicolor	2
A. nidulans	1
A. oryzae	1
A. glaucus	1

TABLE 12.4 Predisposing factors for invasive aspergillosis

Neutropenia
Transplantation
Bone marrow transplant
Liver transplant
Lung transplant
Heart transplant
Graft versus host disease
CMV infection/reactivation
Corticosteroids (prednisone > 1 mg/kg/day)
HIV (CD4 cell counts < 50/mm^3)
Chronic granulomatous disease
Intravenous drug use
Occasionally may coexist with Gram-negative bacterial pneumonia

PATHOGENESIS

Aspergillus is acquired by inhalation of airborne spores; these spores (conidia) are small enough to reach alveoli or sinuses (45–48). Occasionally, conidia in operating rooms may enter the implantation site of prosthetic valves. Exposure is universal, but disease is uncommon, since host factors are very important. Keeping the compromised host away from dusty hospital renovation or construction areas is useful, as is keeping potted plants out of their hospital rooms. *Aspergillus* species, as with many other molds, are considered angioinvasive pathogens. In other words, they have a tendency for vascular invasion, producing thrombosis, ischemia, infarction, and tissue necrosis (46–48).

Most infections originate in the respiratory tract and then subsequently disseminate via the bloodstream to other tissues, including other respiratory tract sites, central nervous system, kidneys, eyes, skin, liver and spleen (45–48). Accordingly, the respiratory tract is the most commonly involved site (56%), followed by the central nervous system (6%) and the upper respiratory tract (sinuses) and skin (5%) (45–48). Multiorgan involvement or disseminated infection is found in approximately 20% of the patients (45–48). Prognosis depends upon the type and severity of disease as well as the underlying immunological status of the patient (45–48, 51). Invasion from a cutaneous source, such as central venous catheters, rarely occurs.

The outcome of infection also varies, depending on the site of infection and the status of the underlying immunosuppressive disease (45–48, 51).

CLINICAL MANIFESTATIONS

Aspergillus infection can manifest in a variety of ways, ranging from colonization to life-threatening invasive disease (45–48, 52). Moreover, the clinical manifestations are varied, depending on the route of infection and the underlying disease. The overall mortality rate depends on the underlying immunosuppressive state and can vary from 40% to 90% (45–48, 52).

MOLECULAR TYPING OF ASPERGILLUS

Several phenotypic and genotypic typing techniques have been developed to investigate the epidemiologic relationship between the environment and clinical isolates by being able to distinguish among individual *Aspergillus* isolates (Table 12.5) (40). By being able to differentiate *Aspergillus* isolates, the understanding of genetic and environmental relationships between environmental and clinical isolates can be improved. Understanding pathogen distribution and relatedness is important for determining the epidemiology of nosocomial infections and aiding in the design of rational pathogen control methods. With the development and implementation of molecular typing techniques based on DNA rather than on phenotypic characteristics such as multilocus enzyme electrophoresis, the typing methods have greatly evolved (40, 53).

Multilocus Enzyme Electrophoresis Multilocus enzyme electrophoresis (MLEE) takes advantage of protein-derived differences among the different strains of *Aspergillus*. MLEE has been used to fingerprint different species and strains of *Candida* (2, 16, 18). MLEE assesses isoenzymes or alloenzymes using the codominant markers for each locus. The power of MLEE can discriminate among gene products of different alleles for a number of loci. The methodology uses multiple enzymes usually between 21 and 29 enzymes and evaluates the similarity coefficients between isolates. MLEE appears to be as good as RAPD with probes to delineate strains of *C. albicans* (31). The main drawback to this method is that it is relatively time-consuming because one must combine the data form at least 10 enzymes that provide variability among isolates.

Randomly Amplified Polymorphic DNA In conventional PCR reactions, two primers anneal to genomic DNA under stringent conditions. The RAPD technique is also called

TABLE 12.5 Overview of different strain delineation techniques used in *Aspergillus* species

Typing methodology	Discriminatory power	Reproducibility	Ease of use	Species-specific	Interpretation
Biotyping	Poor	Poor	Moderate	Yes	Difficult
Serotyping	Poor	Good	Easy	Yes	Moderate
Restriction enzyme analysis	Poor	Poor	Moderate	No	Difficult
RFLP with DNA probes	Moderate	Good	Moderate	Yes	Good
RFLP Afut1	Excellent	Good	Moderate	Yes	Difficult
RAPD	Limited	Poor	Easy	No	Moderate
PFGE	Moderate	Good	Moderate	Yes	Good
PFGE with REA	Good	Good	Moderate	Yes	Good
AFLP	Good	Good	Moderate	No	Difficult
RAPD	Good	Good	Moderate	Yes	Good
MLST	Excellent	Good	Moderate	Yes	Good
MLEE	Moderate	Moderate	Difficult	Yes	Moderate

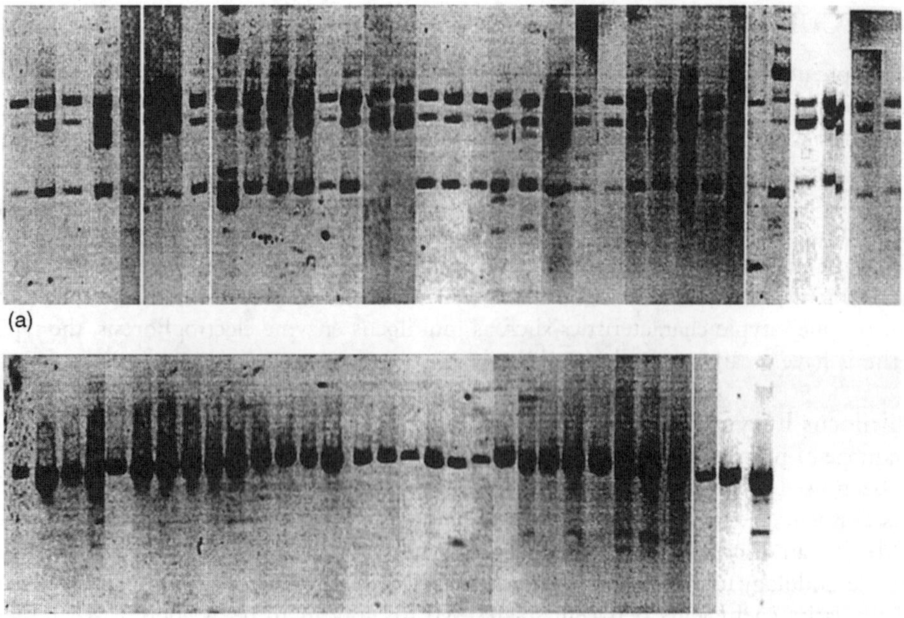

FIGURE 12.4 **RAPD fingerprinting of independent isolates of *Aspergillus flavus* (A) and *A. fumigatus* (B) amplified with primer CX-10.**

arbitrary primed PCR (AP-PCR). The repetitive extragenic palindromic PCR (rep-PCR) or interrepeat PCR are techniques similar to RAPD but with only little modifications (2, 54) (Figure 12.4). Aufauvre-Brown et al. (55) tested 44 different primers on three different *A. fumigatus* isolates. A frequently used primer is "R108," which also appears suitable for other *Aspergillus* species. Several other primers suitable for typing *Aspergillus* spp. have also recently been described (40).

Restriction Fragment-Length Polymorphisms without Hybridization Up to 10,000 different DNA fragments are generated when genomic DNA from an *Aspergillus* isolate is cleaved with a restriction endonuclese that has a 6-bp recognition sequence (1, 2, 15). Some of these fragments are approximately 4000 bp in length. Most of these fragments cannot be distinguished from each other. By restricting the analysis to only large fragments (10–50 kbp), different isolates may show different banding patterns. Denning et al. (56) evaluated different restriction enzymes for their ability to delineate a collection of 31 *A. fumigatus* isolates. The authors determined that two enzymes *Xho*I and *Sal*I seemed to yield the highest discriminatory power with this approach. This technique has also been used to evaluate *A. flavus* on mitochondrial DNA. It clearly identified *A. flavus* in a heterogeneous group of *Aspergillus*, but isolates from identical species could not be distinguished from each other (57).

Restriction Fragment-Length Polymorphisms with Hybridization The primary difference of RFLP with hybridization is that a specific subset of restriction fragments are analyzed (2, 7, 15, 17). The obtained fragments are separated by size and are transferred to a nylon filter by Southern blotting. A subset of the restriction fragments is then detected by hybridization with a labeled probe. The application of repeated sequences as probes will yield a multiple banding pattern. Differences in patterns between unrelated isolates can be expected because of variations in copy number and/or flanking sequences of target regions.

Different restriction enzyme and probe combinations have been analyzed for discrimination between isolates from several *Aspergillus* species. Girardin et al. (58) evaluated multicopy elements in the *A. fumigatus* genome and tested them in combination with the restriction enzyme *Eco*RI for its utility as an effective typing technique. The probe *Afut*1 possesses specific characteristics of a retrotransposon-like element and has been used in most RFLP studies thus far (59). Other probes used for the DNA fingerprinting of *A. fumigatus*, which are based on retrotransposon-like elements, are *Afut*2 and AF4A.

James et al. constructed and characterized a species-specific probe for *A. flavus*, named pAF28. This probe has been used to delineate clinical and environmental isolates in a neonatal intensive care unit (60). To discriminate *A. flavus* isolates from the outbreak and non-outbreak-related situations, an RFLP analysis of *Sma*I digested DNA using RAPD-generated probes were performed.

In a simpler method of this technique, the analysis is peformed on only one specific PCR-amplified target. This fragment is then cleaved by a single or, alternately, several restriction enzymes, and the obtained fragments are separated by electrophoresis. This is often referred to as PCR-RFLP. This approach is generally suitable for discriminating among different species, but has insufficient discriminatory power to distinguish among unrelated isolates within a species.

AMPLIFIED FRAGMENT-LENGTH POLYMORPHYISMS

The amplified fragment-length polymorphyism (AFLP) method was first described by Vos et al. (61). In this method, genomic DNA is cut with two restriction enzymes, one with an average cutting frequency and a second one with a higher cutting frequency. Synthetic double-stranded DNA fragments are ligated to the obtained sticky ends to serve as primer binding sites in a successive PCR reaction. The ligated fragments are subsequently amplified in a PCR reaction using stringent annealing temperatures. The number of fragments that are generated can be modified by extending the amplification primers at the 3′ site with one or more selective nucleotides. The PCR primer that spans the average frequency restriction site is labeled. Although the probes were initially radiolabeled, fluorescence is currently used as the method to identify fragments. A complex DNA banding pattern of 50–500 bp is obtained. Variations between different isolates originate by differences in the number and location of restriction recognition sites in the genome.

Investigations by Warris et al. demonstrate that AFLP is an excellent strain delineation method to differentiate at and below the species level among *Aspergillus* species (72).

Microsatellites or Short Tandem Repeats Microsatellites or short tandem repeats (STRs) are short, repetitive sequences that are abundantly present in the genomes of most of the higher organisms and to a lesser extent in several prokaryotic genomes as well (40, 53). Different isolates can be distinguished from each other based on differences in repeat numbers. Microsatellite markers are easily amplified by PCR using primers based on their flanking sequences. If one of the primers is labeled, the strains can be sized very accurately using high-resolution electrophoresis platforms. The number of repeats in each marker can be deduced from the sizes of the fragments. Microsatellite-based typing schemes yield unambiguous strain types and highly portable data. Microsatellite-based assays are also referred to as microsatellite-length polymorphisms (MLP), microsatellite polymorphisms (MSP), or polymorphic microsatellite marker (PMM). Using four different nucleotide markers, Bart-Delabesse et al. (62) were able to identify approximately 30,000 different genotypes in *A. fumigatus*.

De Valk et al. (40) described another microsatellite panel called STRAf (STR for *A. fumigatus*). By expanding the number of markers to nine, a large number of genotypes can be differentiated.

Multilocus Sequence Typing Multilocus sequence typing (MLST) compares a series of genes (6–10) that are "housekeeping" genes present in all isolates of a particular species (63). Each isolate tested is defined by the alleles at each sequenced housekeeping loci, which together compromise the allelic profile or sequence type (ST). MLST is the molecular alternative to MLEE by targeting the variation present in multiple housekeeping loci. The advantage of MLST compared to MLEE is that DNA is more variable than protein-encoded and fewer loci need to be examined in MLST. Since MLST has now been used worldwide, this typing method enables international comparison of banked clinical isolates. Bain et al. (64) used an MLST scheme with seven genes in *A. fumigatus* to genotype a panel of 100 clinical and environmental isolates. Among the 100 isolates, 30 STs were identified.

In general, due to the high genetic variability of *A. fumigatus*, fingerprinting methods with high discriminatory power have to be applied to discriminate between unrelated isolates (65). Several typing techniques have been described for *A. fumigatus*. On the one hand are the pattern-based techniques like random amplified polymorphic DNA (RAPD) analysis (55, 66), restriction fragment-length polymorphism (RFLP) analysis (58, 67) and amplified fragment-length polymorphism (AFLP) (20). On the other hand are the more exact typing methods based on short tandem repeats like microsatellite-length polymorphism (MLP) (62) and short tandem repeats (STRs) for *A. fumigatus* (also referred to as STR*Af* typing) (40). Among the major problems associated with pattern-based methods are often poor intra- and interlaboratory reproducibility. These issues seriously complicate interpretation of the data (65). Exact fingerprinting methods based on STRs or sequence-based typing schemes such as multilocus sequence typing (MLST) may resolve these issues, provided that they have sufficient discriminatory power.

Infections due to *Aspergillus* species have become an extremely common cause of morbidity and mortality in the high-risk immunosuppressed host (45–48). In fact, aspergillosis has become one of the leading causes of mortality in HSCT recipients as well as solid organ transplant recipients (47–50). It is important to understand the difficulty in establishing a definitive diagnosis of aspergillosis due to the lack of laboratory tests and the broad spectrum of disease manifestations. In many cases, the clinician will have to rely on a high index of suspicion in the high-risk patient to initiate early and appropriate antifungal therapy (52, 68). Because of the difficulty in establishing a correct diagnosis and the rapid and recent development in newer diagnostic techniques and new antifungals, it is of utmost importance for the primary care physician to obtain an infectious disease consultant's opinion in any patient who may be suspected of having a diagnosis of aspergillosis.

Conclusions

Several molecular methods have been described for typing various *Aspergillus* species. Most of the techniques are developed to analyze *A. fumigatus* isolates, which is the most common species. Fingerprinting techniques have been used to gain insight in the colonization patterns of CF patients. Different colonization patterns are found and the meaning of these patterns concerning the development of an infection should be evaluated further by analyzing more patients. Fingerprinting isolates collected from respiratory samples and from the environment showed that a high extent of genetic variability can be found in *A. fumgatus*. Therefore, typing techniques with high discriminatory power are necessary, techniques that fulfill this criterion are RFLP in combination with the Afut1 probe, AFLP, and microsatellites. An additional advantage of the microsatellite methods is the high reproducibility, because of the unambiguous typing data, which make them eligible to analyze epidemiological relationships between large amounts of isolates over a longer period of time. Another exact method is MLST, but the loci described so far are probably not discriminating enough to identify a true source in an outbreak situation. The RAPD method has been used most, probably because this technique needs less equipment and no genomic sequence information is necessary to perform this assay. Fingerprinting techniques with lower reproducibility and lower discriminatory power can still be useful, especially when nosocomial aspergillosis occurs in highly protected areas with small amounts of isolates.

Therefore, the preferred typing technique depends on the epidemiological question and the equipment of a laboratory. The sequencing of more genomes of other *Aspergillus* species may provide more exact high-resolution fingerprinting techniques in the future.

The ideal epidemiologic typing technique applicable to a wide range of fungal pathogens is not yet available (70). However, several molecular-typing methods based on restriction endonuclease analysis of genomic DNA, PFGE, and DNA fingerprinting by Southern hybridization analysis may permit rapid, simple, and sensitive discrimination of specific strains among the most clinically important species of fungi. The combination of these typing methods with standardized studies of *in vitro* antifungal susceptibility will provide new insights into the epidemiology, pathogenesis, and treatment of fungal infections.

REFERENCES

1. Pfaller MA, Pappas PG, Wingard JR. Invasive fungal pathogens: Current epidemiologic trends. *Clin Infect Dis* 2006;**43**:S3–14.
2. Soll DR. The ins and outs of DNA fingerprinting the infectious fungi. *Clin Microbiol Rev* 2000;**13**:332–370.
3. Vazquez JA, Sobel JD. Candidiasis, In Dismukes W.E., Pappas P.G., Sobel J.D. (eds.), *Clinical Mycology.* Oxford University Press, New York, 2003, pp. 143–187.
4. Bodey GP. Candidiasis in cancer patients. *Am J Med* 1984;77(Suppl 4D):13–19.
5. Bross J, Talbot GH, Maislin G, et al. Risk factors for nosocomial candidemia: A case–control study in adults without leukemia. *Am J Med* 1989;**87**:614–620.
6. Kullberg BJ, Filler SG. Candidemia. In Calderone RA. (ed.), *Candida and Candidiasis.* ASM Press Washington, DC, 2002, pp. 327–340.
7. Pfaller MA, Diekema DJ. Epidemiology of invasive candidiasis: A persistent public health problem. *Clin Microbiol Rev* 2007;**20**:133–163.
8. Abi-Said D, Anaisse E, Uzun O, Raad I, Pinzcowski H, Vartivarian S. The epidemiology of hematogenous candidiasis caused by different *Candida* species. *Clin Infect Dis* 1997;**24**:1122–1128.
9. Banerjee SM, Emori TG, Culver DH, et al. Secular trends in nosocomial primary bloodstream infections in the United States: 1980–1989. *Am J Med* 1991;**91**:865–895.

10. Hedderwick SA, Lyons MJ, Liu M, Vazquez JA, Kauffman CA. Epidemiology of yeast colonization in the intensive care unit. *Eur J Clin Microbiol Infect Dis* 2000;**19**:663–670.
11. Hidron AI, Edwards JR, Patel J, Horan TC, Sievert DM, et al. Antimicrobial-resistant pathogens associated with healthcare-associated infections: annual summary of data reported to the national healthcare safety network at the centers for disease control and prevention, 2006–2007. *Infect Control Hosp Epidemiol* 2009;**29**:996–1011.
12. Sanchez V, Vazquez JA, Barth-Jones D, Dembry L, Sobel JD, Zervos MJ. Epidemiology of nosocomial acquisition of *Candida lusitaniae*. *J Clin Microbiol* 1992;**30**:3005–3008.
13. Vazquez JA, Sanchez V, Dmuchowski C, Dembry LM, Sobel JD, Zervos MJ. Nosocomial acquisition of *Candida albicans*: An epidemiologic study. *J Infect Dis* 1993;**168**:195–201.
14. Pfaller MA, Messer SA, Boyken L, Tendolkar S, Hollis RJ, Diekema DJ. Selection of a surrogate agent (fluconazole or voriconazole) for initial susceptibility testing of posaconazole against *Candida* spp.: Results from a global antifungal surveillance program. *J Clin Microbiol* 2008;**46**:551–559.
15. McEwen JG, Taylor JW, Carter D, Xu J, Felipe MSS, et al. Molecular typing of pathogenic fungi. *Med Mycol* 2000;**38**(Suppl 1):189–197.
16. Pfaller MA. Epidemiologic typing methods for mycoses. *Clin Infect Dis* 1992;**14**(Suppl 1): S4–S10.
17. Sullivan DJ, Coleman DC. Molecular approaches to identification and typing of *Candida* species. In Calderone RA. (ed.), *Candida and Candidiasis*. ASM Press, Washington, D.C, 2002, pp 427–441.
18. Zervos MJ, Vazquez JA. DNA analysis in the study of fungal infections in the immunocompromised host. *Clin Lab Med* 1996;**16**:73–88.
19. Vazquez JA, Beckley A, Sobel JD, et al. Comparison of restriction enzyme analysis versus pulsed-field gradient gel electrophoresis as a typing system for *Candida albicans*. *J Clin Microbiol* 1991;**29**:962–967.
20. Vazquez JA, Beckley A, Sobel J.D, et al. Comparison of restriction enzyme analysis and pulsed-field gradient gel electrophoresis as a typing system for Torulopsis glabrata. *J Clin Microbiol* 1993;**31**:2021–2030.
21. Schmid J, Voss E, Soll DR. Computer-assisted methods for assessing *Candida albicans* strain relatedness by southern blot hybridization with repetitive sequence Ca3. *J Clin Microbiol* 1990;**28**:236–243.
22. Lasker BA, Page LS, Lott TJ, Kobayashi GS. Isolation, characterization, and sequencing of *Candida albicans* repetitive element 2. *Gene* 1992;**116**:51–57.
23. Wilkinson BM, Morris L, Adams DJ, Evans EG, Lacy CJ, Walmsley RM. A new, sensitive polynucleotide probe for distinguishing *Candida albicans* strains and its use with computer assisted archiving and pattern comparison system. *J Med Vet Mycol* 1992;**30**:123–131.
24. Dembry LM, Vazquez JA, Zervos MJ. DNA analysis in the study of the epidemiology of nosocomial candidiasis. *Infect Control Hosp Epidemiol* 1994;**15**:48–53.
25. Bostock A, Khattack MN, Matthews R, Burnie J. Comparison of PCR fingerprinting, by random amplification of polymorphic DNA, with other molecular typing methods for *Candida albicans*. *J Gen Microbiol* 1993;**139**:2179–2184.
26. Pontieri E, Gregori L, Gennarelli M, Ceddia T, Novelli G, et al. Correlation of *Sfi*I macrorestriction endonuclease fingerprint analysis of *Candida parapsilosis* isolates with source of isolation. *J Med Microbiol* 1996;**45**:173–178.
27. Holmberg K, Feroze F. Evaluation of an optimized system for random amplified polymorphic DNA (RAPD)-analysis for genotypic mapping of *Candida albicans* strains. *J Clin Lab Anal* 1996;**10**:59–69.

28. Odds FC, Jacobsen MD. Multilocus sequence typing of pathogenic *Candida* species. *Eukaryotic cell* 2008;**7**:1075–1084.
29. Maiden MCJ. Multilocus sequence typing of bacteria. *Annu Rev Microbiol* 2006;**60**:561–588.
30. Borman AM, Linton CJ, Oliver D, Palmer MD, Szekely A, Odds FC, Johnson EM. Pyrosequencing analysis of 20 nucleotides of internal transcribed spacer 2 discriminated *Candida parapsilosis, Candida metapsilosis,* and *Candida orthopsilosis. J Clin Microbiol* 2009;**47**:2307–2310.
31. Pujol C, Joly S, Lockhart S, Noel S, Tibayrenc M, Soll DR. Parity of MLEE, RAPD, and Ca3 hybridization as fingerprinting methods for *Candida albicans. J Clin Microbiol* 1997;**35**:2348–2358.
32. Maki DG, Alvarado CJ, Hassemr CA, et al. Relation of the inanimate hospital environment to endemic nosocomial infection. *N Eng J Med* 1982;**307**:1562–1566.
33. Stern WH, Tamura E, Jacobs RA, et al. Epidemic postsurgical *Candida parapsilosis* endophthalmitis. Clinical findings and management of 15 consecutive cases. *Ophthalmology* 1985;**92**:1701–1709.
34. Weems JJ, Chamberland ME, Ward J, et al. *Candida parapsilosis* fungemia associated with parenteral nutrition and contaminated blood pressure transducers. *J Clin Microbiol* 1987;**1925**:1029–1032.
35. Weems JJ. *Candida parapsilosis:* Epidemiology, pathogenicity, clinical manifestations, and antimicrobial susceptibility. *Clin Infect Dis* 1992;**14**:756–766.
36. Isenberg HD, Tucci V, Cintron E, et al. Single-source outbreak of *Candida tropicalis* complicating coronary artery bypass surgery. *J Clin Microbiol* 1989;**27**:2426–2428.
37. Phelps M, Ayliffe GAJ, Babb JR. An outbreak of candidiasis in a special care unit: The use of resistogram typing method. *J Hosp Infect* 1986;**7**:13–20.
38. Vaudry WL, Tierney AJ, Wenman WM. Investigation of cluster of systemic *Candida albicans* infections in a neonatal unit. *J Infect Dis* 1988;**158**:1375–1379.
39. Burnie JP, Matthews R, Lee W, et al. Four outbreaks of nosocomial systemic candidiasis. *Epidemiol Infect* 1987;**99**:201–211.
40. De Valk HA, Meis JF, Curfs IM, Muehlethaler K, Mouton JW, Klaassen CHW. Use of a novel panel of nine short tandem repeats for exact and high-resolution fingerprinting of *Aspergillus fumigatus* isolates. *J Clin Microbiol* 2005;**43**:4112–4120.
41. Pittet D, Monod M, Filthuth I, et al. Contour-clamped homogeneous electric field gel electrophoresis as a powerful epidemiologic tool in yeast infections. *Am J Med* 1991; **91**(Suppl 3B): 256S–263S.
42. Reagan DR, Pfaller MA, Hollis RJ, et al. Nosocomial candidemia: characterization of the sequence of colonization and infection using DNA fingerprinting and a DNA probe. *J Clin Microbiol* 1990;**28**:2733–2738.
43. Soll DR, Sangtimm CJ, McDowell J, et al. High frequency switching in *Candida* strains isolated from vaginitis patients. *J Clin Microbiol* 1987;**25**:1611–1622.
44. Soll DR. High frequency switching in *Candida albicans. Clin Microbiol Rev* 1992;**5**:183–203.
45. Denning DW. Invasive Aspergillosis. *Clin Infect Dis* 1998;**12**:781–805.
46. Latge JP. *Aspergillus fumigatus* and aspergillosis. *Clin Microbiol Rev* 1999;**12**:310–350.
47. Patterson TF, Kirkpatrick WR, White M, Hiemenz JW, Wingard JR, Dupont B, et al. Invasive aspergillosis: Disease spectrum, treatment practices, and outcomes. *Medicine* 2000;**79**:250–260.
48. Patterson TF. Aspergillosis. In Dismukes WE, Pappas PG, Sobel JD. (eds.), *Clinical Mycology.* Oxford University Press, New York, 2003, pp. 221–240.
49. Marr KA, Carter RA, Crippa F, Wald A, Corey L. Epidemiologic and outcome of mould infections in hematopoietic stem cell transplant recipients. *Clin Infect Dis* 2002;**34**:909–917.

50. Ribaud P, Chastang C, Latge JP, Baffroy-Lafitte L, Parquet N, Devergie A, et al. Survival and prognostic factors of invasive aspergillosis after allogeneic bone marrow transplantation. *Clin Infect Dis* 1999;**28**:322–330.
51. Lin S, Schranz J, Teutsch SM. Aspergillosis case-fatality rate: Systematic review of the literature. *Clin Infect Dis* 2001;**32**:358–366.
52. Warnock DW, Hajjeh RA, Lasker BA. Epidemiology and prevention of invasive aspergillosis. *Current Infect Dis Report* 2001;**3**:507–516.
53. Verduyn Lunel F, Licciardello L, Stefani S, et al. Lack of consistent short sequence repeat polymorphisms in genetically homologous colonizing and invasive *Candida albicans* strains. *J Bacteriol* 1998;**180**:3771–3778.
54. Healy M, Reece K, Walton D, Huong J, Shah K, Kontoyiannis DP. Identification to the species level and differentiation between strains of *Aspergillus* clinical isolates by automated repetitive-sequence-based PCR. *J Clin Microbiol* 2004;**42**:4016–4024.
55. Aufavre-Brown A, Cohen J, Holden DW. Use of randomly amplified polymorphic DNA markers to distinguish isolates of Aspergillus fumigatus. *J Clin Microbiol* 1992;**30**:2991–2993.
56. Denning DW, Clemons KV, Hanson LH, Stevens DA. Restriction endonuclease analysis of total cellular DNA of *Aspergillus fumigatus* isolates of geographically and epidemiologically diverse origen. *J Infect Dis* 1990;**162**:1151–1158.
57. Moody SF, Tyler BM. Restriction enzyme analysis of mitochondrial DNA of the *Aspergillus flavus* group: *A. flavus, A. parasiticus,* and *A. nomius*. *Appl Environ* 1990;**56**:2441–2452.
58. Girardin H, Latge JP, Srikantha T, Morrow B, Soll DR. Development of DNA probes for fingerprinting *Aspergillus fumigatus*. *J Clin Microbiol* 1993;**31**:1547–1554.
59. Neuveglise C, Sarfati J, Latge J, Paris S. *Afut*1, a retrotransposon-like element from *Aspergillus fumigatus*. *Nucleic Acid Res* 1996;**24**:1428–1434.
60. James MJ, Lasker BA, McNeil MM, Shelton M, Warnock DW. Use of a repetitive DNA probe to type clinical and environmental isolates of *Aspergillus flavus* from a cluster of cutaneous infections in a neonatal intensive care unit 2000;**38**:3612–3618.
61. Vos P, Hogers R, Bleeker M, et al. A new technique for DNA fingerprinting. *Nucleic Acids Res* 1995;**23**:4407–4414.
62. Bart-Delabasse E, Humbert JF, Delabesse E, Bretagne S. Microsatellite markers for typing *Aspergillus fumigatus* isolates. *J Clin Microbiol* 1998;**36**:2413–2418.
63. Taylor JW, Fisher MC. Fungal multilocus sequence typing — its not just for bacteria. *Curr Opin Microbiol* 2003;**6**:351–356.
64. Bain JM, Tavanti A, Davidson AD, Jacobsen MD, Shaw D, Gow NA, Odds FC, et al. Multilocous sequence typing of the pathogenic fungus *Aspergillus fumigatus*. *J Clin Microbiol* 2007;**45**:1469–1477.
65. Chazalet V, Debeaupuis JP, Sarfati J, Lortholary J, Ribaud P, Shah P, Cornet M, Vu Thien H, Gluckman E, Brucker G, Latge JP. Molecular typing of environmental and patient isolates of *Aspergillus fumigatus* from various hospital settings. *J Clin Microbiol* 1998;**36**:1494–1500.
66. Leenders A, van Belkum A, Janssen S, de Marie S, Kluytmans J, Wielenga J, Lowenberg B, Verbrugh H. Molecular epidemiology of apparent outbreak of invasive aspergillosis in a hematology ward. *J Clin Microbiol* 1996;**34**:345–351.
67. Verweij PE, Meis JF, Sarfati J, Hoogkamp-Korstanje JA, Latge JP, Melchers WJ. Genotypic characterization of sequential *Aspergillus fumigatus* isolates from patients with cystic fibrosis. *J Clin Microbiol* 1996;**34**:2595–2597.
68. Ascioglu S, Rex JH, de Pauw B, Bennet JE, Billie J, et al. Defining opportunistic invasive fungal infections in immunocompromised patients with cancer and hematopoietic stem cell transplants: an international consensus. *Clin Infect Dis* 2002;**34**:7–14.

69. De Valk HA, Klaassen CHW, Meis JF. Molecular typing of *Aspergillus* species. *Mycoses* 2008;**51**:463–476.

70. Singh A, Goring RV, Simjee S, Foley SL, Zervos MJ. Application of molecular techniques to the study of hospital infection. *Clin Microbiol Rev* 2006;**19**:512–530.

71. Van Belkum A, Quint WG, de Pauw BE, Melchers WJ, Meis JF. Typing of *Aspergillus* species and *Aspergillus fumigatus* isolates by interrepeat polymerase chain reaction. *J Clin Microbiol* 1993;**31**:2502–2505.

72. Warris A, Klaassen CHW, Meis JFGM, de Ruiter MT, de Valk HA, Abrahamsen TG, Gaustad P, Verweij PE. Molecular epidemiology of *Aspergillus fumigatus* isolates recovered from water, air, and patients shows two clusters of genetically distinct strains. *J Clin Microbiol* 2003;**41**:4101–4106.

INDEX

Molecular Techniques for the Study of Hospital-Acquired Infection, First Edition. Edited by Steven L. Foley, Anne Y. Chen, Shabbir Simjee, and Marcus J. Zervos.